T0187243

"Most Americans believe healing consists of manipulating the molecules in our body through the use of medications or surgery. It comes as a surprise, therefore, to discover that sophisticated, effective healing traditions exist in other cultures that are based on a different approach. *Spiritism and Mental Health* is a marvelous introduction to the Brazilian Spiritist tradition. It is also a look at how consciousness-based research is transforming scientific medicine in our own culture."

—*Larry Dossey, MD, author of* The Power of Premonitions,
Healing Words, *and* Reinventing Medicine

"*Spiritism and Mental Health* is a heartfelt paradigm-expanding glimpse into the future of mental health care. This book's incredibly rich assortment of articles may seem off-puttingly esoteric at first glance, but the 26 chapters provide a comprehensive and down-to-earth overview of one of humanity's most ancient healing practices—working with spirits—and how this spiritual perspective may help guide psychiatry out of its current psychopharmacological dead end.

Dr. Emma Bragdon provides a great service by building a bridge that brings these timeless ideas and their modern adaptations (i.e. a description of the Department of Spiritual Assistance at a Spiritist Psychiatric Hospital in Brazil) to an American audience, with the help of an all-star lineup that has enough medical credibility to pass muster among the staunchest skeptics (Beverly Rubik, Melvin Morse, Linda Russek, Dean Radin, and Stan Krippner, among others). The book contains invaluable resources—extensive references, a listing of professional associations, and a glossary of terms. Dr. Bragdon is to be commended—two thumbs up!"

—*Eric Leskowitz, MD, faculty member of the Department of Psychiatry,
Harvard Medical School, and Director of the Integrative Medicine
Project at Spaulding Rehabilitation Hospital, Boston, USA*

"In *Spiritism and Mental Health*, psychotherapist Dr. Emma Bragdon, a renowned author and expert on Kardec's Spiritism, assesses the importance of including the spiritual aspects of human existence in mental health care. Drawing on decades of her own experience, and together with an impressive international team of professionals in the field, this scholarly book discusses numerous revealing case studies and stunning results. A must read for health care professionals; a leading-edge contribution toward the new paradigm required in our American mental health care system!"

—*Klaus Heinemann, PhD, Physicist and author*

"Evidence that intuition and inner knowing has a central role in mental health care is keenly substantiated in this ground-breaking book on Spiritism. Brazilian Spiritist medical doctors contribute chapters revealing the rich 150-year-old history of spiritual treatments used in Brazilian community centers and psychiatric hospitals. Modern consciousness researchers and psychiatrists expose the importance of accepting a new paradigm of the mind in order to implement healing. Together in one book they offer a model sure to bring a renewal to the practice of psychiatry and psychology."

—*Judith Orloff, MD, Psychiatrist and author of* Second Sight

"This book is brilliant for all those interested in mental health and the role of spirit. It brings together the current scientific evidence supporting the role of the spirit in mental health and the amazing and ground-breaking experience from integrating psychiatry and Spiritism in Brazil. What an inspiration. Now we need to find a way to bring this into practice."

—*Dr. Haraldur Erlendsson, CMC, DCN, MSc, MRCPsych,*
Psychiatrist, The Dene Hospital, West Sussex, UK

"A brilliant explanation of Spiritist practice in Brazil—a tour de force in introducing consciousness and spirituality to psychiatric treatment. I highly recommend this book for those wishing to practice truly holistic medicine."

—*John L. Turner, MD, Neurosurgeon and author of* Medicine, Miracles
and Manifestations: A Doctor's Journey Through the Wolds of Divine
Intervention, Near-Death Experiences, and Universal Energy

"I recommend reading this book wholeheartedly. I think it is an important contribution to broadening our perspectives and it presents a wealth of information from other cultures. It confronts our fundamental beliefs and asks us to address the spiritual dimensions of mental health treatment. I believe it is our ethical obligation to investigate this to evaluate and revise our own mental health treatment programs."

—*Brian Sackett, PhD, Psychologist*

"Clinicians who are open to exploring transpersonal aspects of mental health and illness will find *Spiritism and Mental Health* absolutely fascinating. This book will also be of interest to anyone who is exploring the deeper processes and meanings of life and the human condition."

—*Daniel Benor, MD (Psychiatry), Editor-in-Chief of* The
International Journal of Healing and Caring

"*Spiritism and Mental Health* opens a new view on psychiatric practices in centers throughout Brazil. A number of chapters in the book have been published in peer-reviewed papers, while others appear here for the first time. Spiritist care in St. Paulo in the area of mental sub-normality is carried out at the Spiritist Hospital André Luiz. I have had an opportunity to visit this hospital and it is one of the best run mental institutions I have ever come across. One reason for this is the high level of compassionate care given by the volunteer Spiritist workers. For anyone interested in mental health, the Spiritist work in the psychiatric field being carried out in Brazil deserves wider recognition as many of the principles involved could with advantage be incorporated into psychiatric practice of other countries. A book which raises many interesting questions and provides some challenging answers."

—*Peter Fenwick, MD, Psychiatrist and author of* The Art of Dying

"*Spiritism and Mental Health* is a must read for mental health workers interested in incorporating into their understandings beliefs and practices from another culture. Editor Emma Bragdon has brought together provocative and stimulating papers by scholars and practitioners working in the tradition of Brazilian Kardecist-Spiritism and those striving to incorporate the Spiritist perspective into their own, more traditional frameworks. The chapters clearly present and analyze the assumptions and therapeutic practices of this distinctive healing tradition while showing how it may be used to complement more conventional healing practices. The book is filled with case studies of patients treated by doctors, psychiatrists and other therapists in hospitals and religious centers in and outside Brazil with combinations of conventional Western and Spiritist treatments. The outcomes for the patients provide a new and exciting direction for scholars and therapists willing to expand their frameworks and approaches to treatment."

—*Sidney Greenfield, PhD, Professor Emeritus of Anthropology, University of Wisconsin-Milwaukee, and author of* Spirits with Scalpels: The Cultural Biology of Religious Healing in Brazil

"This book brings new light to our understanding of mental health and encourages a deeper approach to healing. Emma Bragdon's work shows an insightful and integrated understanding of science, spirituality, and the world of subtle energies. The Foreword by James Lake, MD is a testimonial of great value. As a doctor and healer I found it highly informative reading. It is my belief that this type of understanding will become increasingly important in our next stage of evolution, as more of us work consciously with subtle energies to achieve a greater sense of balance and well-being."

—*Alice Salazar Almeida, MD, a Brazilian who now works at The Hale Clinic, London, UK*

"Author Emma Bragdon's excellent new book, *Spiritism and Mental Health*, adds a new dynamic to the important understanding of how spirituality fits into mental health care. It explains how spirituality not only plays a significant role in mediating deep psychological problems, but also in achieving mental health and personal development. The Brazilian Spiritist practitioners who have contributed to the book's contents represent more than 150 years of experience and decades of professional expertise in this field. This book is ground-breaking and is essential as a reference for all health professionals."

—*Nick Bunick, author of* Time for Truth *and* In God's Truth, *and subject of the bestselling book* The Messengers

"This inspiring and insightful book offers clarity to the philosophy and practice of Kardec's Spiritism. Emma's sensitive and extensive research illuminates subjects such as mediumship, spirit attachment/obsession, spiritual disease and the merging of Spiritism and medical science. The testimonials of recovery from spiritual conditions which are frequently misunderstood and misdiagnosed were profound. This book is a powerful read and excellent resource."

—*Heather Cumming, co-author of* John of God: The Brazilian Healer Who's Touched the Lives of Millions *of related interest*

Mutual Support and Mental Health
A Route to Recovery
Maddy Loat
ISBN 978 1 84310 530 5
Community, Culture and Change series

Reflective Practice in Mental Health
Advanced Psychosocial Practice with Children,
Adolescents and Adults
Edited by Martin Webber and Jack Nathan
ISBN 978 1 84905 029 6

Social Perspectives in Mental Health
Developing Social Models to Understand and
Work with Mental Distress
Edited by Jerry Tew
ISBN 978 1 84310 220 5

SPIRITISM AND MENTAL HEALTH

Practices from Spiritist Centers and
Spiritist Psychiatric Hospitals in Brazil

EDITED BY

EMMA BRAGDON, PHD

FOREWORD BY JAMES LAKE, MD

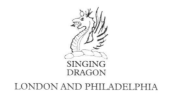

SINGING
DRAGON
LONDON AND PHILADELPHIA

Copyright Acknowledgments

We wish to thank the publishers for permission to reprint the following:

Lightening Up Press first published Marcelo's story in Chapter 6 in *Kardec's Spiritism* (2004) by Emma Bragdon, pp.60–63.

Sage Publications first published Chapter 11, "Jung, Spirits, and Madness: Lessons for Cultural Psychiatry" by Joan Koss-Chioino, in *Transcultural Psychiatry 40*, 2003, pp.164–180.

Elsevier previously published Chapter 20, "Compassionate Intention as a Therapeutic Intervention by Partners of Cancer Patients: Effects of Distant Intention on the Patients' Autonomic Nervous System," in *Explore 4*, July 2008, pp.235–243. The authors are Dean Radin, PhD, Jerome Stone, MA, RN, Ellen Levine, PhD, Shahram Eskandarnejad, MD, Marilyn Schlitz, PhD, Leila Kozak, PhD, Dorothy Mandel, PhD, and Gail Hayssen.

Every effort has been made to trace copyright holders and to obtain their permission for the use of copyright material. The authors and the publisher apologize for any omissions and would be grateful if notified of any acknowledgements that should be incorporated in future reprints or editions of this book.

First published in 2012
by Singing Dragon
an imprint of Jessica Kingsley Publishers
116 Pentonville Road
London N1 9JB, UK
and
400 Market Street, Suite 400
Philadelphia, PA 19106, USA

www.singingdragon.com

Copyright © Singing Dragon 2012

Library of Congress Cataloging in Publication Data
Spiritism and mental health : practices from spiritist centers and spiritist psychiatric hospitals in Brazil / edited by Emma Bragdon ; foreword by James Lake.
    p. cm.
  Includes bibliographical references and index.
  ISBN 978-1-84819-059-7 (alk. paper)
  1. Mental health--Brazil--Religious aspects. 2. Spirituality--Brazil. I. Bragdon, Emma.
  RC489.S676S64 2011
  362.196'8900981--dc22
                                                     2011007366

British Library Cataloguing in Publication Data
A CIP catalogue record for this book is available from the British Library

ISBN 978 1 84819 059 7

Printed and bound in Great Britain

*This book is dedicated to those who support the evolution
of mental health care throughout the world*

Medical Disclaimer

The material in this book is for informational purposes only and is not intended for the diagnosis, treatment, cure, or prevention of disease. Please visit a health professional for medical advice. If you have a mental illness or physical condition please recognize the value of seeking many points of view in deciding on a course of treatment.

Contents

Foreword   1
James Lake, MD, Chair, International Network of Integrative Mental Health, Inc.

ACKNOWLEDGMENTS   8

Introduction   10
Emma Bragdon, PhD, Director, Foundation for Energy Therapies, Vermont, USA

PART I THE SPIRITIST UNDERSTANDING OF MENTAL HEALTH   21

1   A Brief History of Spiritism   22
Emma Bragdon, PhD

2   A Brief Overview of the Philosophy and Development of Spiritism's Methodologies   29
Alexander Moreira-Almeida, MD, PhD, Professor of Psychiatry, Medical School of Juiz de Fora, University of São Paulo, Brazil

3   The Spiritist View of Mental Disorders   37
Alexander Moreira-Almeida, MD, PhD

4   The Relationship of Mediumship to Mental Disorder   47
Marlene Nobre, MD, President, International Medical Spiritist Association; President, Brazilian Medical Spiritist Association; President, Cairbar Schutel Spiritist School, and President of "Lar do Alvorecer" Day Care Center, São Paulo, Brazil

5   Case Studies of Those with Serious Diagnoses   55
Emma Bragdon, PhD

PART II SPIRITIST TREATMENTS: PRACTICE   71

6   Three Spiritist Psychiatric Hospitals   72
   A The Spiritist Hospital André Luiz   73
Roberto Lucio Viera de Souza, MD, Director, Spiritist Hospital André Luiz, Belo Horizonte, Brazil, and Jaider Rodrigues e Paulo, MD, Psychiatrist, Spiritist Hospital André Luiz, Belo Horizonte, Brazil

   B The Spiritist Psychiatric Hospital of Porto Alegre   82
Emma Bragdon, PhD

C João Evangelista Hospital   88

*Candido Pinto Vallada, MD, Vice President, Council of Directors and General
Coordinator, Spirituality and Mental Health Integration Program, Hospital João
Evangelista, São Paulo, Brazil, Camilla Casaletti Braghetta, MA, Occupational
Therapist, HOJE, São Paulo, Brazil, Giancarlo Lucchetti, MD, Research Executive
Coordinator, Spirituality and Mental Health Integration Program, Hospital João
Evangelista, São Paulo, Brazil, Frederico Camelo Leão, MD, PhD, CEO, Hospital
João Evangelista, São Paulo, Brazil, and Homero Vallada, MD, President, Council of
Directors at the Hospital João Evangelista, and Associate Professor, the University of
São Paulo Medical School, São Paulo, Brazil*

7   Magnetic Healing, Prayer, and Energy Passes   97
     *Gilson Roberto, MD, Medical Director, Spiritist Psychiatric Hospital of Porto Alegre,
     Brazil*

8   Psychotherapy and Reincarnation: A Necessary and Fruitful
     Encounter   104
     *Julio Peres, PsyD, PhD, Clinical Psychologist and Researcher at the Program for
     Health, Spirituality and Religiosity, Psychiatry Institute, University of São Paulo
     School of Medicine, São Paulo, Brazil*

9   The Group Field   113
     Emma Bragdon, PhD

10   Spiritual Counseling and Fellowship in Spiritist Centers   116
     *Carlos Appel, MD, General Practitioner, Porto Alegre, Brazil, and Tania Appel, MA,
     medium and leader, Casa de Dom Inácio, Abadiânia, Brazil*

11   Jung, Spirits, and Madness: Lessons for Cultural Psychiatry   126
     *Joan Koss-Chioino, PhD, Professor Emerita, School of Human Evolution and Social
     Change, Arizona State University, USA*

12   The Practice of Integrating Spirituality into Psychotherapy   140
     Mario Sergio Silveira, PhD, Administrator, Hospital Bom Retiro, Curitiba, Brazil

13   When Medical Doctors Are Mediums   149
     Gilson Roberto, MD

PART III CURRENT SCIENCE,
PSYCHOTHERAPY, AND SPIRITISM   155

14   A Science of Understanding the Mind: The Next Great Scientific
     Revolution   156
     *Alan Wallace, PhD, President, Santa Barbara Institute for Consciousness Studies,
     California, USA*

15   Spirit Attachment and Health   165
     Alan Sanderson, MD, President of the Spirit Release Foundation, London, UK

16   Soul-Centered Psychotherapy   175
Andrew Powell, MD, Founding Chair, Spirituality and Psychiatry Special Interest
Group, Royal College of Psychiatrists, UK

17   Current Research on Survival of Consciousness and Mediumship   189
Linda Russek, PhD, Director, Heart Science Foundation, Arizona, USA

18   The Power of "Magnetized" Water   201
Beverly Rubik, PhD, President, Institute for Frontier Science, California, USA

19   The Positive Potential of Dissociative States of Consciousness   212
Melvin Morse, MD, pediatrician, researcher, and author

20   Compassionate Intention as a Therapeutic Intervention by
Partners of Cancer Patients: Effects of Distant Intention on
the Patients' Autonomic Nervous System   221
Dean Radin, PhD, Senior Scientist, Institute of Noetic Sciences, Sonoma State
University, California, USA, Jerome Stone, MA, RN, Ellen Levine, PhD, Shahram
Eskandarnejad, MD, Marilyn Schlitz, PhD, Leila Kozak, PhD, Dorothy Mandel,
PhD, and Gail Hayssen

21   The Pineal Gland and Its Influence on Body–Mind–Soul Integration   237
Decio Iandoli, Jr., MD, PhD, Professor of Medicine, UNIDERP,
Mato Grosso do Sul, Brazil

PART IV THE INTERNATIONAL
IMPACT OF SPIRITISM   247

22   What Spiritist Centers Offer Outside Brazil   249
Janet Duncan, founding member, the International Spiritist Council, and former
President of the British Union of Spiritist Societies (BUSS)

23   Contributions of Brazilian Spiritist Treatments to the Global
Improvement of Mental Health Care   257
Stanley Krippner, PhD, Professor of Psychology, Saybrook University, San Francisco,
USA, and Emma Bragdon, PhD

PART V EDUCATION AND RESEARCH   267

24   Training Mediums Who Treat Psychiatric Patients   268
Gerald Magnan, past supervisor of the Department of Spiritual Assistance, the Spiritist
Psychiatric Hospital of Porto Alegre, Brazil

25   Teaching Health Professionals How to Support Personal
Transformation in Patients   277
Gelson Roberto, Psychologist and advisor to the Spiritist Psychiatric Hospital of Porto
Alegre, Brazil

26 Researching the Invisible: Entangled Minds, Psychiatry, and
    Psychology   285
    *William Braud, PhD, Professor Emeritus, Institute of Transpersonal Psychology, Palo
    Alto, California, USA*

    THE CONTRIBUTORS   295

    APPENDIX I FURTHER READING AND VIEWING   298

    APPENDIX II ORGANIZATIONS SUPPORTING THE INTEGRATION OF
    SPIRITUALITY AND PSYCHIATRY   300

    GLOSSARY   302

    REFERENCES   305

    SUBJECT INDEX   327

    AUTHOR INDEX   333

List of Figures and Tables

Figure 5.1 Causes and potential outcomes of severe mental illness   66

Figure 18.1 Dark-field microphotograph from live blood analysis of a normal healthy
person's blood sample   202

Figure 18.2 Dark-field microphotograph of the initial live blood analysis of a 55-year-old
man that shows considerable blood congestion   203

Figure 18.3 Dark-field microphotograph from live blood analysis of the same 55-year-old
man (see Figure 18.2) after six months of drinking alkaline water from an ionizer 203

Figure 18.4a GDV photo of induced light emitted from a tap water droplet   205

Figure 18.4b GDV photo of induced light emitted from a droplet of water from a stream in
the High Sierra Mountains of California   206

Figure 18.4c GDV photo of induced light emitted from a droplet of water from an ionizer.
The same tap water whose GDV emission pattern is shown in Figure 18.4a was sent
through the ionizer   206

Figure 18.5a GDV photo of induced light emitted from a tap water droplet   207

Figure 18.5b GDV photo of the same tap water as in Figure 18.5a after a group of six
people project "healing love" to the water   208

Table 19.1 The spectrum of dissociation as seen in healing, health, and mental dysfunction 213

Figure 20.1 Laboratory layout   225

Figure 20.2 Protocol for sender stimulus   226

Table 20.1 Participant demographics for the three groups   229

Figure 20.3 Sender and receiver normalized mean skin conductance levels across all 38 sessions 230

Figure 20.4 Sender and receiver normalized mean skin conductance levels for all motivated
sessions   230

Figure 20.5 Sender and receiver normalized mean skin conductance levels for control sessions 231

Figure 20.6 Comparison of sender and receiver effect sizes measured at stimulus offset for
all sessions, motivated sessions, and for trained, wait, and control groups separately 231

Figure 20.7 Normalized comparison of receiver skin conductance levels in the three groups 232

FOREWORD

James Lake, MD

The roles of healers and priests have overlapped since the beginning of recorded history. Until historically recent times priests and other spiritual adepts were regarded as healers, and gifted healers were elevated to the status of priest or shaman. By the early twentieth century psychoanalysis had pathologized or outright dismissed the psychological dimensions of spiritual experience and the relevance of spirituality in mental health.

Today, biological theories of brain function are accepted with little debate by conventionally trained medical professionals—and by a growing number of our patients—as adequate explanations of the causes of mental illness. Even as science long ago eliminated "spirit" from its discourse, biomedicine has relegated considerations of spirituality and "energy" in health and illness to interesting if clinically irrelevant *new age* fads.

In the face of such skepticism, emerging research findings reviewed in this book suggest that spirituality is not only related to physical and mental health and well-being, but that spiritual beliefs and practices often play a central role in both the prevention and treatment of mental illness. The strong historical relationships between religious and spiritual beliefs and health stand in stark contrast to the failure of contemporary biomedicine to adequately address these issues.

This book presents an integrative model of care centered around the understanding and treatment of spiritual issues that manifest as mental and emotional symptoms. The authors believe that there are complex causes and meanings of mental illness; and agree that the broad goal of mental health care is to provide compassionate care resulting in lasting symptomatic relief while emphasizing safety, respecting each patient's unique cultural values and spiritual beliefs, and contributing to their general physical and psychological well-being.

I believe this book will significantly advance the level of discourse on the role of spirituality in mental health, resulting in greater openness to spiritual models of care in the USA and other countries.

Every system of medicine is constrained by inherent limitations on its theories and clinical methods, and no single interpretive framework or particular treatment approach is ideally suited to *all* patients who report the same symptom. Particular treatments are ineffective or only partially effective when they fail to address the complex biological causes or psychological, cultural, or spiritual *meanings* of mental illness.

Limitations of Pharmacologic Treatment

While contemporary pharmacologic treatments used in conventional mental health care frequently provide temporary symptomatic relief they seldom adequately address—and certainly *do not cure*—the root psychological, biological, or spiritual causes or meanings of mental illness. Biomedical psychiatry continues to accrue important scientific advances in the basic neurosciences, pharmacology, molecular biology, and genetics; however, its successes are limited by many factors, including:

- incomplete understandings of the postulated mechanisms of action of many drugs

- limited efficacy of many drugs in current use

- significant safety problems and related compliance problems caused by toxic side-effects or drug–drug interactions

- unaffordability or limited availability of drugs that are regarded by Western trained physicians as the most effective treatments for a particular mental illness.

Psychopharmacologic treatments are demonstrably not only *inadequate* but the dominant contemporary model of mental health care based on their exclusive use is often inappropriate and may interfere with or delay patient care, especially when significant cultural or spiritual factors manifest as mental and emotional symptoms.

Contemporary biomedical psychiatry becomes even more problematic when one examines its theoretical foundations. The best research evidence from genetics and functional brain imaging studies suggests that multiple indirect relationships probably exist between *functional dysregulation* of the brain at the levels of neurotransmitters and neural circuits and predispositions to develop cognitive, affective, or behavioral symptoms. To date, however, only the most basic mechanisms of brain function at the level of discrete neurotransmitters, single neurons, or simple circuits of neurons in non-human animal models have been clearly elucidated. Taken together these issues have resulted in growing controversy among health care providers and patients over the *appropriate* and *reasonable* uses of pharmacological treatments in mental health care, and there is ongoing dialogue in the general public and the medical community about whether the risks and limitations of psychopharmacologic drug treatment outweigh their potential benefits. Challenges to the conventional biomedical dogma of contemporary Western psychiatry invite systematic, open-minded examination of diverse non-pharmacologic treatment modalities including herbal medicines, other natural products, mind–body therapies as well as postulated "energetic" or spiritual treatment methods.

Religious and Spiritual Beliefs and Mental Health

Almost 80 percent of individuals who seek medical care for any reason feel that their religious or spiritual beliefs are directly related to their health concerns, while only 16 percent of conventionally trained physicians or nurses ever inquire about these important matters (King and Bushwick 1994). Over 90 percent of surveyed family practice physicians (Neeleman and King 1993) believed they were competent to address religious or spiritual issues with patients.

In a large US multi-center trial (MacLean *et al.* 2003), two-thirds of patients wanted physicians to be more aware of their spiritual beliefs and a third wanted to be asked about these beliefs. Not surprisingly, patients want to share their spiritual beliefs, but only if they feel physicians will respect their values (Hebert *et al.* 2001).

Research findings suggest that religious practices and spiritual beliefs probably have both indirect and direct effects on mental health and general well-being. Epidemiologic studies suggest that religious beliefs have a primary protective effect on mental health (Levin 1996, 2003). Social, behavioral, and psychological models have been advanced in efforts to explain observed relationships between religious or spiritual practices and mental health. Religious or spiritual values are correlated with health-promoting lifestyle choices, including exercise, diet, and moderate alcohol use (Hamburg, Elliott and Parron 1982). Findings of a large survey study suggest that religious and spiritual beliefs are associated with improved self-management of symptoms in patients with bipolar disorder (Mitchell and Romans 2003). Findings from the NIMH Epidemiologic Catchment Area survey (N = 2969) support the view that regular weekly attendance at religious services is associated with significantly lower incidences of most anxiety disorders including agoraphobia, generalized anxiety disorder, and social phobia in general, but a relatively higher incidence of obsessive-compulsive disorder in younger individuals with strong religious beliefs (Koenig *et al.* 1993).

Religious beliefs and practices are an important source of encouragement, social support, and insights to individuals who suffer from chronic severe mental illness, including schizophrenia (Sullivan 1993). Support groups built around shared spiritual themes have beneficial effects on self-esteem, quality of life, and community involvement in schizophrenics (Sageman 2004).

Spiritual Practices and Mental Health

In addition to established social, cultural, and psychological advantages of religious involvement and spiritual belief systems, there is emerging evidence that prayer and other forms of spiritual healing have direct beneficial effects on health. A systematic review of 23 controlled trials of different healing approaches concluded that beneficial outcomes are reported almost 60 percent of the time when distant healing intention alone is employed to treat a particular medical or psychiatric disorder (Astin, Harkness and Ernst 2000). Over 2000 case reports or research studies have been published on different forms of healing including prayer and other forms of spiritual healing (Jonas and Crawford 2003).

Functional brain imaging studies suggest that deep meditative states achieved through yoga and other spiritual practices are associated with metabolic changes in brain regions involved in sustained attention (D'Aquili and Newberg 2000). Several studies have shown above-chance correlations in electrical brain activity between pairs of individuals separated by electromagnetic shielding who are instructed to "communicate" through intention (Schlitz and Braud 1997; Standish *et al.* 2003). Preliminary findings suggest that healing intention is associated with subtle changes in brain activity in patients who are empathically bonded with spiritual healers (Achterberg *et al.* 2005).

Prayer

Almost 40 percent of family practice physicians (Olive 1995) disclosed that they had prayed with patients, and 9 out of 10 of those believed that praying with their patients had beneficial effects on the medical problem or psychiatric problem that was being addressed. A large national poll found that almost 50 percent of patients would like to share in prayer with their physicians during medical office visits (Yankelovich Partners Inc. 1996).

A general population survey of over a thousand respondents found that almost 80 percent of adults believe that prayer can help people recover from disease (Sloan, Bagiella and Powell 1999). For example, approximately three quarters of cancer patients who use alternative therapies believe that prayer is an effective treatment of cancer (Samano *et al.* 2004). Only 11 percent of individuals who pray in efforts to improve their health disclose this fact to their physicians.

In terms of mental health, survey findings (Astin *et al.* 2000) show that a significant percentage of severely depressed or anxious individuals engage in regular prayer in efforts to address their mental health problems, and approximately one-third believe that prayer is very helpful in improving their symptoms. Significantly, the same survey findings suggest that only 10 percent of individuals who self-treat any mental health problem using prayer had approached a psychiatrist or family physician for treatment at any time during the previous year (Anderson, Anderson and Felsenthal 1993; King and Bushwick 1994).

Differing Views on the Causes of Mental Illness

In spite of ongoing progress in the neurosciences the causes of mental illness remain obscure. This is due to the fact that contemporary biomedical psychiatry rests on philosophically and scientifically ambiguous ground. In conventional biomedicine foundational theories from physics, chemistry, and biology form the basis of an explanatory model of physical and mental illness. Biomedicine claims that "causes" of illness—and by extension the mechanisms of action underlying *legitimate* treatments—rest on biological processes that can be described in the reductionist language of science. While discrete "causes" of some medical disorders have been confirmed as specific metabolic or genetic problems or discrete disease-causing microorganisms, in the domain of biomedical psychiatry there are no simple identifiable "causes" of disorders and no single model adequately explains the complex and subtle "causes" of mental illness. There is no "unifying" theory of mental illness because no particular explanatory model has been confirmed as *more valid* or *more adequate* than any other.

What remains are competing social, psychodynamic, genetic, endocrinological, and neurobiological models of symptom formation reflecting disparate assumptions about the nature and causes of symptoms, and a correspondingly diverse set of perspectives that inform the theories and clinical methods of psychiatrists, psychologists, social workers, and other mental health professionals.

In contrast to conventional biomedicine, basic concepts of health, disease, and healing are conceptualized in Chinese medicine, Ayurveda, and other healing traditions in ways that differ from the reductionist tenets of science. In Chinese medicine and Ayurveda, for example, symptoms are interpreted as indicators of imbalances of postulated fundamental energetic principles. In these healing traditions the causes of illness (including mental illness) cannot be reduced to discrete physiological changes in terms that are understandable in conventional biomedicine.

As biomedicine evolves, emerging paradigms may eventually result in an expanded interpretation of illness phenomena that will permit rigorous scientific explanations of the kinds of "energetic imbalances" postulated by Spiritism and other healing traditions that expand beyond the confines of biomedicine.

The Emerging Paradigm of Integrative Mental Health

As the authors of this book compellingly argue, mental health care is being shaped by an emerging synthesis of theories and clinical perspectives from cutting edge research in physics and the basic neurosciences, biomedicine, and the world's traditional healing practices. A future *integrative paradigm* will incorporate understandings from genetics, the neurosciences, consciousness research, complexity theory, and quantum field theory in addition to the evidence for the role of human intention in healing that is now emerging from studies on "energy medicine" and spiritual healing methods. The result will be rapid evolution away from the limited bio-psycho-social model based on simplistic understandings of "treating" neurotransmitter "imbalances" with prescription drugs, into a broader, more inclusive paradigm that starts from, but is not limited to, the conventional biomedical view and acknowledges the central relevance of "energy" and human intention to health and wellness.

The new integrative paradigm of mental health care will lead to better and more adequate understandings of the disparate causes and *meanings* of symptoms combining multi-modal therapeutics from biomedicine and healing traditions with the wisdom of the world's great spiritual traditions.

The authors of this unique volume argue for a broad integrative vision that subsumes both empirically based scientific methods and intuitive or spiritual approaches. They persuasively assert that the best model of care should honor both biomedicine and diverse alternative perspectives. In other words, there are reasonable and appropriate roles for both conventional pharmacologic treatments and the range of non-pharmacologic—including spiritual—therapies in medicine and mental health care.

Novel explanatory models of mental illness causation will emerge from the rigorous open-minded examination of methods used in systems of medicine not limited to biomedicine as well as ongoing advances in the basic neurosciences. Future *more complete* theories that conceptualize symptoms as manifestations of complex dynamic relationships at biological, energetic, informational, and *spiritual* levels will lead to more effective treatment approaches addressing the causes and meanings of symptoms at multiple inter-related hierarchic levels. Increasing openness around the globe and in biomedicine to the world's healing traditions will accelerate the evolution of conventional biomedical psychiatry toward a *truly integrative* model of mental health care directed at the whole person in the context of his or her cultural identity and spiritual beliefs. This evolution will result in increased uses of cost-effective integrative approaches that will translate into reductions in long-term costs associated with expensive conventional pharmacological treatments and improvements in safety in mental health care.

Spiritism: A Unique Integrative Model of Care

As you will read in these pages, the Spiritist movement in Brazil is a truly integrative model of mental health care that addresses the core issues of mental illness taking into account patients' medical, social, cultural, and spiritual needs. The successes of the Spiritist movement demonstrate what can be achieved in the alleviation of human suffering when hospitals, clinicians, and patients collectively embrace a model of care that acknowledges the inter-related roles of body, mind, and spirit in mental health.

The expert authors of this unique volume have made a compelling case for the central role of spirituality in mental and emotional well-being. Clearly the time is right for open-minded discussion of the role of prayer and other spiritual approaches in health and healing in medicine and mental health care. It is my hope and expectation that pilot programs borrowing from the innovations of Spiritism will come about in the USA and other countries, and that from these small beginnings mental health care will evolve into a paradigm and model of care that is more effective, safer, and more accessible.

James Lake, MD
Monterey, California
January 2011

Acknowledgments

A book of this kind is obviously a team effort, with each player making a particular contribution and essential to the success of the whole.

The financial sponsors of this work have come through the Marion Foundation and the Rudolf Steiner Foundation. It's hard to find words big enough to communicate the depth of my appreciation for your years of trust, support, guidance, and friendship.

Of course, I am profoundly grateful to the authors who contributed their work through the chapters—and all they have done in preparation. Alexander Moreira-Almeida, MD, was a contributor as well as my consultant when I was developing the idea of this book, and without his kind introductions to many of the contributing authors in Brazil this book would not have come to be. I must also thank Stanley Krippner, PhD, who first introduced me to Alexander.

One of the intentions of this book is to further dialog between Brazilians and those outside Brazil about Spiritism and its practical applications. This has meant that authors who have Portuguese as their native tongue had to entrust their work to translators, so we can benefit from their thoughts in English. This is not such an easy task when it comes to translating esoteric terms or spiritual practices when there are no words in the English language that accurately convey the concepts. There were a number of well-informed translators, most of whom are Spiritist mediums themselves, who have helped in this task: Rogerio Severo, PhD, Amantino Ramos de Freitas, Elza D'Agosto, Horatio Monteverde, Juliane Silveira, and Melissa Varga, PhD. Some of the translators are not known to me, so I take this opportunity to acknowledge their important contributions. Thank you!

Some of the chapters were sent out for peer review after I received them to ensure accuracy and explore the logic, and wisdom, of the viewpoints expressed. I am grateful to Vernon Neppe, MD, Julie Beischel, PhD, Glen Aldochine, MD, John L. Turner, MD, Immanuel Tjiong, JSM, JSD, Barbara Strong, Horatio Monteverde, Joan Koss-Chioino, PhD, and Alexander Moreira-Almeida, MD, for adding valuable perspective.

My heart-felt thanks to those clients and contacts who have shared their journeys with me, in some cases allowing me to participate during their inner transformation as they were confronting their inner shadows. This includes the participants in all the 45 and more groups I have led to visit John of God in Brazil since 2001. The deep longing that inspired you to go to Brazil, and the courage you have had to show to do your inner work, have spoken to my heart, and now bring heart and soul to this book. Namaste. (I bow to your Deep Self.)

Special thanks to Jessica Kingsley for her vision and enthusiasm in taking on this book and shepherding it personally as my Editor at Jessica Kingsley Publishers. Your insight is keen, your vision wide, and you are ever respectful. Your professional production team has also been front and center with their work. Much appreciated! I am grateful to Marc Micozzi, MD, PhD, for having such energy about the book proposal that he introduced me to Jessica Kingsley.

My personal support team has been superb: I can name some, but many who have contributed must go un-named, as that list goes on forever. My friends and family in Vermont and especially my son, Jesse, and his wife, Allison, and children (Sam and Rowan) in Boston lovingly gave me companionship, support, soup, and…space to hole up and concentrate, as needed. Deep thanks. Paula Sellars and Phil Roth, Esq., the other members of the Board of Directors of the Foundation for Energy Therapies, have been consistently generous, caring, and resourceful. They have carried the light when the sun was behind dark clouds. My dear friends living in or frequenting the community of Abadiânia, Brazil, have fed me with important information, inspiration, and help in the development of my understanding and practice as a medium, and kept me laughing as well: the medium João Teixera de Faria (known as John of God), Dorothy Cooke, Marisa and João Restle, Tania Appel, Jorge Daher, MD, Catherine Tucker, Sara Jane Kingston, Raymond Cadwell, Beth Pereira, Grainne McEntee, and João Vasco. Medical anthropologist Anna Jessica Theissen, PhD, was the first to inspire me about Spiritist Psychiatric Hospitals when we met on several occasions in Abadiânia. Jessica introduced me to a few of the contacts she had developed while completing her PhD dissertation for UC Berkeley: "The Location of Madness: Spiritist Psychiatry and the Meaning of Mental Illness in Contemporary Brazil." Eduardo Kurashiki is the first Brazilian to facilitate a visit to one of the Spiritist psychiatric facilities. He embodies the kindness that radiates from Spiritists who volunteer their time in such places.

The painting on the front cover was done by a patient at Casas André Luiz by the name of Alex Sandro de Lima. Casas André Luiz is a Spiritist Hospital providing room, board, and care for people who are significantly impaired cognitively and will be living in the institution for the rest of their lives. On arrival, Alex did a painting that was all dark colors, reflecting what appears as deep despair. Several months later he did the painting on our cover which shows balance and light: a true testimony to what he is receiving at Casas André Luiz.

Last, but by no means least, I must give thanks for what I receive from my own spiritual guidance. Dona Marta Thomas, an exemplary Spiritist teacher, medium, and healer in São Paulo (introduced by Julika Kiskos, PhD), told me with a twinkle in her eye in 2001, "You have so many guides helping you in your work, you need at least two taxis just to bring them with you from place to place when you do your study of Spiritism." "They" are truly the endless source of inspiration and energy for the book. At the beginning and at the end, putting this book together has been a sacred task, in which I was given much help.

INTRODUCTION

Emma Bragdon, PhD

We are currently facing a sharp increase in the cost of health care, as well as an exponential increase in the number of people on disability because of mental health issues. In the USA, our conventional medical establishments have the resources to administer excellent emergency medical care, but, according to the World Health Organization (Tandon *et al.* 2000), our overall health system performance ranks 37th, and Americans rank 72nd in overall level of health compared to 191 countries—even though we have the most expensive health care system in the world. We can extrapolate that our knowledge and practices regarding the healing of mental illness and chronic degenerative physical disease are not exemplary.

This obviously signals a need to look outside our borders for ideas about how to improve our health care systems, to prevent disease and maintain wellness. Possibly we can also learn more about the causes of illness.

> The precise causes [etiology] of mental disorders are not known.
> (US Department of Health and Human Services 1999)

Robert Whitaker (2010), an award-winning medical journalist, reflects that our top medical authorities still do not know the real cause of mental illness. While many benefit from conventional psychotropic drugs, the majority of individuals who use these powerful medications do not experience significant or sustained improvement or are unable to tolerate their long-term use because of associated toxicity and serious adverse effects including weight gain, loss of libido, gastro-intestinal distress, and, in some cases, worsening of the mental health problem for which they are being treated. Whitaker suggests that conventional psychiatry relies too heavily on psychotropics and too little on viable non-pharmacologic alternatives:

> The drugs may alleviate symptoms over the short term, and there are some people who may stabilize well over the long term on them, and so clearly there is a place for the drugs in psychiatry's toolbox… However, [given the long-term outcome research] psychiatry would have to admit that the drugs, rather than fix chemical imbalances in the brain, perturb the normal functioning of neurotransmitter

pathways... [Psychiatry has to figure out] how to use the medications judiciously and wisely, and everyone in our society would understand the need for alternative therapies that don't rely on the medications or at least minimize their use. (Whitaker 2010, p.333)

Recent systematic reviews of quality placebo-controlled trials bear out Whitaker's observations and provide confirmation that available pharmacologic treatments do not adequately address common mental health problems including major depressive disorder (Fournier *et al.* 2010; Kirsch 2008; Thase 2008), bipolar disorder (Fountoulakis 2008), schizophrenia and other psychotic disorders (Dixon *et al.* 2010; Tajima *et al.* 2009), dementia (Birks and Harvey 2006; Lam *et al.* 2009), obsessive-compulsive disorder (Shoenfelt and Weston 2007), post-traumatic stress disorder (Berger *et al.* 2009), and generalized anxiety disorder (Katzman 2009). In spite of compelling evidence to the contrary, we continue to treat symptoms as if they are caused by a "broken brain" in which deficiencies or "imbalances" of serotonin and other neurotransmitters are regarded by modern psychiatry as sufficient explanations of mental illness.

In 2009 one out of eight adults in the USA was taking psychiatric medication, most believing that medications are necessary for bolstering brain function in the way that insulin is essential for the diabetic. The results to society have not been positive. In 2007 the disability rate due to mental illness was 1 in every 76 Americans.[1] That's more than double the rate in 1987 (a year before Prozac was introduced), and six times the rate in 1955 (before psychotropics were being used) (Whitaker 2010, p.10). The tremendous increase in the number of people claiming disability for mental illness is an indictment of contemporary biomedical psychiatry and points to serious unresolved problems of efficacy and safety with available psychotropic medications.

In other words, when psychiatric medications are used *as the sole sources of healing* and do not address the root cause of illness, they may be ineffective or result in worsening, to the point where patients turn to more potent synthetic medications, sometimes resulting in debilitating adverse effects that interfere with their ability to function socially and at work. Research on the long-term effects of psychiatric medications reported by the Director of the National Institute of Mental Health in 1996 reveal that they compromise brain function rather than enhance it (Hyman 1996).

We have hunted for big simple neuro-chemical explanations for psychiatric disorders and have not found them. (Kenneth Kendler, Co-Editor in Chief of *Psychological Medicine*, quoted in Lacasse 2005)

These circumstances signal a need to look outside our borders to cultures and healing traditions that offer effective therapies, other than psychotropic drugs, that can add to our toolbox for improving mental health and promoting wellness.

In order to transform mental health care into a more effective, more humane model it is incumbent on physicians to remain rigorously open-minded about the range of alternative therapies and integrate those that work and are safe into the current model of biomedical psychiatry. Only in this way can the general population achieve a higher level of wellness.

It is also timely to consider: Is there a spiritual imbalance in our way of life signaled by the fact that so many people are seeking help for mental illness, and overall the level of health of our population ranks 72nd amongst 191 nations? Shealy and Church (2008, p.25) reviewed the research to find that spiritual practice and belief have a marked positive influence on longevity and health. They have been found to:

- improve the survival rate of patients after operations

- ameliorate pain

- raise levels of pleasure-inducing hormones in the brain

- improve mental acuity

- reduce depression

- boost immune system function

- reduce the time it takes wounds to heal

- reduce the frequency and length of hospital stays

- increase marital happiness in men

- reduce alcohol consumption and cigarette smoking

- reduce the incidence of cancer and heart disease

- improve the health of older adults

- add years to the average life-span.

Spirituality involves each of us in the quest for ultimate meaning and purpose in life. It supports connection to and relationship with the sacred dimensions of life and with each other. A life directed by one's spiritual intention is more likely, then, to move a person towards wellness.

Exploring a Resource in Brazil

From 2001 to 2011 I immersed myself in studying Spiritism, spending three to six months each year in Brazil participating at various Spiritist Centers, visiting Spiritist Psychiatric Hospitals, and learning from direct contact with Spiritist leaders who are mediums, teachers, and hospital administrators. Why? I found

Spiritism a unique, safe, and powerful way towards helping people address chronic mental and physical problems through healing that complements conventional health care. It encourages people to take steps to manifest their highest potential for wisdom, peace, and creativity. It has been involved with this task for 150 years and its popularity among the most well educated and wealthy in Brazil is currently growing at a rapid rate.

This book is written for an audience of health professionals, students of the health professions, and those involved with all aspects of health and healing who want to understand Spiritist therapies, how they work, and contemplate how they might help our ailing health care system. Although this book is not oriented towards proselytizing Spiritism, it is timely to consider how we might use effective components of Spiritist treatments to treat the mentally ill, as well as foster well-being.

An Accessible Path for Growth and Well-Being and a Model for Integrative Health Care

Spiritism not only supports mental health and spiritual growth, but does not deplete anyone's bank account. It is not an arm of government, or any church. It is wholly supported by private donations.

Anyone can attend and make use of the services of a Spiritist Center. Spiritism is a community-based, grassroots social movement that is available to people of every religion, race, economic status, and age. It has been effective and has continued developing since 1860. The community centers, now numbering 12–13,000 and serving 20–40 million people in Brazil alone (a country of 200 million), seem to have sprung up around every corner, as common as convenience stores, offering the daily bread of spiritual inspiration, community support, and laying-on of hands to balance the energies of the body and mind. Almost every center also has optional training programs for those who want to develop their psychic and/or healing abilities. Fifty Spiritist Psychiatric Hospitals in Brazil help those in profound states of mental illness who need inpatient care.

More than 45 groups of individuals from the USA, Israel, China, Europe, and Africa have come with me to visit these centers. All are amazed at the resources the centers and hospitals provide and wonder how we might create something similar to benefit them at home. It seems obvious to us that the Spiritist Centers and hospitals are giving us a model of integrative health maintenance for physical and mental health. We have nothing like them in the USA or Europe.

I was so excited by what I discovered, and wondered why I hadn't learned about this in graduate school. Then I noticed the dearth of documentation on this fascinating topic and felt inspired to report to both the general audience and health professionals what I had learned. With the help of generous grants, I wrote a book about the work of John of God's sanctuary, *Spiritual Alliances* (2002), and produced a 30-minute documentary film about his work, *I Do Not Heal, God Is the One Who Heals* (2006). Next, I wrote a book documenting Spiritism titled *Kardec's Spiritism* (2004), followed by another 30-minute documentary film, *Spiritism: Bridging Spirituality and Health* (2008). On November 17, 2010, Oprah Winfrey dedicated her internationally acclaimed afternoon TV talk show to stories about John of God, opening the door to many people internationally to learn about the work of this Brazilian spiritual healer. CNN aired a report on John of God in December 2010. The BBC, ABC, and Discovery Health had produced hour-long reports on him in previous years. Clearly, network attention is pointing to the extraordinary phenomena of Brazil's spiritual healing resources, but rarely has the limelight extended to include anything about Spiritist Centers and hospitals. I was pleased to be invited to report on these to health professionals in a medical journal (Bragdon 2005) and medical school textbook (Bragdon 2010).

In practice, Spiritism (Kardec 2004a, 2004b) has already found a home in 31 countries around the world, and there are 70 Spiritist Centers in the USA alone. Some who participate find it answers a need to acknowledge and develop spirituality as part of mental health without the mandates that became overly rigid and authoritarian in some of the traditional ways of practicing religion.

If we see that Spiritism offers something of value, we do not have to create centers and hospitals exactly like those in Brazil, of course. We can create our own version of these centers and hospitals, to serve our own needs, resonant with our own cultures. However, the models for both hospitals and community centers that Brazil has developed may be of great help to us as we try to integrate Spiritist theories into our own health care system regarding the cause of mental illness as well as its healing practices.

The Cause and Cure of Mental Illness from a Spiritist Perspective

Brazilian Spiritist Psychiatric Hospitals take an integrative approach to mental health care. They are not averse to psychiatric medications, and see them as an important means to helping patients in many circumstances. Their dispensary for medications is just as up to date, just as full and varied, as a similar storeroom in the USA in a conventional hospital. Well-trained psychiatrists prescribe the drugs when they feel it is necessary, for example when a patient is completely overwhelmed and disoriented and needs the comfort of sleep and being buffered from feeling the emotional extremes that made him or her unable to function. Social workers assess and treat social causes of mental illness, just as medical doctors diagnose and treat biological factors that can exacerbate psychological problems. Therapists are also available for occupational therapy, group therapy, physical education, art, music, being in nature, and other "complementary" therapies.

Patients in Brazil, often the disadvantaged, are not so quick to continue use of expensive medications as we are in the USA, nor are the medications seen in advertisements on television and news media, making them appear appealing, even sexy. Thus, the number of people interested in continuing use of psychotropics is not as large in Brazil as in the USA (Whitaker 2010).

When a patient elects Spiritist treatment in the hospital then the conventional treatments are used in conjunction with Spiritist therapies. Highly trained mediums, who have extraordinary resources for empathy, add their medical intuition and facility for understanding and treating the subtle bio-psycho-social and spiritual dynamics of the illness. They are often able to pinpoint that the cause of the illness originated in past lives or particular circumstances of the current life—and help the patient release it. Other Spiritist treatments put patients into closer connection to spiritual resources for their healing through prayer, blessed water, and laying-on of hands. When patients receive these treatments in the context of being one in a group of other patients receiving treatment a "group field" emerges that improves the ability of each person to be receptive to higher spiritual forces. Attending to the subtle body as well as the bio-psycho-social needs of the patient is a level of integrative care we do not typically have in our clinics and hospitals.

Spiritist psychiatrists do not believe that the brain is the home of the mind and the spirit. Thus they cannot embrace the notion that finding the right chemical for the brain will be the most essential antidote to imbalance of the mind, spirit, and emotions. They believe that vast aspects of the mind and spirit reside outside the physical brain in the "perispirit," a subtle body that envelops the physical body and holds the blueprint of the body and the seeds of illness. The perispirit changes as it is worked with in Spiritist therapies—seeds of illness are dissolved and the receiver becomes spiritually uplifted.

Allan Kardec, the founder of Spiritism, described the perispirit as "a subtle, ethereal, nearly massless covering…a kind of energy body that serves as a blueprint for the human form" (Kardec 2004a). This etheric body permeates the physical body in every detail, creating an exact duplicate of every organ and limb. Its main function is to transmit energy to the physical body. Congestion of energy in the perispirit, or a weakening caused by stress, negative thinking, being overly judgmental, lack of forgiveness of self or others, or depression, can link to a particular organ or system in the body, causing a physical manifestation of illness. In the perispirit one finds not only the karmic consequences of negative behavior in past lives, but the seed of uncharitable acts and negative thinking in the present life.

> The soul…forms a single unity with the perispirit, and integrates with the entire body, which constitutes a complex human being… We can

imagine two bodies similar in form, one interpenetrating another, combined during life and separated at death, which destroys one while the other continues to exist. During life, the soul acts through the vehicles of thought and emotion. It is simultaneously internal and external—that is, it radiates outwardly, being able to separate itself from the body, to transport itself considerable distances, and there to manifest its presence. (Kardec 2004b)

When Spiritist mediums do "psychic surgery" they open the subtle body (not touching the physical body) and begin clearing the "miasms" (that represent congestion in the subtle body) that are the root of the illness. Intervention through focusing a high vibration (associated with pure love) in the "laying-on of hands" also changes the blueprint in and around the physical body and strengthens the foundation for the physical body of the patient to become healed. This kind of spiritual healing is also practiced as preventative care to stop the development of disease states by maintaining an appropriate flow of energy in the perispirit, and in turn to the body.

It is interesting to note here that experiments at the Institute of HeartMath in California demonstrate that consciousness, as expressed in the intentions of individuals, affects the structure of the DNA molecules. HeartMath's team of researchers have concluded that cell-level processes can be influenced by human intention, mediated via energetic interactions (Institute of HeartMath 2003; Shealy and Church 2008, pp.18–20). Thus positive mental and emotional states and laying-on of hands can bring about positive changes in physical and mental condition.

From the Spiritist point of view, after ruling out physical brain damage or disabilities such as significantly impaired cognitive functioning, the cause of most mental illness is embedded in the perispirit, also known today as the "informational body" or "subtle body." Of course, the patient must also change his or her behavior to sustain the changes brought about through the mediums and healers. The cure can be initiated and sometimes completed by Spiritist therapies, but for well-being to be fully realized, the patient him- or herself must be proactive, and transform thought patterns and behavior patterns so they are beneficial to both the patient and others.

Full participation in the Spiritist therapies encourages the patient to educate him- or herself about spiritual principles, become more self-aware of behavior patterns that are positive versus those that are dysfunctional, engage what gives life meaning, and learn how to change thinking in order to create the pathway to healing and well-being. Spiritism is clearly a path of self-responsibility with the assistance of highly empathic helpers.

Results of Spiritist Therapy

Since the late 1960s, with the increased hope (and funding) that biochemistry would find a cure for all mental disease, researchers were not funded to study Spiritist therapies, and thus the successes of Spiritist Hospitals have gone largely unnoticed. However, Spiritist mediums and healers have reportedly been quite effective in helping people heal from mental illness. Dr. Ferreira (1993) wrote about his successes in a Spiritist Hospital in Uberaba, Brazil, in the 1930s and 1940s (Moreira-Almeida and Moreira 2008). He reported that 30 percent of the patients were healed, then released, after Spiritist treatments.

Ivan Hervé, MD (2006), reported about 181 cases he tracked for 20 years of treatment at a Spiritist Center in Porto Alegre, giving a description of their disorders and the results achieved.

- 20 schizophrenics: all improved significantly, with 6 returning to work or to school.

- 18 with autism: 17 improved significantly, learning to communicate and show affect.

- 21 mentally retarded: all improved, with 8 showing exceptional improvement.

- 13 children with panic attacks: all symptoms disappeared.

- 14 with epileptic convulsions: all stopped having convulsions.

- 10 with Down Syndrome: all showed significant improvement.

- 5 with West Syndrome: 3 improved greatly, 2 abandoned treatment.

- 4 with auto-obsession, 5 with bipolar disorder, 4 were drug abusers: their treatment was difficult to assess, as it involved consistent psychotherapy as well as Spiritist therapies.

- 60 classified as "special": all improved modestly to exceptionally.

(Hervé *et al.* 2003)

In addition to the above successes, anecdotal reports, the fact that patients continue to ask for Spiritist treatments both in the hospitals (see Chapter 6) and in Spiritist Centers (described in Chapter 10), and the enthusiasm evident in the increase of Spiritists is testimony to the effectiveness of Spiritist therapies.

Signposts

When we consider the message of some of our most well-trained and pioneering health care professionals who have been leaders in integrative medicine, we see there have been signposts leading us toward an appreciation of the resources of Spiritism:

- Herbert Benson, MD, an Associate Professor of Medicine at Harvard Medical School, began pointing us in the direction of our inner resources for healing in 1996 when he acknowledged that "60–90 percent of all doctor office visits in this country are stress-related and fall within the realm of maladies that mind/body medicine can alleviate" (Benson 1996, p.148). Fifteen years later, we can appreciate the research he did emphasizing the healing inherent in the "relaxation response," and recognize that we can mine more deeply into our innate resources for healing through skillful use of more expanded states of consciousness.

- Peter Breggin, MD (2008, 2010), a full-time consultant at the National Institute of Mental Health, is adamant about the need to find alternatives to the over-reliance on psychotropic medications. Toward that end in 2010 he created an organization that trains mental health professionals in "Empathic Therapy." Breggin writes: "Empathy recognizes, welcomes and treasures the individuality, personhood, identity, spirit or soul of the other human being in all its shared and unique aspects… We begin with fundamentals— the truths that human beings thrive in freedom, grow through personal responsibility, and ultimately yearn to lead creative and loving lives." As forward-thinking as this message is, Breggin does not acknowledge or harness the higher realms of empathy that are associated with mediumship, but training practitioners to be more empathic is certainly a step in that direction.

- Norman Shealy, MD, and Dawson Church, PhD, have proposed the term "Soul Medicine" for an integrative approach to healing, describing it this way: "It harnesses the healing power of consciousness, regardless whether that consciousness is expressed through alternative medicine or conventional medicine… The last six decades of biomedical and pharmacological research have managed almost completely to overlook the study of such crucial factors in healing as consciousness, electromagnetism, faith and quantum processes. Soul medicine simply restores these factors to the equation" (Shealy and Church 2008, pp.17–18). Spiritist therapies are certainly in line with this new terminology, which is an integrative approach.

How This Book Is Organized

Part I begins with the history and philosophy of Spiritism and how Spiritism perceives mental illness. This lays the foundation for a deeper explanation of mediumship and the importance of animating and training this capacity we each have. In Chapter 4 Marlene Nobre details how repressing our psychic abilities can actually lead us into mental illness. Chapter 5 recounts three cases of those with serious diagnoses in Brazil and the USA, and how Spiritist interventions dovetailed with conventional care and contributed to healing.

In Part II you will find more in-depth descriptions of the practical aspects of Spiritist treatments. Chapters 6 and 7 describe the treatments in Spiritist Psychiatric Hospitals. Chapters 8–12 penetrate more deeply into the components of Spiritist treatments and the principles behind magnetic healing, prayer, past life therapy, the group field, fraternal counseling, C.G. Jung's cartography of consciousness, and how to bring spirituality into the practice of psychotherapy. In keeping with the rest of the book, most of the chapters in this part are quite academic, but some incline toward being more personal, as well as reaching beyond the personal to the transpersonal. Many Spiritist health professionals I have met can attune themselves to two paths of knowledge: academic and channeled wisdom that reflects higher intelligence. In Chapter 13 Gilson Roberto, the medical director of a large hospital in Porto Alegre, describes how he weaves together his own capacities as a skilled medium with his well-tutored education and responsibilities as a medical doctor, homeopath, and medical director of a Spiritist Hospital. Dr. Roberto is a model of a practitioner of Soul Medicine.

Part III begins with Alan Wallace advocating the development of a Science of Mind, understanding the vast resources of the mind for healing and self-realization. He believes this is the next step for science to take, and it will be a revolutionary step. Part III continues to reveal the work of scientists well known for their ground-breaking research in bio-physics and the nature of consciousness, as well as our best trained psychiatrists who work with the soul and spirit. Although these people are not dedicated students of Spiritism, each shares a perspective that validates the foundations of Spiritism. In Chapter 17 Linda Russek cites a compelling story that is near perfect in showing evidence of valid mediumship and life after death. This offers a strong anchor point from which to explore the positive potentials of mediums trained in Spiritist healing work.

Kardec, the founder of Spiritism, wrote that Spiritism must be aligned with modern science, or must change to align itself better—so the first three parts of the book make that link.

Part IV reflects on the international impact of Spiritism from the point of view of Janet Duncan, who has been deeply involved with the movement for decades, and lives in England; as well as Stanley Krippner and Emma Bragdon who have been students of Spiritism, and frequented Spiritist institutions in Brazil.

Part V reflects on education and research. An important question is: How can we integrate conventional and Spiritist treatment in hospitals today? Training mediums might be one of the most challenging components of Spiritist work to export outside Brazil. Who is prepared to do this kind of teaching and ongoing supervision in a culture that has not understood that the real work of mediums is to help people? And, how many people are prepared to work as mediums without being paid? A Brazilian psychologist, Gelson Roberto, is teaching about the bridge between spirituality and mental health to other health professionals. He writes about ethics, and how to support patients in their inner transformation. Finally, William Braud charts a course toward more research.

It was difficult to limit the biographies of the contributing authors to a few sentences at the end of the book, as each author is accomplished and influential in his or her own field. Contact information is included to encourage a wider dialogue.

Words that are key to Spiritism, that you may be unfamiliar with, are defined in the Glossary. The vocabulary of the subtle body, and how the invisible realms of spirits interact with the energies (also unseen and usually unable to be measured) of those who are in body, has been well developed in Brazil—but there is a notable lack of words in the English language to describe these subtleties. We hope this book will make a contribution toward this important part of the vocabulary of life.

Finally, there are references from the chapters and resources for further reading and viewing to assist those who want to go deeper in their understanding and also make connections with organizations that are making an effort to teach about the important bridge between spirituality and mental health. An important resource for patients, their families, and health providers is the campaign book to this volume, *Resources for Extraordinary Healing: Schizophrenia, Bipolar and Other Serious Mental Illnesses.*

Note

1. This is the disability rate due to mental illness, meaning that the people were declared eligible for disability because of a mental illness. There are many more people on the disability rolls who were declared eligible for a physical illness but also have a mental illness—I am not counting those people in this number (Robert Whitaker, personal communication, January 6, 2011).

Part I

THE SPIRITIST UNDERSTANDING OF MENTAL HEALTH

Chapter 1

A BRIEF HISTORY OF SPIRITISM

Emma Bragdon, PhD

Communicating and collaborating with benevolent spirits to effect healing has been part of all nature-based shamanic cultures throughout the world for thousands of years (Krippner and Villoldo 1987). Saints and sages of all religions have continued this practice with diverse forms of spiritual healing. Mid-nineteenth-century North America saw the birth of "modern Spiritualism" (Weisberg 2004) when communicating with spirits began to be practiced in a "technologically advanced" society (but was not then used for healing purposes). Separated from the traditions of shamanic culture and the sanctions of a particular church, a modern Spiritualist simply believed that death is a time when the physical body dies, but the spirit of the individual continues on in another form, in another dimension. These Spiritualists developed their own ways to communicate with the spirits within living rooms and assembly halls, using musical instruments, pens, tables, and chairs to facilitate dialogue.

Beginning in 1848, two sisters, both adolescents, Maggie and Kate Fox, of Hydesville, New York, invited the public to witness their extraordinary communications with the spirits. The women put themselves on display in public auditoriums, and submitted themselves to tests by numerous groups of doctors to establish that the rappings, playing of musical instruments, and moving furniture, including heavy tables levitating, continuing about their everyday life came from a non-physical source. Although these might be ascribed to psychokinesis (mind over matter), some of the Fox sisters' meetings divined messages from the departed regarding information they could not have formerly been privy to. Those that found these displays authentic had to engage the belief in life after death, the idea our spirits never die but go on to new life, a life that may intersect with human life. Despite the antagonism of many physicians and religious men who could not accept these ideas, many more found the evidence compelling. Horace Greeley, the famous editor of the *New York Tribune*; Charles Partridge, a publisher; Charles Hammond and R.P. Ambler, both Universalist ministers; Judge John Worth Edmonds, Chief Justice of the New York State Supreme Court; and Nathanial Tallmadge, former governor of Wisconsin, publicly supported Spiritualism and attended Spiritualist activities. Interest in séances (groups gathering for the purpose of communicating with the spirits) began to expand throughout the USA as well as in Europe. By the mid-1850s there were several hundred thousand Spiritualists in the USA; by 1890, there were estimates from 1 to 11 million in the USA.

Like many of his contemporaries in Paris in the 1850s, Léon Dénizarth Hippolyte Rivail (1804–1869) became interested in the phenomena of spirit communication. Rivail was an earnest, intellectual Frenchman, a professor of languages, physics, anatomy, and mathematics, dedicated to improving public education. With the discipline of an academic employing the methodology of a scientist, he began his exploration by crafting over one thousand questions concerning the reason for human life on earth, the nature of the spiritual realms, and the dynamics of spiritual evolution. He then carefully observed, collected, and collated answers to these questions from a variety of ten mediums, each unknown to the others. He was thus in a position to make note of the answers that were "universal," in other words, repeated by all the mediums he questioned. He found that these so-called "universal" answers created a comprehensive and rational philosophy of life—what he named "Spiritism." Soon, he published five books and two booklets under the pen name, Allan Kardec: *The Spirits' Book* (1857), which presents the philosophy, based on the existence, manifestations, and teachings of the spirits; *The Mediums' Book* (1861), which explains the practical, experiential aspects of Spiritism; *The Gospel According to the Spirits* (1865), which illumines the ethical ramifications of Spiritism; *What is Spiritism?* (1865) and *Spiritism in Its Simplest Expression* (1865), which were booklets introducing the basics of Spiritism; and *Heaven and Hell* (1865) and *Genesis* (1868), which elaborate on the concept that heaven and hell are psychological constructs related to the workings of our own conscience. Together they formulate the precepts of "Spiritism"—to distinguish it from other forms of Spiritualism.

Why did he call this philosophy *Spiritism* and not *Spiritualism?* In his time those who were Spiritualists believed it possible to communicate with discarnate spirits, but they didn't categorically embrace reincarnation or notions of spiritual evolution. Spiritists, on the other hand, believe that life is a continuum alternating between life in a body and life as a discarnate, ever progressing toward a spiritual destination, a point of identification as pure love, compassion, and wisdom. Kardec's books advocate a high degree of discipline and perseverance in life— in order to effect personal transformation ("reforma intima" in Portuguese), and transcend the selfish desires of the lower self. Thus, Spiritists take on a rigorously demanding life path. The precepts also advocate communicating with highly evolved spirits for purposes of healing and the study of deeper truths, rather than communing with spirits who are less evolved for the sake of amusement, curiosity, or fascination with phenomena. Thus, Spiritists are attending not only to the regulation of their own behavior, thoughts, and will, but doing what they can to assist spirits to evolve to higher levels. Knowledge of the spiritual worlds, acquired through study, is regarded as *essential* in this task.

Spiritists believe that spiritual healing and the gifts of mediumship originate with God and are given freely to mankind and what is received for free must be given for free. Therefore, all Spiritist healing is without charge or even "suggested donation." Furthermore, Spiritists believe that when a spiritual healer or medium charges money for their services the healer opens the door to less evolved spirits who downgrade the spiritual work, and possibly damage the healer or medium by causing addiction, and mental and/or physical disease. With this in mind, it is interesting to note the downfall of Kate and Maggie Fox, both of whom became victims of alcoholism after making a commercial venture of their mediumship.

Why did Kardec's Spiritism develop in Brazil? In the late nineteenth century it was customary for wealthy Brazilian families to send their male children to European universities. As Kardec's books were in fashion in Europe at the time, they came back to Brazil tucked under the arms of the university students returning home, and then on to the parents and the upper classes of Brazilian society. Kardec's philosophy also found an enthusiastic following in homeopathic physicians, trained in Europe, practicing in Brazil. These physicians had already been trained to accept and use some aspects of spiritual healing as Hahneman (1755–1843), the founder of homeopathy, encouraged the use of intuition in diagnosis, and a form of laying-on of hands for healing. Homeopaths in Brazil were the first to organize groups to study and practice Kardecist Spiritism in Brazil. The upper classes were primed to participate, and the lower classes quickly availed themselves of the charity these Spiritist groups freely offered—free food, free medical services, free dental care, financial and legal advice, orphanages for children and abandoned elders, and institutional living for the mentally challenged or those suffering from dementia.

According to Brazil's 2000 Census, Brazil is 74 percent Catholic, but only a small percentage regularly attend mass. Although impossible to quantify exactly, most Brazilians are practicing "syncretistic religion," participating in spiritual activities of diverse traditions while still attending the high holy ceremonies of the Church, as members of the Church. However, deeply embedded into their approach to life is the golden rule of Christian tradition—to practice charity and goodwill. That Spiritism is infused with this same ethic, and endorses the continued development of moral values associated with Christianity, made Kardec's precepts easy to assimilate by Brazilians.

In fact, Kardec's Spiritist philosophy is considered a path of practical Christianity—but without rituals, priesthood, and churches, and without living in fear of hell and damnation. Spiritists believe in a loving God, the supreme intelligent force, with whom all people may have direct communication. The practice is to attend Spiritist Centers where classroom study is primary, along with laying-on of hands to help one stay balanced, and organized activities dedicated to charitable pursuits. One can take classes to learn mediumship and healing, and continue developing under excellent supervision of those more experienced in these practices.

Since the 1990s Spiritists have been coming from the upper and middle classes in greater numbers and many of them are well educated and have had good scientific training. Spiritism appeals to those who are seeking a path of personal growth.

Kardec said there are three types of Spiritists:

1. Those that are fascinated with psychic phenomena.

2. Those who are too enthusiastic and believe that everything is caused by the spirits. They are apt to make Spiritism into a religion.

3. True Spiritists who study, do research, and are more philosophical and ethical in their approach. They are trying to improve themselves. Spiritism for them becomes a viable path for personal transformation.

The psychiatrists who developed Spiritist treatments out of Kardec's original work, and now maintain Spiritist psychiatric facilities, tend to be of the third type. They empower patients to do the work of personal transformation without proselytizing Spiritism as a religion, or being overly fascinated with its phenomena.

The Spiritist psychiatric hospitals were created by Spiritists in the early part of the twentieth century. There are now 50 such hospitals in Brazil, but none outside Brazil. Many of these hospitals, when they were first created, were managed by Spiritists without collaboration with medical doctors. These original Spiritist hospitals attended those with mental disturbance using only the very humane Spiritist therapies that liberated patients from their obsessions, and reoriented their inner lives on a path of positive thinking and connection to spiritual guidance. When psychiatry became more engaged with diagnosing and treating mental illness from a biochemical perspective in the late 1950s, Spiritist psychiatric hospitals began collaborating with psychiatrists, staffing the hospitals with Spiritist mediums, Spiritist volunteers who practice healing and fraternal support, and physicians. This was in keeping with the idea of offering the patients the most compassionate and effective care possible.

The Spiritist psychiatric hospitals have continued this ideal of integrating the best of medical technology with the best of complementary care, with a strong spiritual base. Incoming patients are assessed for medical issues and social stressors, as well as having the option of being assessed by medical intuitives to define the problems and treatment protocols. Treatments may include: psychiatric medication, individual and group therapy, physical exercise, art and music, occupational therapy, laying-on of hands, prayer, inspired reading, blessed water, and disobsession (a healing at a distance whereby mediums liberate patients from the influence of negative spirits).

Knowledge of Spiritism in the International Community

Kardec was probably the first to attempt to add the study of the life of spirits to the arena of science. However, he has been largely overlooked in history because of some influential but prejudiced people who dismissed him during his lifetime. William James, PhD, considered the father of American psychology, became fascinated with psychic phenomena in 1880 and served as President of the Society for Psychical Research from 1894 to 1895. He felt it was essential that scientists research psychic phenomena and mediumship because it is clearly a branch of human experience that profoundly affects all our lives. Unfortunately, this arena of study is still marginalized, as conventional scientific researchers find it difficult to study a world that is largely invisible and unpredictable.

As a doctoral student at the Institute of Transpersonal Psychology in the 1980s I was not exposed to Kardec's writing or the hospitals and Spiritist Centers of Brazil; nor was this subject part of my undergraduate studies in psychology. Was I asleep during class? No, Kardec and Spiritism have simply not been recognized in psychology, religion, or medicine in North America. Psi phenomena and mediums have been largely dismissed, and one risks being professionally marginalized if one becomes involved in studying these subjects that are still considered a quasi-religious anomaly.

There are doctors in the USA who are sympathetic to what Spiritism offers. Melvin Morse, MD, known for his work with children and near-death experience (Morse and Perry 2001), has been a keynote speaker at the Spiritist Medical Association (AME) (2010). Dr. Morse has also been quite involved in researching remote viewing and the nature of dissociative experiences. See Chapter 19 in this book for his current thinking on the positive aspects of dissociative states of consciousness. Larry Dossey, MD, author of books on the power of prayer (1997), has corresponded with Brazilians around research protocols. Harold Koenig, MD (Duke University's Center for Spirituality, Theology and Health), and Christina Puchalski, MD (Director of the George Washington Institute for Spirituality and Health), have each given presentations for AME. But these outstanding leaders teaching about spirituality and medicine have had little exposure to Spiritism and its hospitals in Brazil.

Rosters of those attending AME conferences in Europe show there are many more doctors there who are interested in Spiritism. In the USA, more paraprofessionals are interested in Spiritism than doctors. In 2008 there were three AME conferences given in European countries and one in the USA.

Spiritism is actually not so foreign to those who study complementary psychotherapy. Rational Emotive Therapy (Ellis and Blau 2000) closely resembles the bedrock of Spiritist therapies that developed out of Kardec's work because it also encourages training the mind to think positively and rationally, but Rational Emotive Therapy does not have the spiritual depth of Spiritism. The shamanic work of "Soul Retrieval" (Ingerman and Harner 2006) has a spiritual viewpoint similar to Spiritism, and it also reconnects patients with fragmented and lost parts of themselves, and encourages reframing one's history in a positive light; however, Spiritism relies more on the work of mediums, and mediums unlock doors to other dimensions—and important sources of information—that are not usually available to practitioners of Rational Emotive Therapy or Soul Retrieval.

International Role of Spiritist Psychiatric Hospitals

Spiritist hospitals have a unique role to play. What other psychiatric hospitals have integrated spiritual healing and mediums as complementary aspects of their program? Acupuncture, Ayurvedic Medicine, Shiatsu, and Tibetan Medicine have a long history of treating the subtle energy body and are all used in some hospitals in the Far East, but are generally only available in clinics outside hospitals in North America. In the USA, Mormon and Catholic hospitals certainly work with prayer but do not tend to be involved with integrative energy medicine, treating the spiritual body, and attending to spirits that may be influencing patients. Sathya Sai Baba created two hospitals (Sri Sathya Sai Institute of Higher Medical Sciences 2008) in India that combine the best of medical technology with serving the patient without charge, in service to God, in a spiritual environment. These hospitals stand as a model example to humane treatment, but they are oriented toward physical problems, not mental disease.

Spiritist psychiatric hospitals have an important role to play in offering Spiritist therapies while continuing to deliver other forms of humane, integrative mental health care—a model for the rest of the world—as well as encouraging the education of health professionals interested in integrative health care. In June 2009, the annual conference for the Spiritist Medical Association of Brazil (AME-Br) convened in Porto Alegre in the state university's largest auditorium. This was an international conference attended by 1500 professionals who are sympathetic to integrating spiritual perspectives into health care, organized by the Spiritist Psychiatric Hospital of Porto Alegre and their study groups. The keynote address was given by Alan Wallace, a North American who founded and directs the Santa Barbara Institute of Consciousness Studies (an excerpt of his talk comprises Chapter 14). In this way, the stage is being set for increasing meaningful international dialogue.

Harold Koenig, MD, wrote that we now know through research that spirituality has a positive impact on health and healing but "it appears that not all spiritual healing practices are equal in terms of benefits. No spiritual interventions, either individual or group format, have yet to be objectively and rigorously tested for efficacy and safety in randomized clinical trials" (Koenig 2007, pp.95–104). It is time for clinical research comparing which forms of spiritual practice have what particular impact on patients.

Dossey advocates researchers to "familiarize themselves with the accomplishments of parapsychology," and he suggests that "experiments be done in surroundings that are cordial to the idea and possibility of healing" (Dossey 2008, p.349).

I believe that Spiritists are particularly well positioned to help in these endeavors because they have been respectfully bringing together science, healing, and parapsychology for 150 years. It is simply up to us to engage and learn from them through the international conferences, published works, and, on site, in their centers and hospitals. They are open to sharing what they know. Are we open to learning?

Chapter 2

A BRIEF OVERVIEW OF THE PHILOSOPHY AND DEVELOPMENT OF SPIRITISM'S METHODOLOGIES[1]

Alexander Moreira-Almeida, MD, PhD

Introduction

Despite the growing discussion about the relationship between science and spirituality many problems remain in integrating spirituality and scientific knowledge. This debate has often been characterized by radicalism and mutual denial. As a consequence of the contemporary emphasis on rationality and empirically based knowledge, building a strong and acceptable base to support the spiritual aspect of life as well as ethics has remained a huge challenge.

Although the current debate on science and spirituality has discussed several important topics, it usually does not touch the scientific investigation of certain claims about the spirit (its existence, survival after bodily death, reincarnation, etc.). However, this was not always the case. During the nineteenth century, through the vehicles of Spiritualism, Spiritism, and psychical research, many researchers tried to use a scientific approach to investigate spiritual experiences. Of special interest among these three related groups was the investigation of evidence that suggested the personality's survival after death (Aubrée and Laplantine 1990; Gauld 1968; Kardec 1860; Myers 2001). The scientific investigation of the existence of a non-physical or spiritual realm, a fundamental claim of many, if not most, spiritual traditions (Hufford and Bucklin 2006), was a main goal of those investigators.

This effort involved numerous high-level scientists and scholars who provided many contributions to topics such as the dialogue between religion and science, and between faith and reason, and even a new approach to metaphysics. However, these works are virtually unknown by contemporary authors in those fields.

Despite often dealing with the same subject (spiritual/psychic experiences), Spiritualism, Spiritism, and psychical research frequently differed from each other regarding views of science, research methods, and success in formulating a comprehensive theory. Spiritism, developed by Allan Kardec, developed a more inclusive philosophical system based on a research program of spiritual experiences. Stressing a rational and empirical investigation, Spiritism developed a theory of the self, including its survival after death—the concepts of reincarnation and unlimited spiritual evolution that formed the basis for a new empirical foundation of ethics, i.e. the founding of moral precepts on experimentally observed facts. Studies in Spiritism also could contribute to topics such as metaphysics, the science and religion dialogue, and the rediscovery of human meaning and purpose. However, these implications of Spiritism have not been the subject of systematic study. The relatively few academic studies of Spiritism usually focus largely on the religious aspect that became prominent in the Spiritist movement later in its history. Currently, the principal ideas of Spiritism have led to a developing social movement spawning study groups, healing centers, charity institutions, and hospitals utilized by millions of people in dozens of countries, but most of them found in Brazil (Aubrée and Laplantine 1990; CEI 2011; Moreira-Almeida and Lotufo Neto 2005; Sampaio 2004; Stoll 2003).

However, we will focus our present discussion on the philosophical aspects of Spiritism and its historical development. The purpose of this chapter is to provide a short overview on the history of the development of Spiritist philosophy, as well as a brief exposition of its content.2 Some contributions of Spiritism to the religion and science dialogue and its relevance to spiritual transformation and a foundation for ethics will also be discussed. To better provide readers with a first hand contact with Kardec's original ideas, we will base this chapter largely on direct quotations from Kardec's writings on Spiritism.3

Development of Spiritism

Allan Kardec (1804–1869) was one of the first scholars to propose a scientific investigation of psychic/spiritual phenomena. During his initial investigation, Kardec raised and discussed most, if not all, of the main hypotheses that were later put forth in psychology, psychiatry, and parapsychology to explain mediumship: fraud, hallucinations, a new physical force, unconscious mental activity, extra-sensory perception (including telepathy, clairvoyance, and super-psi), disincarnate spirits, and several other theories. However, he stated that, before accepting a spiritual or paranormal cause for some phenomena, it would be necessary first to test if ordinary material causes could explain it (Kardec 1860). Based on his studies, he accepted that fraud, hallucination, unconscious mental activity, telepathy, and clairvoyance could explain many phenomena regarded as mediumistic. However, when mediumistic phenomena were studied as a whole (taking into account all kinds of observed mediumistic experiences), the best explanation, for at least some sorts of mediumistic phenomena, would be the Spiritist hypothesis—a spiritual origin for the phenomena (Kardec 1986, 1996, 1999; Moreira-Almeida 2008).

Evidence produced by mediums convinced Kardec that personalities that had survived death could be the source of at least some mediumistic communications (some of this evidence is listed below).

1. Mediums providing accurate information (e.g. personal information about some dead person) unknown to themselves and to any sitter at the mediumistic séance.

2. Mediums showing unlearned skills such as:

    (a) mediumistic writing by illiterate mediums

    (b) writing with calligraphy similar to the alleged communicating personality when alive

    (c) speaking or writing in a language unknown to the medium (xenoglossy and xenography).

3. Mediumistic communications showing a wide range of personal psychological characteristics (such as character, humor, conciseness, choosing of words, likes, dislikes, etc.) related to the alleged communicating personality.

After Kardec became convinced that mediums could put him in touch with spirits (human personalities who survived bodily death), he worked to develop a scientific research program to study this subject and called it Spiritism, defined by him as "a science that deals with the nature, origin, and destiny of spirits, and their relation with the corporeal world" (Kardec 1999, p.6).

> Spiritism has not discovered nor invented the spirit, but was the first to demonstrate its existence by undeniable proof. It has studied it, analyzed it, and made evident its action. (Kardec 1868, p.12)

Spirituality and Science: Spirits as Components of the Natural World

Spiritism does not accept miracles or the supernatural. According to Spiritism, spirits (like matter) are components of the natural world, thus regulated by natural laws and suitable for scientific investigation. Kardec stressed that considering the interaction between both elements of the universe (matter and spirits) would make it much easier to understand and accept many phenomena, mainly those described by spiritual traditions:

> Spirit and matter are the two elements, or forces, governing the universe… Spiritism, in demonstrating the existence of the spiritual world and its relations with the material world, provides the key

to a multitude of hitherto unknown phenomena, which have been considered as inadmissible by a certain class of thinkers. (Kardec 1868, p.3)

Until now, the study of the spiritual principle, considered as belonging to metaphysics, has been purely speculative and theoretical; but in Spiritism it is treated as entirely experimental. In mediumship, currently more developed, generalized, and better studied, mankind has found a new observation tool. Mediumship is, with respect to the spiritual world, what a telescope is for the astronomical world, and the microscope for the microscopic world, helping us to explore, study, and—we might say—eyewitness the relationships of the spiritual world with the corporeal world. In the mediumistic phenomena, we can observe the intelligent being separately from the material being. (Kardec 1868, pp.65–66)

According to Kardec, we should be "on guard against the exaggeration from both credulity and skepticism" (1858, p.2). He stressed that we should be very careful in attributing to spirits all sorts of phenomena that are unusual or that we do not understand:

I cannot stress this point enough, we need to be aware of the effects of imagination… When an extraordinary phenomenon is produced— we insist—the first thought should be about a natural cause, because it is the most frequent and the most probable. (Kardec 1860, p.77)

Kardec, despite being a contemporary of positivism, developed epistemological and methodological guidelines for his investigation that are in several aspects in line with later developments in the philosophy of science throughout the twentieth century. He advocated, and actually used, research methods appropriate to the subject matter he was interested in investigating, namely the spiritual element. Thus, for instance, he pointed out the relevance of well-attested reports of spontaneous cases, in contrast with a misplaced attempt to mimicking physics, which, in many cases, appeals to quantitative measurements and laboratory experiments. Kardec also stressed that just collecting experimental data is not enough to make a science, for which it is essential to develop a comprehensive, logically consistent theory. In his pioneering exploration of the new field, he succeeded in allying a sense of rigor to a salutary openness to the novel (Chibeni 1999; Kardec 1860, 1986, 1999; Moreira-Almeida 2008).

Kardec often emphasized the need for a comprehensive and diversified empirical basis for spiritual experiences. To enlarge the range of observed phenomena, he asked that reports of mediumistic manifestations of several sorts be sent to him (Kardec 1858, p.6). He reported having received "communications from almost a thousand serious Spiritist centers, scattered over highly diversified areas of the Earth" (Kardec 1987, p.8). Fernandes (2004), investigating the amplitude of Kardec's correspondence, surveyed Kardec's publications on Spiritism and found published references to contacts related to Spiritism from 268 cities in 37 countries (including Africa, Asia, Europe, and from the three Americas).

> Spiritism proceeds in the same way as the positive sciences,4 by using the experimental method.5 When facts of a new kind are observed, facts that cannot be explained by known laws, it observes, compares and analyzes them. Reasoning then from the effects to the causes, it discovers the laws which govern them. Then it deduces their consequences and seeks for useful applications. Spiritism proposes no preconceived theory... Thus, it is rigorously correct to say that Spiritism is an experimental science, not the product of imagination. The sciences have not made real progress before they adopted the experimental method. This method has hitherto been taken as applicable only to matter, but in truth it is equally applicable to metaphysical things. (Kardec 1868, pp.10–11)

In his revolutionary approach to spirituality, Kardec frequently compared mediums to microscopes, since both were instruments that revealed and put humankind in contact with invisible worlds that, despite being previously ignored, have always had a strong impact on human lives (Kardec 1860). Following Kardec's analogy, the empirical observations provided by mediums and microscopes would allow the investigator to "see" how these invisible worlds are, making possible to formulate and to test hypotheses regarding the natural laws governing them.

Based on his investigations, Kardec developed a comprehensive theoretical framework to account for the whole body of observed phenomena. This resulted in the Spiritualist philosophy called Spiritism. As a philosophical system, Spiritism has many concepts that have been proposed by other philosophies and religions. Some of Spiritism's core concepts are: survival of consciousness after death, communication between incarnate and discarnate minds (mediumship), reincarnation, and unlimited spiritual evolution. According to Kardec, a scientific basis and the coordination of these concepts in a single and comprehensive theory were the main difference between Spiritism and previous philosophies that hold similar notions.

A New Ground for Ethics

Kardec strongly stressed the ethical implications of his studies. Spiritism neither has any ritual nor claims to be the only way to spiritual evolution and happiness. However, Kardec proposed that Spiritism could provide a much larger perspective to evaluate consequences of a behavior. Through Spiritism, one would be able to evaluate the long-term consequences of our actions, not just during one terrestrial life, but also postmortem and in future lives.

This represents a crucial reinforcement of an approach to ethics known as "utilitarianism," whose main exponents were Jeremy Bentham and John Stuart Mill (in the eighteenth and nineteenth centuries). In this approach moral norms are not taken on the basis of authority, or pure intellection, but as following from a scientific appraisal of the consequences of human actions with regard to the attainment of happiness of the whole of humankind.

> Spiritism has, furthermore, a particularly strong moralizing power, to the extent in which it clearly shows…the consequences of good and bad actions, which become so to speak palpable. (Kardec 1868, p.21)

> What Spiritism adds to the Christian moral is the knowledge of the principles governing the relationships between alive and dead men, thus completing the vague notions he gave of the soul, its past and future. It thereby grounds the Christian doctrine on the very laws of nature… Charity and fraternity he before did by pure sense of duty, now he does it by conviction and does it better. (Kardec 1868, pp.30–31)

A Call for Spiritual Transformation

Kardec stressed that an experimental demonstration of survival after death would have a high impact on humanity:

> The very possibility of communicating with the beings inhabiting the spiritual world has very important, incalculable consequences… It represents a complete revolution in our ideas. (Kardec 1868, p.13)

> Had Spiritism just eliminated man's doubt concerning future life, it would already have made more on behalf of his moral amelioration than all disciplinary laws, capable of bridling him in certain circumstances, but which do not really transform him for the better. (Kardec 1868, pp.19–20)

Reincarnation would also have large implications:

> The plurality of existences…is one of the most important laws revealed by Spiritism, since it shows the reality of this law and its need for progress. This law explains a lot of apparent anomalies of human life; differences in social position, premature deaths that, without reincarnation, would make useless to the souls such short

> existences; the inequality of moral and intellectual abilities, by the antiquity of the soul who has progressed and learned more or less, and who, being reborn, brings what has been acquired in his previous lives. (Kardec 1868, p.19)

The cognitive framework provided by Spiritism would be a strong call to spiritual transformation:

> Communication with the beings of the world beyond the grave enables us to see and to comprehend the life to come, initiates us into the joys and sorrows that await us therein according to our deserts, and thus brings back to Spiritualism those who had come to see in man only matter, only an organized machine; we are therefore justified in asserting that the facts of Spiritism have given the death-blow to materialism. Had Spiritism done nothing more than this, it would be entitled to the gratitude of all the friends of social order; but it does much more than this, for it shows the inevitable results of evil, and, consequently, the necessity of goodness... The future is no longer for them a vague imagining, a mere hope, but a fact, the reality of which is felt and understood when they see and hear those who have left us lamenting or rejoicing over what they did when they were upon the earth. Whoever witnesses these communications begins to reflect on the reality thus brought home to him, and to feel the need of self-examination, self-judgment, and self-amendment. (Kardec 1860, pp.421–422)

Conclusion

Despite being virtually absent from the academic debate on the relationship between spirituality and science, Spiritism has developed several contributions to the field that may provide new insights to the religion and science dialogue. A major aspect of Spiritism is the project of pursuing a fact-grounded scientific investigation of topics previously considered metaphysical. Most of the Spiritist ideas discussed here are not new; Kardec did not create them, but they were submitted to experimental investigation and organized into a comprehensive theory through Spiritism. By proposing an investigation of spirituality based on a rational analysis of facts, Spiritism aims to provide a basis for spirituality in the contemporary world, as well as to foster the pursuit of ongoing spiritual transformation.

Notes

1. This chapter is largely based on the paper "Spiritism, Its Research Program on Spirituality and Implications for Spiritual Transformation," published in *The Global Spiral 9*, 5, 2008. Metanexus Foundation.

2. Kardec wrote a brief brochure, *Le Spiritisme a sa plus simple expression* (1862) (available at www.ssbaltimore.org/Resources/SEE.pdf), and a short book, *Introduction to Spiritist Philosophy* (*Qu'est-ce que le Spiritisme*) (1859), that provide good brief introductions to Spiritism and its principles. They provide answers to the most common philosophical and religious questions.

3. Quotations were extracted from published English versions of Kardec's works where available. Otherwise, I translated from the French original. When necessary to improve fidelity to the French originals, I amended quotations from published English versions.

4. "Positive science" means, in the philosophical parlance of that time, inquiry thoroughly based on facts (Kardec 1864).

5. An "experimental method" should not be taken as simply a laboratory method, but a research method based on empirical observations, i.e. on every kind of fact attestable by careful observation.

Chapter 3

THE SPIRITIST VIEW OF MENTAL DISORDERS

Alexander Moreira-Almeida, MD, PhD

Introduction

Several authors argue that Spiritism was "an event of major importance as a source of understanding unexplainable phenomena" in the history of dynamic psychiatry and psychology (Almeida and Lotufo Neto 2004; Ellenberger 1970; Janet 1889). Ellenberger and Janet also admitted that there is evidence that the late nineteenth-century dynamic theories of the unconscious were in part a result of the translation of the communication of the principles of the spirit world into the language of orthodox medicine. Hess (1991) identifies more objective signs of this translation in Myers' "subliminal self" and in Pierre Janet's, William James', and Jung's writings. Koss-Chioino (2003) recently showed several parallels between Jungian and Spiritist views in the structure and content of human consciousness. Chapter 11 in this volume is a reprint of this article.

Spiritism itself developed a comprehensive theory to explain mind, and its relationship with the body and its disorders. This chapter will briefly review the Spiritist view of mental disorders based mainly on Allan Kardec's writings, but also revise it using some later contributions developed by Brazilian Spiritists such as Divaldo Pereira Franco, whom I quote extensively later in the chapter.[1] More detailed analyses have been published elsewhere (Almeida and Moreira-Almeida 2009; Moreira-Almeida and Lotufo Neto 2005).

Allan Kardec was the founder of Spiritism and, for 12 years, the chief editor of *Revue Spirite—Journal d'Études Psychologiques* (Spiritist Review—Journal of Psychological Studies). The objective of this journal was to collect facts and test hypotheses about different spiritual phenomena. Kardec attempted to give rise to a new science and to avoid "the exaggerations of credulity and skepticism" related to spiritual phenomena. Kardec used the subtitle *Journal of Psychological Studies* as he believed that "to study the nature of the spirits is to study the nature of mankind" (Kardec 1858). The *Spiritist Review* is rich in case reports and analyses that illustrate and support the Spiritist philosophy. Kardec often wrote about behavioral disorders, suicidal thoughts, and alteration of sensory perception.

Etiology

Spiritism does not deny the bio-psycho-social causes of mental disorders; it fully acknowledges them. Kardec always emphasized that Spiritism does not come to deny well-established scientific knowledge; it comes to complement it, adding something new—the spiritual element—to our understanding of nature. Several times he compared Spiritism with microbiology: both reveal and investigate dimensions of reality that are invisible to the naked eye but are part of the natural world and can affect our lives (Kardec 1986, 1996). In the same way the acceptance that some mental disorders may be caused by microorganisms or spiritual factors does not deny the possibility of other etiological factors acting within the same patient. This is especially true in exploring and defining the causes of mental disorders.

Allan Kardec discusses the causes for severe mental disorders in the introduction of his first publication in 1860 (1996). He defended a model similar to the "diathesis-stress" model, which has been proposed for schizophrenia (Jones and Fernyhough 2007), where stressors may trigger insanity in those subjects who are already biologically predisposed to mental illness. He also suggested that the content of symptoms in the mentally ill are strongly influenced by cultural factors of the patient:

> The predisposing cause for madness resides within the predisposition of each unique brain. Where there is a tendency that renders the brain more vulnerable to certain impressions; and, where a predisposition to insanity already exists, the brain's manifestation takes on the character of the pursuit to which the mind is most addicted, and it then assumes the form of a fixed idea. (Kardec 1996, p.51)

Mediumship itself might be a triggering factor in individuals predisposed to madness. Therefore, people "who show the slightest symptoms of mental eccentricity or weakness should be dissuaded from its exercise by every possible means; for there is, in such persons, an evident predisposition to insanity, which any and every species of excitement would tend to develop" (Kardec 1986, pp.221–222).

As far as the relationship between body and mind is concerned, the foundation of Spiritism operates on a pragmatic dualist interactionist model. Although not defending a definitive position regarding the ultimate ontological relationship between matter and consciousness, for practical purposes, matter and consciousness are considered as different elements (Kardec 1996). Kardec's investigations of mediumistic communications convinced him that personality (also called mind or spirit) can survive bodily death, so mind is not understood as a product of the brain, but having an independent existence (Moreira-Almeida 2008). However, in order to manifest itself, while incarnated, the spirit needs to make use of the body. The body and the soul, i.e. the unique spirit, exercise a mutual influence on each other that constitutes an interactionist dualism. However, there is supremacy of the spirit over the body as Spiritism bestows a great importance on free will. The body, and especially the brain, are significantly shaped by the influence of an incarnated spirit. More developed brain areas linked to some specific brain functions are the result of the action of a spirit that is particularly skilled in that specific area. Likewise, the corporeal humors are altered according to the tendencies of the spirit:

> A man is not choleric because he is bilious, but the man is bilious because he is choleric. Similarly, with all the instinctive dispositions… if he is active and energetic, his blood, his nerves will have very different qualities… What triggering factor could alter the blood other than the moral dispositions of the Spirit? (Kardec 1869, p.64)

It is recognized, however, that someone's temperament may in part derive from organic imbalances. These imbalances might affect the spirit itself. As the incarnated spirit uses the body to manifest itself, the spirit might have difficulties if this instrument, the body, is disordered. This is the case of a mental illness due to an organic origin.

> A spirit,…when incarnated, is…compelled to act through the instrumentality of special organs. If some or all of those organs are injured, his actions or his impressions, as far as those organs are concerned, are interrupted. If he loses his eyes, he becomes blind; if he loses his hearing, he becomes deaf; and so forth. Suppose that the organ which presides over the manifestations of intelligence and of will is partially or entirely weakened or modified in its action, and you will easily understand that the spirit, having at his service only organs that are incomplete or diverted from their proper action, must experience a functional perturbation about which he is perfectly conscious, but cannot stop. (Kardec 1996, p.375)

The spirit regulates the functioning of the neuro-endocrine and immune systems and the central nervous system. This regulation is understood as the tool used by the spirit to act upon the body. An imbalance in these systems is clearly present in several mental disorders. The imbalance of the spirit is germane to the cause of these specific body disharmonies (Franco 1997, 1999, 2000a). The influences of the spirit over the body generate either a harmonious or unhealthy functioning of the body spurring mutations and several physiologic changes. Thus the body and mind/spirit are in an intense relationship.

Obsession

One spiritual factor Spiritism describes as a component to the causes of mental disturbances are the "obsessions": "the persistent action that a disturbed spirit exerts over an individual" (Kardec 1868, p.45). These harmful influences can happen when an obsessing spirit exacerbates negative feelings and thoughts in the patient through a kind of telepathy.

> Obsession one day will be recognized as a cause of mental disorders, just as is accepted today the pathologic action of microscopic living creatures whose existence nobody even suspected, before the invention of the light microscope. (Kardec 1863, p.35)

Obsession ultimately originates in the moral imperfections of the patient. The patient's own negative feelings, thoughts, and behavior allow the obsessing spirit to mentally tune into the individual, as well as make the patient accept its influence. The obsessing spirit is motivated most of the time by a vengeful feeling against the victim. However, it is important to emphasize that the person can choose to accept or reject the obsessing influence, i.e. the subject has the free will to follow the obsessor's suggestions or not. The more a patient accepts the obsessor's influence, the stronger the psychic/spiritual tie between them, making the obsession more severe. In the most severe cases, such as in possession states, the patient may entirely lose his or her capacity for self-control.

Kardec suggested three levels of severity in these types of obsession:

- *Simple obsession*: the person feels an influence via thoughts and pernicious feelings but these do not alter his or her judgment or free will.

- *Fascination*: makes a person accept the most preposterous statements and theories as truth. [Fascination is] an illusion which is produced by the direct action of a spirit on the medium's thought, which paralyzes his judgment…to make him value the most ridiculous nonsense.

- *Subjugation or possession*: is a constraint which paralyzes the will of its victim, and makes him act in spite of himself… Subjugation may be moral or corporeal in nature. In the first case, the subjugated victim is often drawn to do things that are foolish or reprehensible… In possession, the spirit acts on the material organs of the victim, provoking involuntary movements… and forces the victim to do the most extravagant things.

(Kardec 1986, pp.237–240)

In cases of possession, the obsessing spirit ultimately determines the type of behavior the patient will display. The obsessing spirit momentarily takes over the incarnated body, acting as if it is incarnated. "Whoever had known the patient previously, would not now recognize his language, his voice, his gestures and even his features… He blasphemes and insults and as the obsessing spirit, brings those around him to criticize him. The obsessing spirit surrenders to eccentricities and characteristically acts with furious madness" (Kardec 1868, pp.47–48).

Kardec characterized the difference between the madness of an organic origin from the madness resulting from an obsession:

> Let's not confuse pathological madness with obsession. The latter does not derive from any brain damage but it derives from the subjugation that malevolent spirits exert over certain individuals even though the obsession often has the appearance of madness itself. This change is very frequently independent of any belief in Spiritism and it has always existed. (Kardec 1999)

> Among those individuals considered mad, there are many who are only subjugated… When your doctors understand Spiritism, they will be able to distinguish between these two classes of madness; and they will then cure many more patients than they now do. (Kardec 1986, p.254)

However, the difference between these two types of conditions may not be very simple. Obsession may cause mental disorders, but obsessions may also be triggered by mental disorders (Kardec 1868):

> The depressive condition that brings about pessimistic and nefarious thoughts…opens breaches for the settlement of harmful obsessions, or any other phenomena that deteriorate the cell machinery, favoring the settling of different disorders. (Franco 1999, p.59)

One should also employ caution in order to avoid the mistake of considering the spiritual etiology in an excessive manner:

> Men have often mistaken for cases of possession what were really cases of epilepsy or madness, demanding the help of the physician rather than of the exorciser. (Kardec 1996, p.474)

The hypothesis that obsession might have a role in phenomena associated with hysteria was also proposed by Kardec (1863).

Previous Life

In addition to obsession, there is another kind of spiritual cause of mental disorders proposed by Spiritism: the influence of habits and memories related to previous lives. The self would be composed of a conscious part and an extensive unconscious part that includes the memories of current and past lives (Franco 1995, 2002).

Phobias may result from traumatic events; depression results from a guilty conscience over unfortunate past actions (Franco 1997). That is why ethical behavior is highly regarded and, instead of continuously disturbing guilt feelings, the concept of responsibility is emphasized. "The crop derives from plowing without any predetermined expression of the suffering that must be expressed" (Franco 2000a, p.43).

As for the content of delusions: the hypothesis is that delusions may, in part, be due to vague recollections from past lives. In the specific case of mental disorders, these recollections might not be so clear due to an ongoing organic derangement. Recollections from past lives become mixed up with recollections of the present life (Kardec 1861b, 1866).

The possible impact of experiences from previous lives in certain behavior patterns and problems has also been discussed recently. According to some authors (Haraldsson 2003; Stevenson 1977; Tucker 2008), phobias, "philias" (special likes), skills not learned early in life, problems in the child–parent relationship, and changes in sexual gender identity could have their causes, in some cases, in past lives.

Hallucination

Kardec (1861a) designed a detailed study about changes in perception that are the mark of something out of the ordinary. He proposed a hypothesis that there are three kinds of perceptual changes in the realm of vision:

- *Imagination*: what are currently called illusions are distorted perceptions of a real external stimulus, often caused by fatigue or a low level of illumination and/or suggestion.

- *Hallucinations*: are sense perceptions originating from within one's inner life. Kardec wrote, "An hallucination is a vision from the past of an image that was recorded in the brain, and typically created by the soul during an illness."

- *Apparitions or true visions*: result from real spiritual perception. Apparitions occur in two ways: "it is either the spirit appearing to the person who sees him, or it is the person's spirit who is transported and goes to meet the other incarnated spirit." True visions and apparitions convey unknown information to the individual, that is later confirmed as accurate. Those visions produced by the imagination and hallucinations cannot be confirmed as accurate. This is the main difference between them. According to Kardec, the difference between apparition and hallucination is: "every apparition that does not give any intelligent warning signal may definitely be listed as an illusion." This classification is very similar to another proposed more recently by Ian Stevenson (1983) in the *American Journal of Psychiatry*.

Kardec wrote about numerous examples of apparitions. Apparitions are far more frequent at the time of death. For instance, an apparition of someone who was previously healthy is witnessed stating he or she has died in an accident with a detailed description of the event and the accident, and all details described by the apparition were subsequently confirmed.

Treatment

The commitment to consider the spiritual etiology of mental disorders without rejecting all possible bio-psycho-social causes is emphasized by Spiritism. The essential element for the treatment of obsessions is a beneficial change in the patient's behavior, stemming from moral growth. This strategy seeks to avoid the disturbing thoughts of the obsessing spirit and replaces these thoughts with positive, charitable thoughts.

Additionally, laying-on of hands ("*passés*" in Portuguese) and prayers are given, also aimed at balancing the spirit of the obsessed subject. As for the obsessing spirit, Kardec recommended to try and dissuade the spirit away from his purpose of doing harm by means of dialogues between a counselor and the obsessing spirit in mediumistic meetings, called disobsession (Kardec 1868). Kardec described several case studies showing that a cure was achieved by means of deliberately evoking and then counseling the spirit to stop his destructive thinking and behavior (Kardec 1864, 1865a). Kardec denies that the cures achieved were spontaneous cures, because there were numerous cases of cure through disobsession:

> The proof of the participation of an invisible intelligence, in those cases of cure, derives from chief facts: the multiple and radical cures that were obtained in some Spiritist centers induced only by the evocation and redirection of the obsessing spirits, without magnetization or medications, and often, in the absence of the patient and at a great physical distance from the patient. (Kardec 1868, p.33)

Spiritists also consider the reports of the expulsion of inferior spirits in the New Testament where Jesus and his disciples expelled evil spirits from affected individuals (Mark 1:21–27 and 9:13–28; Matthew 9:32–34 and 12:22–28) as evidence favoring spiritual cures. However, "the real and ultimate healing could only come about by the intellectual and moral improvement of the spirit along several incarnations" (Franco 1999, pp.65–69).

Nevertheless, this search for virtue should be brought about by a real desire for growth and development and not by mechanisms of repression (Franco 2000b). Spiritism emphasizes that religion should not serve as a "psychological departure for the individual to spare himself from confronting life's conflicts, and the processes of liberation from suffering" (Franco 2002, p.178). The search for self-knowledge is a fundamental step for the total unfolding of the spirit.

> No one would be found reincarnated on Earth had not their physical existence possessed a superior purpose... Step by step, progress is constructed and it grows permanent through the habits that are incorporated in the individual... Mistakes and rightful achievements are resources for the unfolding of consciousness to greater achievements. (Franco 1997, p.27)

> A psychologically mature man lives in the greatness of aspirations for the good, the beautiful and the true, and, freed from his ego, he reaches the Self, becoming an integral, ideal man, on the way to infinity. (Franco 1993, p.28)

Prophylaxis

Kardec contends that the Spiritist point of view of life (providing meaning and purpose for life and suffering, as well as evidence for life after death) can provide a cognitive framework that can help one cope better, acting as a buffer against life's stressful events:

> Spiritism...when correctly understood, preserves us from insanity. Among the most common causes of mental disturbance and suicide are the disappointments, misfortunes, blighted affections, and other troubles of human life. But the enlightened Spiritist looks upon the things of this life from so elevated a point of view, they seem to him so petty, so worthless, in comparison with the future he sees before him. Life appears so short, so fleeting, that its tribulations are, in his eyes, merely the disagreeable incidents of a journey. What would produce violent emotion in the mind of another affects him but slightly; besides, he knows that the sorrows of life are trials which aid our advancement, if borne without complaining, and that he will be rewarded according to the fortitude with which he has borne them. His convictions, therefore, give him an acceptance and surrender that preserves him from despair, and consequently from a frequent cause of madness and suicide. (Kardec 1996, p.51)

How does Spiritism prevent the "*tedium vitae*," that is, the negative aversion to life misfortunes and thus melancholy? Despite thoroughly recognizing an organic predisposition to melancholy as a real disorder (Kardec 1862a), Spiritists encourage each individual to clearly articulate and be aligned with his life goals, and motivate him to improve himself further and further. Spiritism would also decrease the number of cases of insanity by advising against the abusive use of alcohol (Kardec

1865b). In these ways Spiritism gives individuals greater "moral courage," and every Spiritist has several philosophical reasons to refrain from suicide:

> The certainty of a future life…the certainty that the abbreviation of life results in something completely opposite to what is originally expected; that he is freed from one evil to endure something that is much more severe…that in the other world he will not be able to see the objects of his preference that he wished to become united with. Thus, suicide is totally against his own interests. (Kardec 1862a, pp.200–201)

Kardec's theory of how Spiritism can play a role at preventing mental disorders (helping to cope with life's difficulties and acting as a buffer against stressful vital events) is in line with the cognitive-behavioral approach used by Koenig, Larson and Larson (2001) to explain how religion helps patients to cope.

Conclusion

Spiritism has developed a comprehensive theory about mental disorders that has influenced patients and health care professionals, most notably in South America, and especially in Brazil. So the possibility of a spiritual cause is proposed to broaden and complement the bio-psycho-social factors commonly part of etiology. This spiritual cause would have its origins in previous incarnations and spiritual influences, the so-called obsessions. The Spiritists argue that the acceptance of this bio-psycho-social-spiritual model could facilitate the development of medicine and psychology and answer many questions and problems.

The academic study of this subject is of great importance due to its practical implications and the interest many cultures have in the subject. At this time, more investigation is needed to further study 1) the effectiveness of Spiritist therapies, and 2) the impact and acceptance of these treatments among Brazilians and those of other cultures.

Kardec emphasized several times that the admission of a "spiritual reality" would be a great advance to the sciences, especially medicine:

> Spiritism opens new horizons in every science, and also clarifies the very obscure question of mental disorders suggesting spirits as a cause that has not yet been fully considered. Disembodied spirits could be a real cause, and in the future, it will be established, through experience, as true…as we find evidence of action of the invisible world over natural phenomena. Once we get on this road, science will possess the key to the mysteries and shall overcome the most formidable hindrances detaining progress: materialism that restrains the full possibilities of observation rather than enlarges them. (Kardec 1862b, p.110)

Note

1. Divaldo Pereira Franco is a male medium born in Bahia (northeastern Brazil) with more than 200 published psychographed books (8 million copies translated into 16 languages). He has also been a Spiritist public speaker, with numerous talks given in Brazil and in 64 foreign countries. He states that his spiritual mentor is a female spirit named Joanna de Ângelis, who has written several works on mental health since 1990. See www.divaldofranco.com/biografia.php.

Chapter 4

THE RELATIONSHIP OF MEDIUMSHIP TO MENTAL DISORDER

Marlene Nobre, MD

Background

Since the 1970s the "Medicine and Spirituality" movement has been proposing a new health paradigm with growing emphasis that is based on the concept of the whole human being, inclusive of body, mind, and spirit (Larson, Swyers and McCullough 1998).

Several important authors have written about the role spirituality plays in health. For more than 30 years, Herbert Benson, founder of the Mind/Body Medical Institute at Massachusetts General Hospital, has been writing and teaching about the positive influence of faith in people's lives (Benson and Stark 1996). Harold G. Koenig, at Duke University's Medical Center, has carried out important scientific studies (Koenig 2005; Koenig, McCullough and Larson 2001) on the role of religion in the healing and prevention of illness.

Other specialists, such as William Miller (1999), Christina Puchalski and Anna Romer (2000), and many others from diverse religious denominations, have been involved in research trying to bring spirituality into medical care. They use the results of this research to complement the courses they teach at their respective universities. Since publishing the book *The Turning Point* (1982), physicist Fritjof Capra has been advancing his innovative proposal for "Holistic Health Care," which calls for the urgent need to adopt this new paradigm that forwards the practice of Integrative Medicine. Professor Amit Goswami of the Institute of Theoretical Physics, University of Oregon, also defends this concept. In his books *The Self-Aware Universe* (1995), *Physics of the Soul* (2001), and *The Quantum Doctor* (2004) he presents a new theory about consciousness, stating that it is the creative source of the physical world but located outside the physical world.

The Spiritist vision of health (Nobre 2006) is also integrative. We believe that all disease processes are essentially governed by the spirit and thus we must attend to the spirit along with the body and mind, in creating well-being. All phenomena—biological, psychic, social, cultural, and spiritual—act upon the spirit. The spirit metabolizes them and integrates them. Working with the spirit itself will thus further positive integration of every aspect of our life experience. Our treatments complement conventional protocols for the body and mind.

It is only natural that Spiritist medical associations around the world find a common ground with all movements that seek to integrate spirituality and health.

Current Consciousness Research

Research done on death-bed visions and near-death experiences (NDEs) today give us robust scientific evidence that the soul survives bodily death. Researchers who have studied NDE, such as cardiologists Michael Sabom (1982) and Pim van Lommel (see van Lommel *et al.* 2001), neurologists Sam Parnia and Peter Fenwick (2001), psychiatrists Raymond Moody, Jr. (1977) and Elizabeth Kübler-Ross (1996), pediatrician Melvin Morse (1990), and psychologists Bruce Greyson (Greyson and Flynn 1984), Kenneth Ring (1984), and Margot Grey (1985), among many others, describe what patients went through after being declared clinically dead. On the basis of such complex subjective experiences, scientists have discussed the real site of consciousness and the mind, since these functions continue even when the patient is in deep coma and there is no record of brain activity. In these situations, the brain structures that provide support to the mind and enable the patient to have subjective experiences become severely damaged. How could the patient retain clear consciousness outside the body when the brain stops working due to heart failure and the electroencephalogram shows a flat line?

The explanation given by the Spiritist–medical paradigm for NDE is the one that makes the most sense and that can be readily accepted from a rational point of view. According to this explanation, the soul (unique spirit) would detach itself from the body but would keep its perceptual ability by means of another body, lighter and less materialized, that would still function despite the fact that the brain in the physical body became inactive. Thus, consciousness and mind would be considered attributes of the soul that could express themselves through the functions of the physical brain or, as described by near-death survivors, through the functions that are also present in the brain of the other body, more subtle and less materialized (Xavier 1947).

Based on the results of research such as that carried out by the scientists mentioned above, and also on the robust evidence gathered from mediumship studies, Spiritist physicians are convinced that thoughts are a product of the soul and not just a result of a chemical–electrical secretion of the brain (Xavier and Vieira 1958).

Spiritist researchers also look into the human mind for the origin of positive and restoring forces that can provide equilibrium to trillions of cells in the physical organism as well as for negative forces that can be highly destructive to them. These researchers also study mediumship (Kardec 2003; Xavier 2005).

The Spiritist–medical paradigm considers that the human being is made up of three parts: soul, physical body, and subtle envelopes—thus, far beyond the biological or psychological dimensions that are perceived by current medical technology. We also believe the psychic component of the human being is much more complex than commonly imagined. The brain, as the organ by which the spirit manifests itself (Xavier 1947), has special neurons to capture impressions and perceptions of the objective/exterior world, as well as those from the interior/subjective world. This way, the spirit is able to exert its specific action upon the world and to leave its co-creative mark. Therefore, the psychic apparatus that is available to the incarnated spirit by means of the physical brain enables it to react to the external world on the objective plane and also offers it the resources to act upon the subjective plane. It is this plane that generates mental creations that are unique to each human being and the innate ideas related to past lives that surface as intuition. In addition, through mediumship, the psychic apparatus allows communication with compatible incarnate or disincarnate intelligences.

The advent of Spiritism on April 18, 1857 was an invitation to better understand the endless web of life in which we live—a web made up of intertwined thoughts, words, and actions, where everything works together. Thoughts, an attribute of the spirit (Xavier 1986), are formed by atoms of another vibrational scale, still unknown to us, and are molded by feelings, which give them shape and character. Mental atoms obey quantum energy laws and may function as waves or particles.

Due to the fact that electromagnetic waves follow the principle of non-locality, as described by the Bell Theorem (and proven by practical physicist Alain Aspect [2007]), and that their speed is greater than the speed of light, thoughts can be transmitted instantly regardless of space or time.

Due to their mental induction property, thoughts may be reproduced in another mind that is in harmony with the same vibration. This is the basis of the mediumship phenomena, inherent to all human beings. "We are connected in spirit with all other incarnate or disincarnate spirits that think the same way as we do" (Xavier and Vieira 1958, p.86). Therefore, spirits can be in tune for good or for evil purposes.

Mediumship Abilities and Dysfunction

The following definition is by the spirit author Emmanuel through the medium Chico Xavier:

> Mediumship: a faculty that is inherent in all human beings that allows them to communicate with other dimensions of spiritual life; a mental force; the interpretation and communication ability of the

spirit. Intuition is the oldest faculty of mediumship. (Emmanuel, cited in Xavier 1986)

Mediumship amplifies our abilities to communicate with other spiritual dimensions and enables us to interpret the life lessons we have learned, so we can apply them for constructive, beneficial actions. Thus, when well used, the mediumship faculty represents an equitable and effective contribution to our spiritual evolution. However, its repression or improper use may result in various types of negative associations, known as "obsessions."

Forms of Obsession

Obsession, which is the domination some spirits may have over certain people (Kardec 2003), is one of the main areas of study of the Spiritist–medical paradigm. Obsession can occur at various levels, from a simple influence without any external sign that propels someone to act in an amoral or immoral way, to a complete disturbance of the person's organism and mental faculties. These pathologies are much more frequent than people think.

When we speak of obsession, most of the time we are referring to the type that is caused by disincarnated spirits who act upon us, causing obsession. They can absorb the vitality and share the life of incarnate persons, as in cases of symbiosis. We also have cases where the disincarnate spirits remain attached to their houses and to the vital fluids of the family, participating in home activities as they did when they were alive. They take part in meals with relatives and sleep in the same rooms they used before leaving the physical body (Nobre 1997).

In her interview in the spiritual plane at the Memorial Park Cemetery with Humberto de Campos (a deceased Brazilian writer), Marilyn Monroe considered obsession as one of the worst calamities affecting mankind (Xavier 1969). According to her statements she was induced by her obsessors to take an excessive dosage of sleeping pills and was unaware that her life was in danger.

Animistic Obsession

A human being is also able to produce an "animistic" kind of obsession, that is, obsession caused by the individual person him- or herself. In these cases a thought pattern or attitude of the individual's own soul acts like an obsessor on his or her own personality. Alternatively, the shadow of an individual's personality can act like an obsessor. In both cases, the obsession can be felt by the person as if it came from an outside source and the individual may thus be confused about the source of the obsessor.

Animistic obsessions include cases of negative and persistent recollections of past lives, which are situations of mental crystallization or fixation of hate or feelings of an inferior nature (Nobre 1997). In this type of animistic obsession, the negative R Agents (see p.53) are endogenous—the person him- or herself is responsible for the negative mental creations and for remaining in an obsessive state. It is worth noting that hateful feelings are a process of self-obsession.

The Shared Obsession

This is the most prevalent type among people plagued by destructive habits like alcoholism or drug addiction, whereby disincarnates avidly absorb the sensations of the physical body of their incarnate victims and remain attached to them (Nobre 1997). Their victims temporarily lose their common sense and equilibrium by, for instance, a weakness for getting high, when they leave themselves open to external influences.

Telepathic Obsession

We believe that the soul can leave the body and function as a free spirit that can generate pathological behavior in others. In this way, incarnated souls influence each other through telepathic obsession. "Millions of homes could be compared to trenches in a war, where thoughts fight thoughts, filled with anxiety and repulsion" (Xavier 2005, p.170). Problems of antagonism among members of the same family reflect this pattern. Very often, within the same home and same family, or even within the same organization, terrible enemies meet again. "Domestic antagonism, apparently irreconcilable divergence among parents and children, husband and wife, brothers and relatives are the result of successive clashes of the subconscious that is forced to rectify problematic situations of a distant past" (Xavier 1943, p.36).

In all cases of neurotic pathologies, such as hysterical disorders, phobias, and anxiety, there are components rooted in obsession (Nobre 1997).

Vampirism

We must also consider organic pathologies caused by severe cases of vampirism (Nobre 1997), where a negative spirit can act like a parasite, drawing energy from the mind in such a way as to cause serious neurological diseases and different levels of epilepsy.

Poltergeist

Obsession may also involve physical effects, also known as poltergeist (Andrade 1983), when mischievous spirits use ectoplasm to hurt and scare people by making loud and persistent noises, causing spontaneous combustion and other dramatic effects.

Spirit Possession

The scientific literature on spirit possession, the most profound kind of obsession, is limited. Currently available are references to only two studies: spirit possession and trance case reports, and epidemiological studies from African and Asian countries showing spirit possession prevalence ranging from 1.5 to 18 percent of the population (Igreja *et al.* 2010; Venkataramaiah *et al.* 1981).

Repressed Mediumship

We are very concerned with pathology that can appear in some mediums who become victim to obsession, which may have serious implications for the origin or further deterioration of illness. Although such cases are rarely considered by psychiatrists when treating mental disorders, mediumship abilities that are repressed, and the obsessions that derive from them, have reached the scale of a social tragedy today. Therefore, such pathologies are a permanent subject of study and research for Spiritist physicians because there is a strong need to properly distinguish them from other mental disorders.

Our thesis is quite clear: when someone is endowed with mediumship ability and does not use it to the fullest, which is to pursue goodness and do charitable work for others, they may end up with serious illnesses and mental disorders (Xavier 1947, 2009). Fear of learning about, developing, or using one's abilities as a medium is very common in many cultures that negate the existence of mediumship, equate it with mental disorder, or are oblivious to the positive potential inherent in mediums to elicit healing in others. Therefore, individuals who choose to repress their abilities in mediumship are common in such cultures.

In the study of repressed mediumship abilities, it is important to consider mental fixation (Nobre 1997), when the mind becomes locked onto an object or a person and cannot change or function properly. The fixation can become so intense that it totally corrodes mental life. This aspect is often observed in cases of chemical and other types of dependency and addiction.

In Brazil, Spiritist physicians have been studying the relationship between mediumship and mental disorder for about 150 years. We are not yet in a position to estimate the number of mediums with mental disorders based on the views and opinions of health professionals who have studied Spiritism (Almeida, Neto and Cardeña 2008). There is still no serious assessment of mediumship in scientific literature. Due to the lack of scientific studies, at the present moment the correlation between mediumship and dissociative disorders cannot be easily defined.

The Dynamics of Disobsession

It is through our aura that we are recognized and contacted by disincarnate spirits. The way obsession works is somewhat similar to an allergic process: the victim's mind produces the antibody against the antigen that the obsessor's mental vibration represents. These mental radiations are called "R Agents." They may have a deleterious character if the feelings they express are of rage, irritation, cruelty, sadness, apathy, etc. There are many types of negative relationships that produce negative R Agents (Nobre 2007), such as partnerships established with evil purposes; a destructive association based on vindication or revenge; and partnerships in vices such as the symbiosis involving habitual overindulgence in eating, sleeping, sexuality, etc.

Healing from these negative influences is achieved when positive R Agents, based on thoughts of love and solidarity, are produced and can neutralize any negative R Agents. The production of positive R Agents can be stimulated by praying, meditation, and also giving or receiving spiritual energy therapy: laying-on of hands and energized water. Of course, another important protocol to resolve conflict is the therapeutic dialogue carried out in disobsession.

It is of fundamental importance to talk to the patient undergoing treatment for obsession about morals, encouraging him or her to engage in constructive study and increasing self-knowledge. In fact, the patient must make a great effort to overcome his or her bad tendencies and dedicate him- or herself to practicing charitable deeds. This is the reason why it is so important that the therapist in disobsession is able to lead the obsessor and his or her victim to mutual forgiveness and changes in their attitudes and feelings. This brings them both enormous benefits. Both need to be convinced that only the heart that loves is able to reach the full power of renewal. In fact, only love conquers hate and goodness overcomes evil.

Spiritist Treatment and Its Effects

Psychiatrist Inácio Ferreira, in the Spiritist Psychiatric Hospital in Uberaba, in the state of Minas Gerais, from the 1930s to the 1980s, was one of the pioneers in the use of spiritual treatment to complement traditional psychiatric therapy. Dr. Ferreira was able to enlist a number of dedicated trained mediums for his studies. In his book *Novos Rumos à Medicina* (New Trends in Medicine) (Ferreira 1993), he states that physicians "must deviate a little from their search for material causes of disorders and focus on studies and experimentations in the spiritual field" (p.47).

In his clinical practice Ferreira facilitated the cure of many mentally ill patients and was able to conclude:

70 percent of these tragedies faced by mankind which result in mental disorders are the consequence of psychic actions with origin in a world that is invisible to our physical eyes, but that are sensed and felt by mediums, people endowed with a sixth sense. (Ferreira 1993, p.47)

Conclusion

The results obtained in Brazil using spiritual treatments like disobsession may be very different from those in other countries. In fact, very few studies have addressed this issue. Obviously, the cultural conditions in Brazil are not the same as those found outside, but aside from the obvious cultural differences researchers have pointed out:

- lack of formal scales and instruments to differentiate mediumship from dissociative disorders

- important methodological flaws while carrying out studies

- challenges in conducting epidemiological studies due to the fact that many religions do not recognize mediumship as a legitimate practice

- lack of evidence regarding life after death and past life memories.

This field of research is therefore wide open, with many unsolved questions.

It would be a very positive step if psychiatrists and health specialists could open their minds to take into consideration mediumship and its numerous implications in the field of mental health.

Chapter 5

CASE STUDIES OF THOSE WITH SERIOUS DIAGNOSES

Emma Bragdon, PhD

Spiritists believe that the causal roots of mental illness are apparent in the subtle, spiritual body, and complete healing can only occur when these roots of illness are attended to, along with alleviation of the biological, psychological, and social stressors. This means that the problems may originate in circumstances of past lives as well as negative habits of thinking in this life. Practically speaking, Spiritist therapies:

- use mediums who can clearly see into the spiritual body and report what they perceive; these mediums offer both "medical intuition" and an ability to channel discarnate spirits who expose the nature of the problems

- use diverse treatments that address the unique spiritual body of each person and facilitate healing the spiritual body

- confer responsibility to the patient for ongoing changes in both thinking and behaving, and encourage ethical behavior that is both compassionate and wise.

As described by Marlene Nobre, MD, in the previous chapter, sometimes patients are hospitalized because they have unusual abilities as healers or mediums and have not identified or trained these abilities. Psychic phenomena can, under these circumstances, take over, uncontrolled. Intense spiritual experiences can be overwhelming and severely disorienting, obstructing the ability of the person to organize his/her thoughts and work, and maintain relationships. Well-trained Spiritist mediums can identify such patients and offer them the supervision they need to harness their abilities. This means that, in Brazil, the Spiritist Hospitals provide a safe haven for those in "spiritual emergency," undergoing an evolutionary process that can be misdiagnosed as an acute psychotic episode, and treated inappropriately with only the use of anti-psychotic medication and psychotherapy.

As we contemplate the human potential that may be crying for attention in spiritual emergency, it is interesting to read the words of Jesus, from the Gospel of Thomas, 45:29–33, taken from the Nag Hammadi Library (Robinson 1977, p.126): "If you bring forth what is within you, what you bring forth will save you. If you do not bring forth what is within you, what you do not bring forth will destroy you." Those with special psychic sensitivities, who resist or repress them, may actually be contributing to the creation of symptoms of psychosis.

In the USA we have no residential facility for patients who are undergoing this kind of transformative process, sometimes called "spiritual emergency," and need care and supervision. Rarely do such patients even meet a person who can help them define the process they are in very generally, much less offer help specific to their circumstances. Rudolf Steiner, the founder of Anthroposophy and the Waldorf School system, forecast that at the turn of the millennium, 2000 and beyond, there would be millions of people in spiritual emergency and very few practitioners suitably trained to provide them with the help they needed to make sense out of their spiritual experiences. The potential evolution of the patient in emergency would thus likely be perceived as a breakdown (rather than a breakthrough), treated as an illness, and the prognosis would be poor.

Marcel's Story in Brazil[1]

Marcel Teles Marcondes came to Palmelo in the Spring of 2002. Although he had enjoyed a normal life (with no significant early trauma) with satisfying work as a travel agent, and many friends, he began to experience emotional problems when he was in his late twenties (in 1996). His father, Arnoldo Marcondes Filho, a bank manager for the Bank of São Paulo State, Banespa, was able to afford excellent medical care for his son, and took Marcel to the best psychiatrists in São Paulo.

Marcel was first diagnosed with depression, then schizophrenia. Antipsychotics were prescribed as well as sleep medication. The prognosis: Marcel would have to manage his symptoms with these strong medications for the rest of his life.

But he never felt well when taking the medications. When he was committed to a psychiatric clinic for 20 days, the hospital environment only added to his stress. His parents then tried touring Brazil with Marcel for eight months in a motor home, to help him relax. Marcel continued to experience bizarre delusions: seeing and feeling crabs and spiders crawling all over him, grabbing at him. He could turn unpredictably aggressive and hostile for periods of time. Sometimes he would hear two to three voices in his head talking to him, simultaneously.

Although the family was Catholic and had been advised by their physicians not to trust the services of Spiritist healers, they took a chance and drove Marcel to Palmelo. He was committed to Euripedes Barsanulfo Hospital, a psychiatric facility, and stayed there as an inpatient for 100 days.

As an inpatient, Marcel continued on anti-psychotic medication, under the care of a licensed psychiatrist. Marcel also participated in the mainstream modes of therapy offered at the hospital: physical activity (playing soccer or gardening), doing occupational therapy, and attending group therapy three times a week. He also participated in the Spiritist activities, including private "energy passes" performed by trained healer/mediums once a week, who transmitted healing energy to Marcel without touching him. He also had private sessions of medical intuition once a month.[2]

"Disobsession" was performed by mediums three times a week in a group format to rid him and other patients, individually, of negatively motivated disincarnates who had attached themselves to the energy field of the patients. This was not an exorcism as we know it, as there were no special rituals or incantations performed by a priest.

All of the Spiritist work was either supervised or done directly by Bartolo Damo, the spiritual head of the hospital. Soon after his arrival, Marcel was told by some of the hospital's mediums that he was being troubled by spirits who had known him in past lives. Although initially disconcerting, this perspective proved to be very helpful, pointing him in the direction of very specific work he had to do to forgive himself and others, make amends, and regain his stability.

From Mental Illness to Mediumship

After several weeks of medical intuitive reading and disobsession Marcel's periods of violent aggression stopped, as did his delusions. He then began studying Kardec's philosophy in the first books, *The Spirits' Book* (Kardec 1996) and *The Mediums' Book* (Kardec 1986). Damo was continually monitoring Marcel's emotional stability, and also his understanding of Kardecist philosophy. Damo could see, by indicators in Marcel's subtle energy field (aura), that Marcel was a medium with healing abilities. This became more evident as disincarnate entities causing his obsessing were liberated. Marcel needed more study and supervision to gain conceptual understanding of spiritual realms and the practice of mediumship. Marcel also needed to come to terms with how his prior lifetimes had contributed to the internal stresses of the present lifetime.

I met Marcel twice in 2003, after he had done a considerable amount of study and skill building as a medium, under the direct supervision of Damo. Marcel was then functioning as a member of a team of healing mediums performing disobsession through energy passes, and was still taking a minimal dose of medication.

Johann Grobler, a psychiatrist from South Africa traveling with me, asked Marcel: "Why does a person get possessed by a disincarnate entity?"

Marcel answered, "When the etheric body (a subtle energy field around the physical body) is weakened by stress or depression, spirits driven by negative emotions, like anger, greed, lust, addiction, fear, and vengeance, can take possession of him or her. The weakened person is unable to over-ride the willfulness of the negative disincarnates, in this case, and he or she is driven to irrational behavior. The undeveloped spirits may come to hurt the person or his family, in response to hurt they felt in other lifetimes at the hand of that same individual. These entities get trapped in obsessing and part of releasing them is to help them be free to go on to their next step of development."

Marcel's current inner balance and peacefulness is obvious and clear testimony to his having successfully confronted his "demons." His healing depended on "inner transformation," called "reforma intima" in Portuguese, which necessitated his making amends for prior wrong-doing (acting in a way that is not compassionate to oneself or others) in this and other lifetimes. His dedication to be of service to others through healing is a significant way that he is making amends.

The negative patterns of the mind brought about by obsession take time to heal. Marcel has been asked by Damo to stay for two years in Palmelo, to study Kardec and other Spiritist teachers, and to continue his service work, receiving spiritual healing, and living a life in which stress is minimized. According to Damo, "This will completely restore his balance."

I had the opportunity to visit Marcel at the home he shares with his mother and father. The love that flowed among them all was palpable, and obviously contributed to Marcel's healing. The three reported that they had been through a lot of soul-searching together, including sharing the events from past lives, where various difficulties had arisen among them, causing conflict that had continued into this lifetime. Marcel's reforma intima had involved all three of them resolving these issues and making a deeper commitment to treat each other with compassion, in brotherhood, that transcends the roles of this lifetime: as mother, father, and son. I feel sure the simple diet, with plenty of acerola juice (high in Vitamin C), also contributed to Marcel's healing.

When I first met Marcel he was ushering visitors as they prepared to have a personal session with Vania Damo, wife of Bartolo Damo. She is gifted in channeling spirits through automatic writing. ("Dona Vania" is one of the most well-respected teachers in the community, as well as the main person who performs the service of automatic writing, to assist those who want to communicate with loved ones who have died.) I had also watched Marcel giving "energy passes" during disobsessions at the hospital. At his present level of development he is learning to deliberately "incorporate," that is, allow a highly evolved discarnate to use his body for a specific period of time, to transmit helpful information or do psychic healing.

Arnoldo, Marcel's father, has come to believe that the majority of cases of schizophrenia are caused by disincarnates possessing a person, or causing an individual to obsess. As he and his wife witnessed their son improving dramatically, they felt they had to accept the principles of Spiritism. Arnoldo told me, "I got back my son. I thought he might be gone forever."

Even as Catholics, the family began believing in reincarnation and the necessity of making amends for mistakes in previous lifetimes. Like Marcel, they learned to strengthen their focus on peace and love, and control the images and thoughts in their minds, to deliberately be more positive. Kardec's Spiritism considers this discipline is essential to healing. It helps individuals separate from the negative influence of undeveloped discarnates—and paves the way for those entities to be "educated," learning that they too are free to develop.

I asked Marcel and his mother and father what they would want others to know about Marcel's healing, if they could address the world. His mother said, "What makes healing possible is our faith in God's goodness, and our ability to see life from new perspectives, getting over our prejudice against Spiritism." Both parents agreed, "The patient must actively participate in his healing through study and other activities of a Spiritist Center, like Palmelo." Marcel said, "My story is concrete evidence that medication in combination with Spiritism works. You need both."

Gerry's Case in Brazil

Gerry is an engaging, personable, and bright American woman, with a master's degree in psychology, who lives in the state of Washington, USA. Her parents called me in 2007 to ask for my help, as Gerry, then aged 28, was going through what they thought was a "spiritual emergency," but was being treated for psychosis. I had written two books on spiritual emergency in the past (Bragdon 2006 [1988], 1990) and am considered an expert in this area.

Gerry was being seen weekly by a Harvard-trained psychiatrist who felt that her case was out of the ordinary. She did not have any significant trauma in her early life, and her family was consistently supportive of her. Gerry's psychiatrist had prescribed anti-psychotic medication for her, but Gerry did not like the side-effects, and her mother and father were afraid that the long-term side-effects would be even more harmful. They wanted to explore alternatives.

Gerry had had a few manic episodes where she had acted in an irrational way, for example removing all her clothes and walking around a lake in a large city in the middle of the night, interacting with the people she chanced to meet. She had been hospitalized during two such episodes and medicated to stop the manic behavior and thought processes. It seemed that her episodes would come upon her every 90 days, and then subside ten days later, leaving her clear-headed and able to return to work. This unusual pattern led her psychiatrist to believe she might need the help of a qualified shaman, which was not part of his skill set.

On hearing the details of her life I suggested that Gerry and her parents come to Brazil and consult with John of God for 12 days as part of a group I was leading there. They did this. During that time span, Gerry was away from her boyfriend, eating a very simple diet of fresh vegetables and fruits and organic meat, and meditating under the guidance of mediums at John's Spiritist Center. A few times when it appeared she might be going into an episode, she was given a small amount of anti-psychotic medication by her parents (under the advice of the psychiatrist), but that seemed to make her agitated and she would attempt to sneak out to roam the streets at night (obviously not safe for a young, disoriented North American woman in a poor village she did not know). She was given feedback by mediums at the center that she was highly sensitive, and could choose to develop her potential as a medium. More important to Gerry was her realization, on her own, while meditating, that her boyfriend was not a good influence on her and she had to sever that tie, which she did.

I learned from Gerry that her first psychotic break happened shortly after smoking marijuana, and I came to believe that this form of socializing was exacerbating her imbalance. With abuse of alcohol and use of marijuana and other stronger recreational drugs the subtle bodies become open and negative entities often enter in, exerting their negative influence on the individual. This can lead to very irrational behaviors as well as addictions, with the person not understanding either that they are being manipulated by entities, or what to do about it.

After understanding that she was likely too sensitive to use marijuana because it led to her getting flooded with psychic experiences, Gerry elected to stop smoking pot and not hang around others who were using drugs or abusing alcohol. All of her negative symptoms stopped. She also looked for supportive friends and a teacher who could help her develop her intuitive abilities in the USA. She found a highly skilled acupuncturist who was also a medium. A small amount of medication was used if she felt she was going into an episode—but this was, for the most part, rarely needed after she returned home.

Almost a year later, Gerry "missed being a normal young woman," and fell back into going to bars to play darts and socialize, even starting up her past relationship again. Again the psychotic symptoms emerged. Her psychiatrist wanted to turn to stronger psychiatric medications; Gerry's mother decided to come back to Brazil with Gerry to help her get off all psychotropic medications completely and address the roots of the illness once and for all.

I was personally hired to guide Gerry and her mother for this second stay, helping them to make use of the resources of John of God's Spiritist Center and employing my own skills as a highly intuitive psychotherapist. Gerry's acupuncturist was also present for the initial two weeks, and was given permission by John of God to continue working with Gerry, as part of her treatment. Shortly after arrival and newly off all psychotropic medication, Gerry began to experience the symptoms of an episode. This time it manifested as catatonia. She lost interest in eating, drinking, sleeping, communicating, using the toilet, and bathing. She wanted to remain standing still, not speaking, staring in one direction. Her condition worsened over time, of course. After several weeks she became severely dehydrated; her lower legs and feet blue with pooling blood. She was also losing a lot of weight. With John of God's full support, a nurse was called in twice to administer fluids intravenously (IVs) to rehydrate her. Gerry reacted like a scared child, at first unable to understand that her life was in danger if she didn't take in liquids. She seemed unable to engage her will to survive, but, with encouragment, finally submitted to the IVs.

From a Spiritist perspective this was an extreme case of possession. Gerry had lost all power over her own functioning, even her desire to survive, and this state of consciousness was with her 24 hours a day.

In the next days Gerry's mother read prayers for psychic protection to her, disobsession was practiced by highly trained mediums for Gerry, and she started to come out of the catatonia. I was invited to be part of the group disobsession meeting when one medium became almost totally overwhelmed by the strength of the negative entitites that had possessed Gerry. It was very moving to later hear from her how much that medium had been able to perceive about Gerry's condition, even though she had never met her and was not part of John of God's Center. The medium and the group completed the work of disobsession for Gerry—reporting it as an especially intense experience. Gerry soon came out of the catatonia; her eyes became brighter and she appeared to re-enter present time, relating more to others. This whole process took six weeks for Gerry, after which her mother took her home to the USA.

At first Gerry lived with her parents, as she was not yet able to take care of herself completely. She again received acupuncture treatments and emotional support from the same acupuncturist who had been in Brazil for two weeks with her, Jessica Randall. Her parents found a psychiatrist trained in orthomolecular medicine,[3] Dr. Brad Weeks, who diagnosed her as highly sensitive. He said she must take care of herself in a very careful manner. She is not psychotic, nor schizophrenic or mentally ill. She was very depleted, and needed a supervised program of supplements of vitamins and minerals. She also needs ongoing care as she learns more about and commits to making lifestyle changes to make sure she does not fall back into the extreme state she can fall into when she doesn't take care of herself properly.

At this time, almost two years after her catatonic episode in Brazil, Gerry is living independently, driving her car, working, and planning on going back to school to become a lawyer in 2011. She has embraced significant lifestyle changes, realizing what her new psychiatrist told her: "Like a Ferrari sports car, she needs the best of fuel and maintenance to keep her in good working order." Gerry is still not sure if she wants to go further in developing her abilities as a medium. This is understandable, given the fact that our culture tends to perceive "mediums" as "odd balls." The term "shamanic practitioner" suits her better and will help her develop her sensitivities to benefit others.

On January 11, 2011, Gerry wrote me an email, excerpted with her permission:

> I have only been really healthy without having to cancel work because of an episode for a year now. I have had minor setbacks, but can handle those. It wasn't until now that I am really starting to grasp the work that is being done in Spiritism and I am so grateful to be a part of it.
>
> I think the most important part of the work in Spiritism is helping me integrate a lifestyle change that I can commit to, with the help of my acupuncturist, my orthomolecular psychiatrist, my psychotherapist, my Shamanism teacher, my mentor at work, and my chiropractor. I really did need this entire team of people and community to help me with this transition. I am now in the second year of my three-year Shamanic practitioner training. Being in a community of other like-minded and sensitive people who are all there to be of service to the land and help the planet with the earth changes has given me wisdom and made me more aware of what I ingest on a daily basis. I stopped drinking alcohol a year ago, and I am also giving up sugar to create a healthy energetic body. I realized that it is an ongoing process of keeping my mind, body and spirit healthy and clean and the more I can do this, the better I can be there for my clients in my private practice. I am currently beginning a new relationship with a man named Paul. He is also a counselor and is supportive on emotional, physical, and spiritual levels.
>
> Thank you, Emma, for all your hard work and dedication to help others with similar mental health problems find God…

A Case Worker in the USA

This story describes the challenge of working in a mental health care system that does not consider that spirits can influence people in adverse ways. Keep in mind that Spiritists believe that schizophrenics are simply sick, ignorant mediums who are heavily indebted because of acting with ill will towards others in previous lives, and misusing their psychic gifts.

Louise is a Brazilian who lives in a suburb of a large city in the USA. She is an esteemed teacher at a local Spiritist Center on most evenings and weekends, and a social worker by day, employed by a US company. This story came to me through an email she sent to me in January 2011. I promised her I would not use her real name or the place where she works. She made it quite clear she is not allowed to use her skills as a Spiritist healer in an overt way with her cases:

> My job as a social worker, although grueling, is just wonderful. It's not easy to deal with the ignorance of and resistance to spiritual matters but I find myself praying nearly every hour on the hour, doing a bit of laying-on of hands when I can, and planting a seed of spirituality wherever there's an opening. All has to be done without anyone's knowledge, including the company and my supervisors.
>
> I see truly heartbreaking cases, 99 percent of them are schizophrenics, delusional, and suicidal with added complications such as mania, psychosis, anti-social behavior, post-traumatic stress disorder, etc. The other 1 percent of the cases have grave and disabling depression, the kind in which the person cannot get out of bed. I see an endless series of painful tragedies: young adults (20–27-year-olds) who have been heavily medicated since age four because they can see and hear spirits, nearly all of them victims of sexual abuse, many victims of gang rape because they live in a suburb of a big city where gangs rule. Not one has any idea of what is wrong with them. Each one talks about his or her "illness" and when I ask "what's your illness?" almost each one says the same thing: "I hear and see horrible things, things no one else can see."
>
> They're scared beyond definition. Some do get "possessed" and become violent, they attack family members, and, when they come back to themselves, they're so horrified by what they have "unknowingly" done (while possessed by a negative spirit) that they gladly ingest anything (medication) to stop it. They'll do anything to solve the problem—without any information about what the problem is or assistance in taking away the root cause. Some try to kill themselves to put an end to the problem, cut themselves, set fire to parts of their bodies, or become alcoholics to numb the pain. You name it; they do it.
>
> Anyway, we have to go to the worst areas in the city to visit them at home or we go to mental wards in the hospital, sometimes even the county jail.
>
> Of course, my concern for them carries into my meetings at the Spiritist Center where I work. There have been nights when we work our whole session for just one of my clients (who never knows

anything about it). One of my mediums got used to reporting: "I've been busy with Louise's clients for two days. I know what we're up against tonight."

In September 2010, I was assigned to work with Tony, who was catatonic—he literally had no reaction to external stimuli, people, or objects. This strapping 6 foot 1 20-year-old spent his days looking at the four walls in his room at his grandmother's house. When he took his prescribed medication he slept nearly 24 hours a day. Apparently the only thing Tony could do was take care of his personal hygiene without help. His grandmother said he hadn't smiled since he had been seven years old, just before his mother died. His hospital diagnosis read "delusional, disorganized behavior, disorganized speech, flat affect, or hallucinations, reacting to internal stimuli, poor judgment and insight...smoked pot in high school."

I couldn't get more than three words out of him when we first met and he looked as if he was thousands of miles away. I took Tony to the psychiatrist and when he filled out the forms he did it in three different types of handwriting. How come no one else noticed? Immediately, I started talking (inside my own mind, telepathically) to the three entities attached to him, acknowledging them, trying to help them.

At my next Spiritist meeting for mediums' work in spiritual assistance, the spiritual mentors brought Tony's soul to talk to me. He was screaming madly, saying that there were snakes wrapped around his head. I calmed him down, the good spirits we work with removed the snakes, and we helped most of the entities with him to detach and go on to the place they could get help.

The next day I talked to Tony's grandmother, who reported that a miracle had happened. She attributed it to my verbal conversations with him. She said that he "connected" with me and would listen to me. Poor lady, there's nothing I can do about her ignorance of the spiritual problems her grandson has had, and the spiritual work that can be done, and needs to be done.

When I went to see Tony two days later, he was on the porch of his house, looked at me, smiled broadly, and came down the steps to shake my hand. He also shook the hand of my co-worker and introduced himself with full first and last name. He invited us to come inside with him, and asked us to sit down, all in full correct sentences. He remembered I had asked him about his doctor and dentist and now he could tell me who they were. He opened his wallet and showed me business cards from his doctor and his driver's license. He showed me his picture and explained that he used to wear dreads but gave them up because kids would pull on them in school.

During our conversation, I told him that I didn't want to sound like a grandmother to him, that I knew that he already had one. He smiled and said, "Well, I don't have a grandmother on my mother's side, you can be that grandmother."

I left his house on cloud nine. It took me a few days to come down I was so happy. I was very grateful that the spirits let me witness their handiwork. Most of the time we work with them but the results aren't always shown to us.

In the next few weeks, during two of our Saturday meditation and spiritual treatments, I did a distance healing for Tony. Distance healing is when someone stands in for the sick person and that person receives treatment by the healers. While I visualized Tony and prayed for his recovery the spirits followed my thoughts and went to his room and treated him. They removed negative spirits, recharged and reshaped his perispirit,[4] and did psychic surgery as they often do. They also cleaned the environment in his home.

Four months have passed since I first met Tony. He no longer takes any psychiatric medication. He is participating at a day program that has a gym, music room, play room with billiards, cards, chess, checkers, ice hockey table, etc. He's picked up in the morning and driven home at night. The program provides group therapy, psychiatric care (as needed), meals, activities, and outings. Tony told me he plays the harmonica and drums, and is learning piano. He may still be "delusional" and "reacting to internal stimuli" because he hears spirits and has no idea what this means. He still has something of the "possessed" look in his eyes (bulging, drooping) and although he looks people in the eye he cannot sustain it for a normal period of time. I don't see any evidence of disorganized behavior, disorganized speech, or hallucinations, poor judgment, or insight. He looks and behaves almost normally now. I still need to have his "developmental problem" evaluated and find him a suitable school.

Tony is such an innocent, sweet young man with no malice, no anger, no drinking, no drugs, no cursing, no dishonesty of any kind in his heart. He believes in God and attends church on his own once a week. I don't know what his potential is and I don't know how much Spiritism can do for him. But I know our mentors know and their plan will continue until Tony reaches his limits, at least for this life. I'll continue doing my part and wondering just how far he can go.

Resources Outside Brazil

There are very few resources in the USA for people undergoing the kind of profound inner transformation that these three young people were guided through. If we take Gerry as an example, one needs to set up a support team of individual practitioners, which can be quite expensive. Fortunately, her parents were able to give her this support. People like Tony (who comes from an economically and educationally poor background) have to rely on serendipity to receive the extraordinary healing he received—in secret. It was also fortunate that his social worker found a program that suited him. The day program Tony participates in is more like a social club, and seems to meet Tony's needs very well.

Sanctuaries and care facilities that offer a caring and safe residential environment, and do not rely mainly on psychiatric drug treatment (which does not work for people like Gerry, Marcel, and Tony), often do not meet with approval by medical authorities or neighbors. A record of one such sanctuary, Pocket Ranch, is documented in *Resources for Extraordinary Healing: Schizophrenia, Bipolar and Other Serious Mental Illnesses* (Bragdon 2012), along with the new sanctuary that replaced it, as well as other alternative residential care facilities.

I have spoken to several Spiritist Psychiatric Hospital administrators in Brazil about the possibility of facilitating English-speaking patients and their families who may want to go to Brazil and have treatment in the Spiritist Hospitals in Brazil. This is a possibility in the near future. John of God's Center in Abadiãnia, Brazil, is not set up to take care of people with serious psychological conditions, unless those individuals are accompanied by qualified caretakers.[5]

Conclusion

Figure 5.1 charts the cause of serious mental illness and paths of being victim to or emerging from that condition. It summarizes the previous sections.

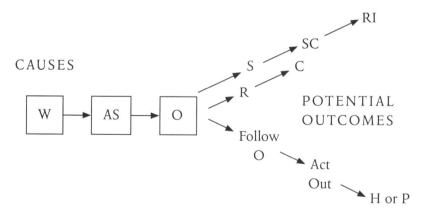

Figure 5.1: Causes and potential outcomes of severe mental illness

Box "W" symbolizes "weaknesses" that cause mental illness. These can be a genetic predisposition, social conditioning which cultivates certain habits of negative thinking or destructive behavior, trauma, lack of discipline, lack of morals, lack of self-care, drug use that leaves one open to negative spirits, an imbalance brought from previous lives, for example residual guilt or anger, or the mismanagement or repression of mediumship abilities.

Box "AS" stands for "attracting spirits" who want to live through the person's weakness, or use the person to take revenge for prior wrongs they feel they were victim to in previous lives.

Box "O" stands for the obsession or attachment of the spirit to the individual. The result is the person hears inner voices that encourage him or her on a path of self-destructive or overly aggressive behaviors.

When the disturbed person "Follows O" he or she follows the dictates of the obsessors without being able to disidentify with them, or say "no" to them. "Act Out" may take the form of abuse of alcohol or drugs, or various other forms of self-destructive or violent behavior. Paranoid feelings and ideation may be apparent. If this reaches crisis proportions, the end result is "H or P," "hospitalization or prison."

Activities in a Spiritist psychiatric hospital will include conventional treatment (supervision, medication, psychotherapy, physical education, adequate rest, balanced meals, and possibly ECT) with the option of Spiritist therapies (prayer, blessed water, laying-on of hands, medical intuition, and disobsession).

Activities in a conventional hospital that does not provide Spiritist therapies may provide respite, and likely initiates a prescription for psychiatric medication to suppress symptoms, possibly for a long period of time, even life. Prison may provide the same. In the worst of cases prison may involve physical restraint and isolation, leaving a person alone without resources to manage the obsession, and thus exacerbating the problem. A return to hospitalization or prison, or living the life of a homeless person, is likely if the individual has not learned how to effectively cope with obsessors, or is weakened by the side-effects of psychiatric medications. In many cases, long-term use of psychiatric medication has led to inability to function in work or family life and the need for support through welfare.

If the disturbed person at the position of "O" opts for "R," then he gravitates to religion. In a religious institution he will have guidance to follow the dictates of the religious authorities and the religious doctrine. That can help him to "Control" ("C") his behavior and say "no" to his desire to follow the dictates of the obsessors. The fellowship and encouragement to practice self-control found in religion can lead to gentler behavior and a better quality of life.

A parallel path is symbolized by "S," or Spiritism. This provides a possibility whereby the individual understands the concept of "working on himself or herself" to become more self-aware, more self-responsible, and more in control of his or her choices. He or she begins to understand the law of karma, that his or her actions have consequences. "SC" represents attending a "Spiritist Center." The activities at the Spiritist Center will include study, blessed water, prayer, fellowship, improving relationships, laying-on of hands to facilitate maintaining balance during stressful times, feedback from mediums to increase self-awareness and improve self-care, appreciation of diversity (as the centers are ecumenical), and organized charity work to reinforce the practice of compassion. The result is "RI," "reforma intima," or personal transformation. As one continues on this path, consistently attending Spiritist activities and working on one's self, the original causes of mental illness can dissolve; negative or obsessing spirits will then no longer be able to gain hold of the person. Positive aspiration and personal connection to spiritual sources have replaced negativity.

The results one achieves through personal transformation are the cultivation of forgiveness, humility, patience, faith, compassion, gratitude, appreciation, self-awareness, and a stronger connection to spiritual guidance and inner wisdom. Some will find that their previous openness to negative spirits is replaced by an ability to channel positive spirits to effect healing for themselves and others.

Of course, the sequence graphed in this map can be short-circuited. If a person has a weakness, and is somewhere on the path that ultimately leads to "H or P," he or she may at any time wake up and understand that he or she can make another choice for a better quality of life, become more self-aware, exercise self-control, and assume self-responsibility. This change may happen at any moment through being exposed to people of goodwill, an interaction with a loved one or a counselor, a dream, a personal prayer, or a vision. It could possibly happen through positive feelings sent in prayer through others, as well. See Chapter 20 for evidence that compassionate intention has a therapeutic effect.

Prayer of Caritas[6]

God, our Father, who is all power and goodness,
give strength to those who go through tribulations;
give light to those who seek the truth,
and fill the human heart with compassion and charity.

God, give the guiding star to the traveler,
consolation to the afflicted, and rest to the sick.
Father, give repentance to the guilty, truth to the spirit,
guidance to the child and a father to the orphan.

Lord, may Your goodness extend over everything that You have created.
Mercy, Lord, to those who do not know You, and hope to those who suffer.
May Your goodness allow the consoling spirits
to spread peace, hope, and faith everywhere.

God, a ray of Your light and a spark of Your love can inflame the earth.
Let us drink from the fountains of this abundant and infinite goodness,
and all tears will be dried, and all pain will be lessened.
A single heart, a single thought will rise up to You,
like a cry of gratitude and love. Like Moses on the mountain,
we wait for You with open arms. Oh, Goodness, Oh, Beauty, Oh, Perfection,
we wish in some way to deserve Your mercy.

God, give us the strength to progress so we may rise up to You,
give us pure charity, give us faith and reason,
and give us the simplicity that will make our souls
the mirror that will reflect your image.

Amen

Notes

1. This is extracted from *Kardec's Spiritism* (Bragdon 2004, pp.60–63). It is one of the clearest cases of a patient being assisted by the Spiritist integrative approach to helping someone diagnosed with schizophrenia.

2. Medical intuitives are able to sense imbalances in the physical and energy bodies of a patient and articulate the nature of those imbalances so as to implement diagnosis and treatment that includes subtle aspects not often perceived by conventional medical professionals.

3. Orthomolecular psychiatric therapy is the treatment of mental disease by the provision of the optimum molecular environment for the mind, especially the optimum concentrations of substances normally present in the human body.

4. Allan Kardec, the founder of Spiritism, described the perispirit as "a subtle, ethereal, nearly massless covering…a kind of energy body that serves as a blueprint for the human form" (Kardec 2004). See page 15 for a further explanation.

5. Anyone interested in participating in programs in the Spiritist Hospitals should write to the Foundation for Energy Therapies, c/o Emma Bragdon, at EBragdon@aol.com. The Foundation intends to update our website, SpiritualAlliances.com, and *Resources for Extraordinary Healing: Schizophrenia, Bipolar and Other Serious Mental Illnesses* (Bragdon 2012) as needed, to facilitate those looking for the kind of help that Spiritism has to offer in its hospitals.

     Those who are drawn to Spiritist therapies, but are not subject to a serious mental imbalance, can find Spiritist Centers in their own locales through the International Spiritist Council (www.intercei.com), which maintains an updated list of Spiritist Centers worldwide, or the United States Spiritist Council (www.spiritist.us).

6. This is repeated in Portuguese before meditation time begins, mornings and afternoons, at the Casa de Dom Inácio, the healing center of John of God in Brazil. "Caritas" does not have a direct translation into English. One might say it encompasses care, compassion, and love of humanity.

Part II

SPIRITIST TREATMENTS

PRACTICE

Chapter 6

THREE SPIRITIST PSYCHIATRIC HOSPITALS

Editor's Note

If the spirit is not acknowledged as existing and real, psychiatrists will only pay attention to effect. They will be impeded from divining the root causes and will never cure effectively... New theories—with solid experimental foundations—point at the spirit, illuminating and unveiling. But, we need courage, not only to acknowledge these theories, but also to examine them.

(Azevedo 1997)

The wisdom of integrating treatments for body, mind, and spirit into health care is becoming obvious to more and more health professionals as well as to those seeking treatment. This chapter highlights three different models currently used in Brazil's Spiritist Psychiatric Hospitals, integrating spiritual treatments to improve mental health care.

I was fortunate to personally see five Spiritist Psychiatric Hospitals in action in Palmelo, Curitiba, Porto Alegre, Anapolis, and São Paulo during site visits, each one lasting a week or more. The Spiritist Psychiatric Hospital in Porto Alegre, HEPA, is particularly large, and has an impressive school for training mediums, as well as continuing education for health professionals onsite. The Spiritist Hospital André Luiz in Belo Horizonte has developed a very strong trans-disciplinary group meeting, where MDs join with mediums for diagnosis and treatment planning. The Hospital João Evangelista in São Paulo is initiating the organization of research collaborating with universities and other Spiritist Hospitals in Brazil. A brief description of the particular program dedicated to helping those with addictions at the Spiritist Psychiatric Hospital Bom Retiro in Curitiba can be found in *Resources for Extraordinary Healing: Schizophrenia, Bipolar and Other Serious Mental Illnesses* (Bragdon 2012).

THE SPIRITIST HOSPITAL ANDRÉ LUIZ

Roberto Lucio Viera de Souza, MD, and
Jaider Rodrigues e Paulo, MD

Brief History of Hospital Éspírita André Luiz (HEAL)

HEAL's founding was the result of direct guidance received from spiritual mentors during meetings held on December 25, 1949, at Grupo da Fraternidade, a Spiritist Center in Belo Horizonte. The guides explained that the geographic region around Belo Horizonte held a lot of mental patients under the influence of suffering spirits, who were either triggering or worsening the patients' psychiatric problems. It took 18 years after it was conceived for the founders to gather the amount of money needed to purchase the land and build the institution.

HEAL started operating as a philanthropic hospital in October 1967. During its initial stages we counted on qualified personnel to apply the academically accepted therapeutics; however, those professionals were not open to applying spiritual therapies, so the Spiritist protocols were relegated to a position of parallel, independent therapeutic options. Integration between conventional therapies and complementary spiritual treatments was only achieved in 1977, after the arrival of new, more open health professionals who accepted the vision of the spiritual aspects of diseases.

From the beginning, we asked Spiritist mediums to cast light on the severe psychiatric cases that presented no effective response to the prescribed conventional psychiatric treatments. The spiritual information about patients' previous lives retrieved by these mediums, who had no previous knowledge about the cases, showed a logical connection to the cases and led to the conclusion that certain spiritual therapies (prayers, magnetization, spiritual studies, and the mediums' intuitive input and interventions) should be applied to complement the formal medical therapy, to produce optimal results.

Since 1977 we have structured an interdisciplinary team, whose members are all engaged and in agreement with the primary objectives of the institution. Our bio-psycho-social-spiritual treatment model involves all therapists, operating as a group together. We discuss specific themes that impact our patients, for example the value of life, relationships, emotional life, and techniques for improving spiritual growth. This process has led to a greater appreciation of the spiritual perspective and to a more solid engagement of the therapists.

The nature of the team's engagement no longer needs to be as intense at present because we have made improvements in our conventional treatments and our Department of Spiritual Assistance, (DAE). Patients are increasingly receiving a more consistent and specific treatment for their needs. In some cases a homeopath is called to join the multidisciplinary team. There are also patients for whom electrotherapy is prescribed. In those cases, an anesthesia risk assessment is performed by a psychiatrist, an anesthesiologist, a nurse, and hospital technicians.

Without losing the free-of-charge character of DAE's therapies, the administration of DAE has become more professional. The group of volunteers has grown to approximately 350 and improved the spiritual assistance provided. We have hired a Director for volunteers and a Coordinator (a Spiritist health care professional with a good level of knowledge and experience as a coordinator as well). We have hired administrative assistants who are all Spiritists. Our administration and therapeutic teams have also found an approach to clinical work that increases our compatibility with Brazil's national mental health policy.

Available Patient Care

Patients are separated in different wings based on the level of care needed and the specific complexity of the disease they are experiencing. Depending on the severity of the case, individualized approaches are applied, leveraging all resources available in an attempt to accelerate patients' recovery. We move patients from one wing to another in line with the evolution of each case, a practice aligned with the most up-to-date approaches of psychiatry.

In addition to the hospitalization and walk-in sections available since October 1967, HEAL now has a Protected Home (for chronic patients who, for diverse reasons, eventually become hospital residents) and two day care sections: one for male addicts and the other for psychiatric patients of both genders. HEAL has 145 beds available, and can provide care for up to 60 addicts plus 120 with psychiatric disorders in its "Day-Care Department" (Therapeutics and Social Assistance Center—CETAS).

The entire administrative management and the Council of HEAL are run by unpaid volunteers. The hospital has about 250 hired workers and 12 paid medical professionals. The institution is not directly supported by any governmental organization, nor directly connected to SUS (the Brazilian Social Security System), relying solely on the profit that results from private and/or private health care plan patients. In spite of that, part of the hospitalization and all day care services are made available free of charge for more than 150 impoverished patients each day. This is only possible thanks to the energetic, sacrificing spirit of our volunteer crew.

Spiritual Assistance

Medicine and religion have walked hand in hand during most of human history. The roles of shaman and doctor, in many cultures and even up to the present day, are positions held by the same individual. The word "saint," which is often used by religions to indicate an enlightened person who reflects or is an intermediate for divine reality, is a synonym for "sound"—i.e. in good health. This intertwines a higher-spiritualized condition with the state of being healthy. The etymology of the word "therapist," which designates a health care professional, is derived from the Greek and refers to "one who leads to wholeness." This is similar to the etymology of the word "religion," derived from the Latin, *religare*: "re" is defined as to return to and "ligare" is defined as to link or bind. Thus, religion binds us again to our Creator.

Medicine in general, and medical schools in the USA specifically, have been showing a growing interest in spirituality's impact on health. This is inferred from the relevant number of publications addressing this subject in the most respected specialized magazines, as well as by the number of courses that are now being offered by American universities. The concept and approach applied there to what spirituality really is may differ substantially from what we offer. At HEAL, it's the Spiritist principles that guide the work of volunteers and the perception of those who are assisted, without proselytizing.

As soon as a patient is accepted into our hospital, inpatients requesting spiritual assistance are given individualized and/or group assistance, and each is told about the spiritual perspective of illnesses according to the Spiritist principles or the patient's original religion. This first conversation not only presents the Spiritist therapies but also reinforces the complementary character of them, making it clear that they complement but do not obstruct conventional therapy.

Therapists at the hospital only bring patients to the Spiritual Assistance Department (DAE) as a result of a request from the patient, or the patient's family members, along with formal written authorization. Patients requesting deeper involvement with DAE are evaluated by a fraternal worker who tells them about the spiritual therapies offered. The free-of-charge spiritual therapeutics include:

- daily prayers transmitted twice a day by a system of speakers, concomitantly with the spiritual activities

- Gospel and Spiritism study meetings, aimed at encouraging reflection and spiritual and moral renewal, with themes varying according to the type of patients present

- spiritual magnetization (laying-on of hands), applied either one to one or by a group working together on one person

- fraternal services, offered to patients and family members whenever needed, during which the Spiritist therapeutics are explained and reinforced; the volunteers are responsible for hearing the patients and their moral pain, as well as for providing guidance about how patients can take greater advantage of the spiritual assistance they can receive at the hospital

- disobsession meetings

- spiritual guidance meetings (medical intuition), for further help concerning the most challenging cases

- library of books with spiritual themes, from which patients can borrow books during their stay at the hospital

- public gatherings for inpatients, family members, and day patients.

Spiritual Guidance Sessions: A Multidisciplinary Approach

Spiritual guidance meetings are an additional tool for health care providers working at HEAL. Each patient is selected to participate by the multidisciplinary team responsible for him or her, according to the severity of his or her mental process. Patients selected are typically found to have mental disorders that are severe, do not respond well to other protocols, and/or when the progress of the infirmity and its consequences are unpredictable, for example a bad prognosis. Patients' families not only receive detailed information about the patient's situation, but must also authorize the spiritual guidance session by means of a written letter of consent.

Meetings are held from 8 to 10 a.m. on Thursday of each week. Seventeen people attend. Twelve are mediums: seven ostensive mediums (five who are clairvoyant plus two who perform healing through magnetization), and five who are supportive of the ostensive mediums. The clairvoyants are able to sense the drama patients are facing presently or have faced in their previous lives, and their current psychological and spiritual condition. Channeling by mediums is rarely used due to the challenging nature of that work. The magnetizers are able to observe each patient's spiritual body, and assess the type of issues that affect the spiritual body through the patient's spiritual associates who are present (the patient's spiritual friends and enemies). The team is completed by three doctors, an event coordinator, and an assistant, who is usually an expert in the area of spiritual assistance. The doctors involved in the meeting assess the medical records of each patient and then share all the relevant details they are allowed to divulge to other team members, respecting privacy and ethical standards of medical practice.

The meeting starts with team members reading an edifying text quietly to themselves. After that, the coordinator asks one of the participants to pray to the Creator of life for blessings and protection.

An assistant from the team is then assigned to bring patients from their units, so that each can participate. Patients then wait their turn with their assistants, and are taken into the meeting room in turns, one after the other, with an interval of about five minutes between patients.

When it is the patient's turn, he or she walks into the room where the 12 mediums are concentrated, sits in a chair that has been previously placed for him or her, and is invited to remain silent, if possible. Two team members responsible for magnetic energy transmission apply magnetic therapy to the patient, following a specific magnetization technique in which they stand beside the patient, palms facing him or her, without touching the body. Meanwhile, the other team members remain concentrated and perform their work, some observing only, some mediums taking notes about the patient, and others keeping their concentration in order to provide the spiritual–magnetic foundation that is needed for the work to be performed.

After all patients have been seen, their medical records are separately analyzed, with all mediums reporting what they have observed or written. Each distinct case is then evaluated to define the type of magnetic transmission each patient needs. The team also sets a few guidelines that assist the multidisciplinary team in reassessing their work with each specific patient.

In every meeting one of the hospital team members also goes through the same process these patients are given. This way the team member not only benefits from the work itself, but also is reminded of the magnitude of the work he or she is performing.

All patients are reassessed weekly, so that the work of the multidisciplinary team can be readjusted according to changes that are noted in the patient. All notes produced are kept in a patient-specific record. The same process is repeated week after week, for as long as the patient is in the hospital. In cases where imminent suicide risk, violence, and treatment sabotage are observed, the team decides how to report to those who need to have the information.

A final analysis of each patient is performed at the time of their discharge from the hospital. Patients receive a formal prescription for the continuation of their spiritual assistance at that time. This continuation can take place in Spiritist Centers independent of the hospital in which patients can continue to receive laying-on of hands, and participate in prayer and in discussion groups to support their living a balanced life and continuing personal growth.

We will now look at two severe cases of inpatients who experienced this process with excellent outcomes.

Case 1

>Patient "Ernesto": 32 years old, married, male, born in Belo Horizonte. Administrative clerk for the secretary of a private university.

Ernesto was admitted to Hospital Éspírita André Luiz on February 16, 2009, coming from a hospital to which he had been taken to treat smoke inhalation caused by the smoke of a fire he set himself, in an attempt to bring his life to an end.

Ernesto's mother reports he had had play therapy sessions at the early age of four for being unruly. According to the responsible therapist, he was very intelligent. Ernesto's father died when Ernesto was six, and his mother got married again soon after. The mother–son relationship was not very good. Ernesto has always been an only child. At the age of 15 Ernesto started the frequent use of cocaine, cannabis sativa, and tobacco.

As a teenager, Ernesto got married for the first time, divorced, and remarried another woman. He did not have a peaceful marital life due to his aggressive temper. He's the father of a girl born with Duchenne muscular dystrophy. Having a bad sexual relationship with his wife, he once tried to attack her with a knife because she was rejecting him.

Six months before being hospitalized, Ernesto started experiencing intense mood changes: aggressiveness, recurrent thoughts of murders and destruction, anger towards himself, and self-destructive thoughts were common. His wife took their daughter back to her father's house after one of the couple's angry exchanges. Police were called on many occasions due to Ernesto's violent acts, which included threatening his father-in-law's life. It was during an outburst that he set fire to his apartment, was rescued by police officers, taken to a hospital for clinical treatment, and finally guided to Hospital Éspírita André Luiz.

Ernesto caused lots of trouble at HEAL. He managed to keep himself clearheaded; however, he acted rebelliously and was even physically aggressive with other patients, engaging in a number of fist-fights. Nurses often had to physically restrain his movements to protect him as he would fall in a way that hurt his body. He was constantly threatening the medical team, beating his head against walls, breaking windows, and inciting other patients to create messes in the ward.

He has also sabotaged and boycotted his own treatment, mocking and threatening to hurt his mother. It was common to hear him say he hated everything and everyone, and that he wanted to kill people, including himself. The multidisciplinary team eventually prescribed electroconvulsive therapy (ECT) after evaluating the specifics of the case and its severity, and with Ernesto's mother's consent.

Ernesto was subject to a total of 12 ECT sessions, with little progress for the first eight sessions. It was then that the health care team decided to assign him to receive spiritual guidance in one of the sessions previously described.

On March 5, 2009, Ernesto participated in his first session. The team noticed that, in spite of the residual constraining effects of ECT, Ernesto had a mocking smile and impatient behavior during the meeting. The mediums could see he was under the control of a herd of rioters of the "spiritual world" who, connected to him by means of their similar pattern of feelings (aggressive temper), were using him as a puppet to create turmoil and aggression. Had it been possible, they had plans to use the patient to commit crimes against society, something that would have been possible due to one of his past lives in which he produced poisons out of plants and roots with the intent to hurt others. He had effectively killed many people. Ernesto's rebelliousness, his tormented childhood, bad familial relationships, and his prior uncontrolled use of drugs fit well into what the rioters wanted him to do. They also intended to cause as much trouble as possible to the hospital, for its Spiritist medical approach was seen as an obstacle to their malignant plans, which included punishing some patients and causing people to speak ill of the medical team.

The clairvoyants found Ernesto's energy centers (chakras) to be congested with dark, unruly energies. His physical brain was poisoned by the effect of drugs and about to suffer an apoplectic fit. He was thoroughly dominated by a group of spiritual villains, who kept repeating in unison that, if he was undecided about fulfilling their demands, he'd better die, because "on the other side" he'd be much more useful to them.

During five consecutive weeks Ernesto was taken to the meeting for spiritual guidance. Each time he received magnetic therapy (chakra cleansing and energy transmission) and during each meeting more negative entities were detached from him. Improvements were observed by the multidisciplinary team from the very first week.

The patient who had consistently refused any treatment approach became more and more accessible. He presented fewer psychomotor crises, developed a better relationship with other inpatients, and started attending occupational therapy and music therapy sessions. Ernesto eventually showed more interest in physical activities and all other treatment options at the hospital. He once talked about how hard it was for him to go through hospital treatment, and expressed the desire of having a normal life once again, even though he accepted that his marital life had already come to an end. He became willing to talk to his mother (which he had been previously unwilling to do), and expressed the need of doing something useful, for it was too tiresome for him to spend so many hours with no responsibilities.

Ernesto's team had a hard time discharging him from HEAL to continue his treatment at home. His wife was afraid of him and did not want to live with him anymore, and his mother also said she was afraid and didn't feel safe living alone with him in the same house. Finally his stepfather, then divorced from his mother, out of pity accepted to host Ernesto in a neighboring city for no more than

30 days. After that period, Ernesto's mother decided to allow him to live with her for a given period, if he followed his doctors' guidelines, and did not cause his stepfather any trouble.

Ernesto had three follow-up medical appointments with a psychiatrist after being discharged from the Spiritist Hospital. Medication was gradually reduced to a single 500 mg dose of sodium valproate at night. This drug is an anticonvulsant used in the treatment of epilepsy and bipolar disorder, as well as other psychiatric conditions requiring a mood stabilizer. By his last appointment, Ernesto was ready to go back to work. He was then referred to a local medical service to continue his treatment. Continued psychosocial therapeutic support was prescribed.

Comments

The use of spiritual treatment has been crucial for this patient. His organic, psychological, and psychic resistance to psychoactive drugs, psychosocial assistance, other chosen therapy (which included arts and physical activities), and even ECT left the medical team a bit perplexed. He resisted all possible approaches until spiritual assistance was offered. Response to this therapy was clearly positive and fast. With a history of the need for physical restraints to control his psychomotor excitement and impulses for self-destructive behavior, the patient increasingly became more self-controlled and receptive from the first spiritual guidance session. From then on he started responding to the treatment as a whole, being eventually discharged from HEAL and, after three months of medical follow-up, he was finally able to return to work.

It's likely that his deeds in past lives have had a strong influence over his actions and tendencies in his present life. As said before, in past lives he made use of poison substances to kill other people. In his present life he has also used illegal drugs, which affected his psychic system, leading him to develop psychotic behavior that caused a lot of suffering. This is the law of karma in action.

Case 2

Patient "Marie": 34 years old, single, female, profession unknown.

Marie checked in to the Hospital Éspírita André Luiz on March 23, 2010, with psychomotor agitation. Eighteen months earlier, during her first pregnancy, she started experiencing episodes of psychomotor agitation with aggressive behavior towards herself. She had been hospitalized in psychiatric hospitals many times during this period.

According to her family, these episodes were characterized by changes in mood from euphoria, to megalomania, to depression, with noticeable loss of weight during the most recent few months. During her psychiatric interview at intake, she presented organized thoughts, delirious content and ideation, and a suspicious, threatening look. From time to time she would let out fragmented sentences such as "A secret organization has brought my aborted kid to Brazil. He's now been raised by my aunt" and "There are criminal organizations." She was involuntarily hospitalized for the risk she imposed to both herself and others. Nothing relevant has been found in her family history to explain the problem she has.

When hospitalized, Marie kept herself isolated in her room, unwilling to accept any clinical approaches. Hostile towards the therapeutic team, she threatened the doctors, saying she would even sue them or call security if they did not leave her alone. She refused to take the prescribed medication and to adopt any treatment. She said she was being persecuted by occult powers.

The spiritual guidance team started working with her on April 6, 2010, in response to a request from her therapists and family. The mediums' research on her past lives revealed she had previously been a nun, the assistant of a mother superior. Markedly cruel with her subordinates, she had been responsible for the death of many nuns in the convent, especially due to the criminal abortions she got involved with to conceal that epoch's common clandestine relationships. The result was that Marie was being persecuted by the spirits of those entities, who claimed revenge for the past suffering she had caused.

A day after her first meeting of spiritual guidance, significant improvement was seen. Marie participated in only three of these meetings, eventually accepting the prescribed therapies. She also developed a better interaction with other patients and her overall situation improved greatly. She has been discharged from the hospital with instructions to continue her clinical and spiritual treatments.

Comments

In this specific case we can observe the law of action and reaction (karma) working. In her previous life, Marie had performed criminal abortions, which often led the subjected nuns to death. In her present life, her first psychotic crisis took place during her pregnancy, which somehow had restimulated her past deeds and brought her karma to the surface to be dealt with.

Marie's case is common at HEAL. We are only able to perform the initial steps of a healing process that should ideally last a long time. Such a process has to be continued outside the hospital, at both the patient's home and in her community. Patients and their families should not see the first results as a miracle or a definitive solution for the problem. The treatment—both medical and spiritual—needs to be continued, with the patient adopting a new, healthier attitude towards life, proactively trying to increase her health.

THE SPIRITIST PSYCHIATRIC HOSPITAL OF PORTO ALEGRE

Emma Bragdon, PhD

History

The Spiritist Psychiatric Hospital of Porto Alegre (HEPA) was founded in 1912 by Spiritists. It is one of about 50 independent Spiritist Psychiatric Hospitals in Brazil, most of which began in the 1930s–1950s. The state where HEPA is located, Rio Grande Do Sul, has many enthusiastic participants in Spiritism. Five hundred Spiritist Centers are in this state alone.

Like all Spiritist Psychiatric Hospitals, HEPA offers conventional treatment protocols (psychotherapy and drugs) that are typical to psychiatric facilities in any developed country with the option of Spiritist treatments as complementary care. Those patients and their families who want to be involved with Spiritist treatments at HEPA must authorize this option, as it is not imposed on patients.

From 1992 to 2002 there were no Spiritist treatments available at HEPA, as medical doctors of that time expected bio-physical treatment to be the most promising and effective mode of therapy. Research has not substantiated that perspective. Since 2000 a new generation of researchers[1] in Brazil are beginning to report that Spiritist therapies do make a noticeable positive difference as a complementary/integrative therapy.

When Gilson Roberto, MD (see Chapters 7 and 13), came to work at the hospital as the Medical Director in 2002, the hospital re-established Spiritist treatments for patients, renewed the training program for mediums, and began to offer evening classes for health professionals concerning the value of spirituality in healing treatments and health maintenance.

Current Profile of HEPA

The hospital sits on six hectares (almost 15 acres) of a wooded hillside in a middle-class residential neighborhood, a 15-minute drive from the center of

Porto Alegre, a major city in the south of Brazil. The grounds include a stream, trails, a garden, soccer fields, and a building for outdoor activities. The hospital is accessible by public transportation.

A small 25-by-50-foot one-story building serves as the facility for Spiritist treatments on site. It has five meeting rooms that serve 15 groups of mediums (150 mediums in total), who meet either to improve their skills in healing and mediumship or to help patients. The building is surrounded by a garden area and is a short two-minute walk to the hospital's reception area. This is also the location for evening classes for health professionals continuing education programs.

According to HEPA's Technical Director, in 2008: The hospital has 700 beds. There are 300–350 live-in patients in 11 different units; 60–90 of these patients are private, the rest are partially sponsored by a government welfare program. The average length of stay is 22–26 days.

Outpatient day hospital resources are offered from 8 a.m. to 5:30 p.m. to 20–30 people for no more than three months at a time. The hospital has an infirmary and offers nutritional support but all emergency medicine for physical problems is handled at a general hospital off-site.

The hospital employs 26 physicians. Twelve psychiatrists work in intake, diagnosis, and placement only. Twelve other psychiatrists are on staff, attending patients directly. Two physicians are specialists in internal medicine. All work part-time only. Of these physicians, two are dedicated Spiritists, four or five do not like the Spiritist perspective, and the rest either tolerate or accept it.

Any MD in the area can have hospital privileges and bring their patients to the hospital to stay. The hospital could also receive patients from abroad, but they are not in a position to accept insurance payments from insurance companies in other countries. The staff, at this time, only speak Portuguese.

The hospital uses a multidisciplinary (or interdisciplinary) approach that includes group therapy and personal therapy with psychologists, art, music, physical education, occupational therapy, and social assistance (charity/volunteer help to those in need). Families of patients are encouraged to be involved, but family systems therapy is not available. Special support sessions are provided for families dealing with family members' drug/alcohol abuse.

As noted above, 80 percent of the patients are partially paid for by the state or federal government. The state provides for an average of 28 days only. The federal government partially pays for care after that, when patients need more extended care. The amount of money paid by government per day per patient is about eight dollars less per day than what is needed to cover their most basic costs. The hospital depends on money from private patients and donations to make ends meet. The financial situation is challenging.

The two wards we visited, accommodating 30–45 patients each (one for women, the other for men), were clean and orderly with 2–4 beds in each bedroom. Food was simple and nutritious with servings of meat, vegetables, and fruits. We were not allowed entry into the private wards of the hospital to protect the anonymity of the patients there.

There is one television per unit in the dayroom of each ward. It is not on all the time. Periodically there is peaceful music, prayer, or inspired talks played on loudspeakers.

Currently the hospital is experiencing changes on many levels. For example, the medical personnel are not in the habit of reporting on each patient's involvement with spiritual treatments but only drug interventions. Nurses make note of behavioral changes they observe on the wards. Both the medical and the technical directors understand that the reporting done in house in each patient's file needs to change to include notations on Spiritist therapies given and their effects. The supervisor of spiritual direction, Gerald Magnan, has begun to make these notations, filing them in the Spiritual Assistance Department. Clearly, in 2008, these and other steps were being taken to further integration between medical personnel and Spiritual Assistance volunteers.

Organizational Structure

The Board of Directors of the hospital, numbering nine, are all mediums. They channel the advice of disincarnate spiritual advisors, also known as "mentors" of the hospital, as part of their process of decision-making. We could say the mentors of the hospital are the highest authority.

In 2008 the President of the Board was 98 years old. There are three vice presidents: Gilson Roberto (Medical Director) and two others who are involved with elements of the hospital related to Spiritism and Finances. The power for making decisions really lies in these three vice presidents and the mentors they channel.

Spiritual Assistance Programs (DAE)

The goals of the DAE are:

- to walk hand in hand with the technical staff to improve the care for the patient

- to develop scientific research with the doctors on staff

- to offer laying-on of hands to patients on all wards (only 5 out of 11 wards consistently offer this now).

Gerald Magnan was Director of the DAE in 2008, when I was visiting the hospital (see Chapter 24 in this volume on training mediums). Gerald supervises all the mediums and they all work exclusively for the hospital. He described their Spiritist activities at the hospital:

> A team of mediums meets twice a week in a private room to pray and radiate energy on a subtle level to cleanse and energize the hospital and all the wards. People with mental illnesses are often beset with negative thinking, and the cleansing meditation helps clear the air and renew the group's intention to embrace a strong connection to positive spiritual energies and the mentors of the hospital.
>
> Spiritist therapies include disobsession, fraternal counseling, magnetized water, as well as special sessions of laying-on of hands. Group discussions of the New Testament's Gospels According to Spiritism are also offered to patients.
>
> All patients in five wards have the option for laying-on of hands as volunteers come to those wards once or twice a week to provide this therapy for all patients who choose to come to the dayroom to receive it. Patients' family members, staff, and family members of those taking part in educational classes at the hospital may also receive laying-on of hands, and disobsession, on request. This support is also made available for hospital staff who have become out of balance, depleted, and seek help. In these cases, the medium works one-on-one with the staff person.
>
> There is a special group of mediums that offer fraternal support for those who are chemically dependent and their families. Recently, an advanced group of mediums has offered disobsession to those requesting it through email.

The Program for Training and Supervising Mediums

In order to function as a medium with patients, one has to initially do 2–3 years of study, followed by practicum and more study in a group. Each group is under the supervision of Gerald. The groups are well organized and Gerald, an exceptionally well-trained medium, maintains the order in each group meeting working with patients. He is interested in research and has been keeping audiotapes and written notes documenting Spiritist treatments of patients.

I viewed a disobsession session at HEPA in April 2008, with a group of eight mediums supervised by Gerald. Four mediums received negative spirits associated with patients who were mentally ill, and were able to voice details of the obsession while channeling the obsessing spirit. Four mediums were available to donate laying-on of hands, and mentally transmit the energy of certain colors to the mediums who were receiving the negative spirits in order to assist them as they worked. A helper took notes and managed the tape recording of the session.

Gerald monitored the energies of each medium to see they were not becoming depressed or depleted by the session. He also counseled the obsessors as they came into the mediums, basically giving verbal psychotherapy, to encourage them to release the attachment they had to the patient and go on in their evolution. No patients were present. The session was offering healing at a distance (remotely) to patients in the hospital wards.

After sessions of disobsession or laying-on of hands, a few ounces of "magnetized" water are given in a small cup to both the mediums and those who received healing who may be present (e.g. a guest). The "magnetized" water is simple bottled water that was infused with positive, healing energy through prayer said by the leader of the mediums.

"Is there ever a bad disobsession session?" I asked. Gerald answered, "No, only a session where some mediums are left sad or depleted. In case someone is depleted: they don't leave. They pray and cleanse more until they are uplifted."

There is no expectation that a patient will be cured by one disobsession session. Instead, treatments are given according to the current problems patients are having and many different types of therapies may be needed as well as more than one disobsession session.

Results of Therapies

It is difficult to validate exactly what impact the Spiritual therapies are having, as clinical research has not been done at HEPA to establish the effectiveness of care. However, nurses report that patients are generally calmer for 3–4 days after they receive the laying-on of hands. Effects of disobsession have only been measured subjectively through reports from staff, mediums, and patients. Anecdotal evidence shows that disobsession provides patients with relief from some self-destructive habits of negative thinking and feeling.

Continuing Education for Professionals
Monday 7:30–9 p.m.

A study group for health professionals who are already part of the Spiritist Medical Association (AME) of Brazil takes place. They study Spiritist texts for one hour, then meditate, and then receive channeling and share as a way to support each person opening spiritually. They have been meeting since 2005.

Tuesday 7:30–9 p.m.

Dr. Gilson Roberto and his brother, Gelson Roberto (a psychologist who is in clinical practice as well as directing a Spiritist Center independent of the hospital), each host study groups in two adjoining rooms. The groups are composed of doctors, psychotherapists, and laypeople interested in the interaction between medicine, spirituality, and psychology.

Gilson's evening class in April 2008 provided a power-point presentation that covered the following:

- thoughts are seeds of illness or health

- different brain wave patterns impact thought content

- the pineal gland's role in mediumship; anatomy and physiology

- alternating between current science and the writing of André Luiz, a disincarnate, to demonstrate that André Luiz predicted medical breakthroughs. This shows that channeled materials (André Luiz channeled 13 books through Chico Xavier)[2] can be scientifically accurate and forecast future events.

Gelson's evening class, in November 2008, focused primarily on the relationship between psychology and Spiritism, specifically how psychology and spiritual realities interface. The foundation of this relationship, as he sees it, is that psychological health requires a moral transformation. He posited that humans are now confused because man has distanced himself from spirituality and that has led to many illusions about the nature of life on earth. An infantile psychological state dominated by pride and selfishness is now more apparent than ever. Spiritism can provide the steps for improving this situation.

Gelson has a gift of meeting his students directly, in an empathic way, while still maintaining a very intelligent grasp of his subject. Both Gilson and Gelson are very professional presenters.

Notes

1. Electronic Library in Spirituality and Health: www.hoje.org.br/elsh.
2. The André Luiz collection, by C. Xavier, comprises 13 books. Many of them have been translated into English, and can be purchased online through a Spiritist bookstore in New York: www.sgny. org/books–2/francisco-xavier-andre-luiz-collection.

JOÃO EVANGELISTA HOSPITAL

Candido Pinto Vallada, MD, Camilla Casaletti Braghetta, MA, Giancarlo Lucchetti, MD, Frederico Camelo Leão, MD, PhD, and Homero Vallada, MD

In Brazil, more than 90 percent of the population has some kind of religious affiliation. Nevertheless, many people do not follow one strict religious code, but express their spirituality, moral values, and faith in different ways, often using diverse religious or spiritual practices. Most individuals consider the spiritual dimension as very important to their lives and understand that spiritual practices can effectively help one cope with adversities, diseases, and mental suffering.

According to Spiritist principles, human diseases are related to the imbalance between body, mind, and spirit. In order to re-establish the harmony of an individual, Spiritist Centers offer resources such as Spiritist "passés" (laying-on of hands over someone else's head or body), prayers, study groups (reading and discussing passages from Spiritist literature), "magnetized" water, and disobsession.

Spiritual Help during Hospitalization

For individuals who become ill and need more intensive care, hospitalization can be a difficult process, not only because of the temporary physical disability, but also because hospitalization causes a disruption of the patient's daily activities: in work, leisure, social support, and spiritual/religious habits.

In the majority of general hospitals, hospitalized patients have access to spirituality through the chaplaincy and other hospital services that schedule religious visits for those patients who request it. However, psychiatric hospitals usually do not have this option due to concerns about the benefits and drawbacks of this assistance.

Among Brazilian hospitals, Spiritist Hospitals in particular have historically been institutions that since their beginnings have addressed the need for spirituality in their patients. Such hospitals have mostly been philanthropic entities (not-for-profit organizations), where health care professionals and Spiritist volunteers have offered spiritual assistance as an optional complementary therapy.

João Evangelista Hospital

João Evangelista Hospital (HOJE) is an independent, non-for-profit, philanthropic institution, which specializes in mental health care, and is located within the city of São Paulo. HOJE has been functioning since 1953 and currently offers care for inpatient and outpatient units, in both a day hospital and 24-hour-care hospital. It has 95 beds, divided into four wards, enrolling private patients and those on public welfare.

The mental health teams at HOJE are composed of different professionals including six psychiatrists, three psychologists, three occupational therapists, two licensed social workers, four licensed technical nurses, seven nurses, 38 licensed auxiliary nurses, one art therapist, one physical education specialist, and two nutritionists.

Conventional psychiatric care and treatment includes medication, psychotherapy, and a range of other techniques such as electroconvulsive therapy. Those modalities and techniques are evidence-based practices which aim to apply the best available evidence gained from the scientific method in clinical decision-making, accepted and promoted by a wide range of representative associations (e.g. the World Health Organization, the American Psychiatric Association, and the Psychiatric Association of Brazil).

HOJE's commitment is to provide integrative care in mental health based on rigorous ethical standards, attending to the foundations of psychosocial well-being through a specialized and well-trained team. The therapeutic process for each patient is individualized and constantly re-evaluated, in order to reintegrate the patient fully into society as soon as possible after hospital treatment.

HOJE started its activities in 1953, under the administration of Ana Gemignani Motta, also known as "Dona Nina." At its beginning, Dona Nina introduced Spiritist assistance to the hospitalized patients, personally leading the group of volunteers who offered this complementary treatment. Among the Spiritist practices that she organized were prayers, meetings of mediums, Spiritist "passés," volunteers' visits to the patient (called "fraternal visits" or "fraternal counseling"), and "healing at a distance" treatments for patients with the most severe illnesses.

Fraternal counseling involves meetings with patients in which the patients talk about their difficulties and receive some help to cope with their problems. The meetings are booked according to the coordinator's assessment of the need, as well as the patient's willingness to meet, the severity of their issues, etc.

Since Dona Nina had abilities as a medical intuitive, she usually participated in the medical evaluations of each patient, transmitting her spiritual impressions of the patient to the psychiatrist.

When Dona Nina passed away in 1978, it became difficult to maintain a satisfactory Spiritist assistance program in the hospital. According to some reports from members of the hospital staff, a period of greater unrest was observed in the hospitalized patients when they did not have Spiritist assistance available.

PRISME

Recently, the Programa de Integração Saúde Mental e Espiritualidade (Spirituality and Mental Health Integration Program) (PRISME) was created to respect and value the spiritual dimension of our hospital program, as well as to reinstate Dona Nina's initial purpose of giving complementary Spiritist therapy to the patients. PRISME has also been created at HOJE to improve and test the efficacy of the complementary Spiritist approach; thus we are committed to research as well.

In medical literature there are few studies regarding the spiritual/religious needs of hospitalized psychiatric patients. The existing research points out that patients hospitalized in psychiatric hospitals have the same needs for spiritual/ religious assistance as those in general hospitals, but have less access.

With this in mind, patients following the Spiritist doctrine or other religions can come to HOJE in order to receive the necessary medical treatment, where their religious/spiritual faiths play an integral role in the treatment. In spite of being a Spiritist Hospital, HOJE takes a broader view and addresses patients with different religions, respecting their faiths and considering their spirituality in general as an important part of well-being.

In João Evangelista Hospital, PRISME is performed by health care professionals specialized in mental health care. When a patient has selected PRISME, these PRISME professionals have access to the information of that patient's file and are connected to the multidisciplinary team treating the patient. We consider this kind of interdisciplinary and interdepartmental communication to be essential to maintaining the high quality of our program.

Intake

After initial registration, the patient is evaluated by a psychiatrist and a social worker. Then a brief spiritual history is conducted by a member of PRISME, identifying the religious/spiritual needs of the patient and verifying if the patient chooses some kind of spiritual assistance during his or her hospitalization.

We make every attempt to be considerate of the vulnerable status of the patient, who has just become both a mental health patient and hospitalized. What the family can tell us about the spiritual needs of the patient is important—but we must also be authorized by the patient, or the family if the patient is not able to make a decision, in order to offer the patient spiritual assistance. Under the Brazilian Federal Constitution (Article 5°, Federal Law n° 9.982/00), religious assistance in hospitals can only be performed with the patient's and/or his or her family's permission. In João Evangelista Hospital, a Relative and a Patient Consent Agreement Form was created in order to allow "spiritual assessment" of each patient during hospitalization. Those patients who choose treatment without spiritual assistance of any kind will receive only conventional psychiatric treatment.

The evaluation of the patient is conducted when most appropriate. In other words, if the patient has severe psychotic symptoms and is confused or very aggressive, the interview will be postponed to another moment, when the clinical team considers it more appropriate. In this assessment, the objective is to understand what the patient's needs are to exercise his or her spirituality. We seek to provide conditions for the patient to perform his or her religious/spiritual activity even when hospitalized. There are several ways of practicing spirituality, through prayers, readings, special television programs, charitable activities to benefit others (such as giving help to other patients who are severely disturbed), practice of physical exercises (e.g. yoga, soccer, volleyball, basketball, and gymnastics), meditation, and contact with nature, among others. During hospitalization, we must assess the possibilities of undertaking these activities, together with each patient's clinical condition, physical space, and materials available.

Most importantly, the patient must be made to feel welcome to practice his or her spiritual or religious belief in a hospital situation, so it can contribute to his or her well-being.

Modalities of Treatment in PRISME

Among the modalities of care that the hospital offers to Spiritists within PRISME is the reading and study of *The Gospel According to Spiritism* (Kardec 1987) or other religious books by Spiritists, and the administration of Spiritist "passés." Mediumistic meetings for disobsession are available but patients are not present, even when one is the subject of the meeting.

Spiritists encourage the habit of reading and reflection on the content of principles of Spiritism as a way to change the pattern of negative thoughts and cultivate positive thoughts and a healthy lifestyle. In the Gospel reading, topics are selected by the PRISME personnel and staff in accordance with the appropriateness to each patient's clinical situation. It is recommended that volunteers do not address issues that stimulate the patient's disorders, such as negative statements: obsession, suicide, and past lives, among others. Instead, the passages should address comforting issues and inspire the patient towards ideas of forgiveness, hope, and spiritual growth to effect a positive future. Therefore, the use of works of the primary Spiritist texts by Allan Kardec, Francisco Cândido Xavier, and Divaldo Pereira Franco are highly recommended.

Another form of assistance are Spiritist "passés" (laying-on of hands) which are a positive transmission of energy from one person to another, with the goal of restoring balance or health to the receiver. During such a session, a team of volunteer Spiritists, coordinated by a leader, performs the work within the hospital wards. These teams have typically already worked together in the administration of "passés" in their local community Spiritist Center and schedule visits to the hospital specifically to help patients.

The sessions with mediums are performed by a group of highly trained Spiritist mediums in two different ways. In both types of meetings one medium on the team leads the group and begins by praying for the patient's well-being with the goal of providing wholesome energy. One type of mediumistic meeting is dedicated to prayer and receiving the occasional communications from the spiritual realm which are channeled to the medium for the benefit of the patient. This does not usually include information on details about their physical or mental status. In the second type of meeting, sessions of disobsession may be held: a type of assistance where the mediums also act to avert negative spiritual influences on the patients. PRISME collects all communications and information generated in these mediumistic meetings to use for the benefit of the patient's treatment.

PRISME's Involvement in the Day Hospital

PRISME also provides special care to the patients served at the Day Hospital at HOJE. The Day Hospital encourages meaningful social interaction of patients, trying to place them and encourage their participation in areas of culture, leisure, and community activities to assist them to integrate into society. This kind of work is carried out by the occupational therapists and social workers in discussion groups, tours to the zoo, museums, and musical performances.

Even though they are in the rehabilitation process, many patients still have difficulties in social interaction and need the assistance and encouragement of staff. Given this need, an intervention was organized to benefit these patients and investigate their spiritual/religious needs. We now offer a "therapeutic group meeting" focusing on the issue of spirituality and promoting the integration (or reintegration) of the patient's spiritual/religious activities adjacent to the area of treatment of mental disturbances. Those patients who desired assistance to practice Spiritism specifically were offered the same Spiritist modalities as were offered to the inpatients (above).

The Role of Volunteers

Every form of spiritual assistance offered in HOJE, as in other Spiritist hospitals (passés, prayers, mediumistic meetings, and fraternal visits), is undertaken by volunteers. Spiritist principles encourage everyone to practice charity in order to grow spiritually, which is why many Spiritists in the area willingly volunteer to undertake this work in hospitals.

All volunteers who work at the hospital receive some basic guidelines that aim to ensure harmony between the spiritual approach and psychiatric treatment:

- It is recommended that the volunteers do not interfere with medical and psychosocial treatment of the patient, nor suggest the use of or termination of medications of any kind.

- They are not to advise the patient or his or her family to change their doctor or other health care professional.

- It is essential to orient the volunteer to observe the importance of conventional therapies in treating the patient in order to avoid interpreting the mental disorders as being only of spiritual origin.

- Should volunteer mediums obtain any information spiritually relevant for the care of the patient (for example, while giving the "passés"), this information is forwarded to the coordinators of PRISME.

- The volunteer is told he or she must not notify the patient or family directly about any opinions regarding patient care. As the technical team and PRISME know the history of each patient more thoroughly than the volunteers, and can assess patients' clinical conditions, it is best that they first confirm the information and decide if it will produce a beneficial effect for the patient, then choose if the information is relevant to the patient or his or her family, and the time at which that information could be passed on.

An advantage of volunteerism is the benefit the volunteers derive from their work. Volunteers often report a change of outlook on life, feeling new motivation, feeling useful. There is even some reduction of prejudice against the mentally ill. The work also offers the possibility of social interaction with other volunteers, who often share the same mindset, also contributing to a better quality of life for these workers.

Expanding Knowledge and Understanding

HOJE also has a partnership with "The Program for Health, Spirituality and Religion" at the Institute of Psychiatry, in the Hospital of the Faculty of Medicine, University of São Paulo (IPq-HC-FMUSP). This project is coordinated by health professionals. The purpose is to advance the issue of spirituality in care for patients and develop new models of care. It aims to address spirituality in a broader sense, not just as it applies to conventional religion, but with a focus on discussion and expression of values, beliefs, and way of life. Later on, the results of this project will be adapted and tested at HOJE.

In addition, some of the most well-respected Brazilian Spiritist Hospitals contribute knowledge gained by years of Spiritist assistance practice. They are sharing these experiences with HOJE to find new ways to care for psychiatric patients, using the approach provided by the Spiritist principles first articulated by Kardec. We are conducting annual meetings of the Brazilian Spiritist Hospitals to exchange experiences in order to improve the care we offer patients.

Given that the complementary spiritual approach as outlined above generates information about the patients, which can often be useful for the health professional or the patient in providing extra information or words of comfort and hope, PRISME has organized the implementation of the Spiritual Care Registry (SCR, or RAE in Portuguese), where all relevant information concerning spiritual needs and approaches is recorded. The need to compile all relevant information in a systematic and standardized way was recently recommended in the meetings of Spiritist Psychiatric Hospitals.

It was suggested that the SCR/RAE, which is comprised of notes from all care providers, information from the mediums, a copy of the informed consent of the patient and family (or guardian), and developments made by the coordinator of spiritual care, should be used by all participant hospitals. In this way, the exchange of experiences and future research investigation involving hospitals that use SCR/RAE will be considerably enhanced.

Another goal to be achieved is to recruit and train more volunteers. Thus HOJE in conjunction with the Spiritist Medical Association of São Paulo is organizing a training course for new volunteers. The course will be standardized, and could be used in other Brazilian Spiritist Hospitals, if they need to expand their assistance activities.

Results

Recent data show that patients have benefitted from the spiritual treatment offered at HOJE. A survey conducted of 96 hospitalized patients observed that, of these, 79 percent had a religious denomination, 53 percent attended some religious institution, 53 percent had sympathy for some other religious group beyond their own, and 90 percent would like to receive religious/spiritual assistance during their psychiatric hospitalization. The data collected in this study suggests that patients have admitted a wish to continue religious attendance which shows the importance of spiritual/religious assistance for patients at the time of their treatments.

Our hospital staff have observed and formally documented that the patients appreciate the spiritual care offered at the hospital. Similarly, most of the patients are observed by hospital staff to be calmer during and after the treatments by Spiritist volunteers. (This data has not yet been analyzed and published.) Of course, an environment that lowers the level of stress and offers comfort, encouragement, and hope can already provide a better condition for recovery.

Research

More recently, PRISME has been developing a study in order to test the efficacy of a Spiritist complementary approach to the drug-dependent inpatients' treatment. A group of patients who receive Spiritist assistance will be compared with a group of patients who receive only conventional treatment. The study will look at clinical aspects such as duration of the hospitalization, improvements of symptoms, etc.

Conclusion

In conclusion, Brazilian Spiritist hospitals attempt to see the patient from a more holistic view, not only as a person who is imbalanced, or ill, but also as a bio-psycho-socio-spiritual being. In this model of care, each aspect of patient care complements the other in order to provide as complete psychiatric care as possible.

Editor's Note

Chapters 7–12 consider more deeply the various components of Spiritist therapies used in Brazil's Spiritist Centers and Spiritist Hospitals, as well as with Spiritist psychotherapists.

> Jesus focuses on the sickness of soul that affects people individually and socially, physically and spiritually. This perception of sickness is central, and healing is his signature activity. Jesus does not teach how to be virtuous, how to be saved, or how to be a good church member. He says nothing about memorizing dogma or following a strict set of moral rules. Instead, he continually demonstrates how to be in this world as a healer... From time to time we are all in need of healing, and we are all called to be healers. (Moore 2010, pp.59–60)

Chapter 7

MAGNETIC HEALING, PRAYER, AND ENERGY PASSES

Gilson Roberto, MD

The utilization of magnetism through prayer and laying-on of hands (passé in Portuguese) as resources for healing have accompanied the history of mankind, practiced all over the world for thousands of years. In the time of Isis (in Egypt), the Chaldean priests utilized the laying-on of hands to re-establish health. In the Gospels, we read about the healings performed by Jesus Christ through the laying-on of hands. From Ancient Egypt to modern times, this knowledge has drawn the attention of countless scholars and researchers. Several studies on the utilization of magnetism, laying-on of hands, and prayer in favor of human health are currently under way.

The idea that there exists in any individual a latent force that can be emitted through an act of will is very old. In the Vedic tradition, this force is called "prana," a Sanskrit word for "primordial energy." Aristotle recognized this notion as "entelecheia," a vital force or energy flow. In China it was called Ch'i or Qi, the energy of life. This cosmic force would be present in every living organism, circulating through the network of meridians, the state of its flow in the human organism being the fundamental basis of acupuncture. The same force or potency can be found under different names in most cultures' respective understandings and applications.

In the fifteenth century, Paracelsus (Michaelus 1983) developed his magnetic theory and his "system of magnetic sympathy" as an attempt to understand the process of becoming ill and healing, in which he maintained that magnets were as capable of attracting certain infirmities and illness as they were capable of attracting iron. In the seventeenth century, Van Helmont (Michaelus 1983) claimed to have obtained significant healings through the use of magnets and metallic plates on the bodies of patients. A contemporary of his, the Jesuit, Hell, who was also a renowned physicist, obtained interesting effects with the usage of magnets not only on humans, but also with animals.

However, Michaelus (1983) reports that it was with the German physician Franz Anton Mesmer (1734–1815) that the idea of magnetism as a form of healing took on greater relevance. Mesmer realized that magnetized iron wasn't necessary, because he seemed capable of emitting this healing magnetic force himself, which he dubbed "human magnetism," and he believed that this force could be transmitted to other people. In 1779 he published the book *Animal Magnetism*, in which he defended the thesis that there exists a fluid that interpenetrates everything, and which gives people properties analogous to those of magnets. He believed that, like a magnet, the hands and eyes of some individuals can radiate a special fluid that comes from the organism itself, and can influence individuals and animals. Although his theory was widely opposed and discredited by the mainstream science of his time, it cleared the way for new knowledge.

Christian Friedrich Samuel Hahnemann (1755–1843), creator of homeopathy, believed that the human being is constituted of the body (matter), the spirit, and life force. This life force is what organizes and gives life to matter, sustaining its functioning and making health possible. Illness is then a consequence of a disturbance of a spiritual nature in that life force. Hahnemann wrote that illnesses are "solely spirit-like (dynamic) derangements of the spirit-like power, the Vital Force that animates the human body" (cited by Filho and Curi 1995, p.xvii).

In order to reach a cure Hahnemann believed we must recompose the regulating dynamism of this life force through the immaterial (dynamic) elements of medicine. In his book, *The Organon of the Healing Art*, he writes:

> In the healthy condition of man, the spiritual vital force (autocracy), the dynamic that animates the material body (organism), rules with unbounded sway, and retains all the parts of the organism in admirable, harmonious, vital operation, as regards both sensations and functions, so that our indwelling, reason-gifted mind can freely employ this living, healthy instrument for the higher purpose of our existence. (Hahnemann 1995, p.4)

In 1784 the Marquis of Puységur, a disciple of Mesmer, discovered "artificial somnambulism," an induced state in which subjects exhibit behavior similar to that displayed by sleepwalkers, and in 1787 Dr. Pététin of Lyons discovered "artificial catalepsy," an induced condition that occurs in a variety of physical and psychological disorders and is characterized by lack of response to external stimuli and by muscular rigidity, so that the limbs remain in whatever position they are placed. By 1841 James Braid (1795–1860) had developed hypnotism. Jean-Martin Charcot (1825–1893) later made a methodical study of it, and Sigmund Freud (1856–1939) utilized it in the creation of psychoanalysis (Michaelus 1983).

The Anatomy of Human Magnetism

To better understand the healing process that uses the magnetic force or vital energy we must go back to a view of the totality of the human being, seeking an understanding of his integral constitution: mind–body/spirit–matter. Spiritism presents us a threefold view of the human being, as being constituted by a physical body, a spiritual body (which we call the "perispirit"), and the soul or unique spirit itself.

Just as the human body has its complexity, being formed by several systems and organs with defined functions, the perispirit possesses an even more complex nature, with countless properties and functions. (It is possible to divide it into other structures with specialized tasks; however, due to the subject's complexity, I will not go into great detail now.) Besides the perispirit, we possess the "etheric double," which is our vital body, mediating the functions of the physical and spiritual bodies.

Spirituality informs us that we are in a constant exchange of mental energies of varied nature, in which each mental wave produces a specific vibratory intention, which carries the wishes, feelings, and ideas of the one who emitted them. All thoughts and feelings which we emit are a part of us, our creations, and are extensions of our souls. These mental manifestations gravitate around each individual, creating a vital halo or magnetic field (aura) that expresses the intimate nature of each of us. We constantly create the psychic atmosphere that we breathe and that accompanies us.

These force currents that form our magnetic field (aura), or bio-field, act on the physical and spiritual bodies' cells, which are closely linked. It is impossible to determine precisely where one begins and the other ends. André Luiz, in the book *Evolução em Dois Mundos* (Evolution in Two Worlds), refers to it thus:

> Considering every cell in action as a living unit, like a microscopic motor, in connection to the power plant of the mind, it's clearly understandable that all cellular aggregations emit radiation, and that these radiations articulate through functional synergies, which are constituted of resources that we can call "force tissues," enveloped and emitted by the body.
>
> In man, however, such a projection appears profoundly enriched and modified by the factors of continuous thought, which, in adjusting themselves to the emanations of the cellular field, model around it, in and around the personality, the well-known vital body (or ethereal double of some spiritualist schools), a more or less radiant duplicate of the creature.
>
> Thus, we have in this conjugate of physico-chemical and mental forces the human aura, particular to each individual, permeating him while seeming to emerge from him, in the manner of an egg-shaped field, in spite of the irregular features of its configuration, working as a sensible mirror in which all states of the soul are expressed, with characteristic signs, and in which all ideas are made evident, shaping living canvases, when they endure in vigor and similarity, like in a common cinematograph. (Xavier 1998a, p.127)

And in the book *Mecanismos da Mediunidade* (Mechanisms of Mediumship):

> It is thus that each creature's vital halo, or aura, remains woven with subtle atomic currents of the thoughts that are particular or habitual, within norms that correspond to the law of the "energy quanta" and to the principles of wave mechanics, which impress upon them their particular frequency and color.
>
> These forces, put in constant synchronous movements or agitation states by the impulses of will, establish for each person a particular mind wave. (Xavier 1984, p.45)

Therefore man also possesses his own magnetism, functioning, metaphorically, as a magnet, being a center of attraction and repulsion, exteriorizing his field of energetic radiation through his mental activity and the use of his will. It is also to be found that certain people seem to radiate peace when we come close to them, while others bring us uneasiness through their presence alone: it's the magnetism with which they are charged, positive or negative.

Magnetic Action

Kardec (1996) states that there are three manners of magnetic action:

- through the magnetizer's fluid (*Human Magnetism*)

- through the fluid of the Spirits acting directly, without any intermediates (*Spiritual Magnetism*)

- through the fluid that the Spirits transmit through the magnetizer, combined with his or her own fluid (*Mixed or Human–Spiritual Magnetism*).

In the laying-on of hands taught by Spiritism, "Mixed Magnetism" is employed, that is, the union of human magnetism (the medium's) under the action of the magnetism of the spirits.

Seeking "syntony" (a harmony equal to being at one with something) with the spiritual plane through prayer, the medium performing the passé uses his will and impresses a mental force that drives the radiating power of his psyche, which expands through the hands towards the recipient. Should the treatment be executed by the human magnetizer alone without the collaboration of the spirits the results would be slower. The spirits, through their spiritual magnetism, are not only capable of influencing someone's vital field, but also hold a transformative and penetrative power capable of performing immediate or fairly rapid healings, according to the spirits' level of evolution.

André Luiz clarifies further:

> Acknowledging the magnetic fluid's capacity for creatures to
> influence one another, with even more amplitude and efficiency
> over the cellular entities of the Organic State—particularly blood
> and histiocytic cells, determining their satisfactory level, migration
> or extreme mobility, the production of antibodies, or, still, the
> improvisation of other combative and immunological resources, in
> the defense against bacterial invasion and the reduction or extinction
> of pathogenic processes… (Xavier 1998b, pp.200–201)

Just as a blood transfusion represents a renewal of physical stamina, the laying-on of hands through Spiritists is a transfusion of physio-psychic energies. This parallel holds true except for the detail that organic resources are taken from limited reserves, and psychic elements are taken from the unlimited reserve of the spiritual forces.

The medium-healer performing the laying-on of hands becomes an instrument of infinite kindness, a channel from which the sublime energies flow, extracted from the celestial sources of the Divine supply.

Prayer

The same healing magnetic force which is put in motion by the laying-on of hands can also be transmitted through long distances through the radiating action of prayer. A prayer for another is the emanation of a thought rich in vibratory content. Allan Kardec affirmed that "thought and will represent in ourselves a power of action that reaches far beyond the limits of our corporeal sphere. To pray for another is an act of that will" (Kardec 2006, p.418).

A prayer benefits the person who says it as well as the person who receives it. Meditation and prayer bring on an elevation of thought, generating waves of a very high frequency, with consequent repercussions in molecular biology. When we pray, we detach our thoughts from mundane, material concerns, and seek inner harmony. This simple attitude promotes a relaxation of psychic tensions, favoring energetic flow. Concentration consolidated by faith, noble feelings, and sublimated mental images all increase the frequency of the mental waves, expanding our perispirit, unlocking psychic channels, removing the accumulated deleterious fluids, renewing tired cells, toning our nervous system, and stimulating all glandular functioning in the maintenance of organic balance. In response to all this comes the divine sustenance from above, this divine medicine that cools our souls, lends us heart and courage, removing woes and disturbing spirits, sustaining our forces so we may proceed on our earthly journey, and handing us inspirations for the answers to our difficulties.

Prayer is one of the greatest therapeutic instruments. It is a great resource that medicine itself is coming to acknowledge. Many people are healed by faith, activating these animistic and spiritual energies. The habit of prayer should be natural for all human beings. Just as we need bodily hygiene and daily nourishment, we need this spiritual hygiene and divine nourishment.

André Luiz states in *Mecanismos da Mediunidade* (Mechanisms of Mediumship):

> In the circuit of forces that is established with prayer, the soul not only predisposes to regenerate the balance of corrupted or exhausted physical cells through the influx of the restoring energies it incorporates, spontaneously, assimilating the rays of the Highest Life which it addresses, but also reflects the illuminating suggestions of the disincarnated intelligences of a nobler condition with which it establishes contact.
>
> Prayer constitutes the basic formula of inner renewal, through which divine understanding flows down from the Heart of Life into the life of the heart. (Xavier 1984, p.179)

Laying-on of hands, along with prayer, constitutes an invaluable resource in the search for healing and in facilitating a renovation of mental attitude, a key factor to reach definitive healing. Along with the receiving of vital forces, it's necessary that we rid our minds of negative thoughts that ultimately reflect in our organic field.

The disorganization resulting from our unbalanced mental patterns is marked on the subtle field of individuality, which is reflected on matter. All mental creations provoke alterations in our energetic field, with consequences for the balance of our cellular structure. Even if all physical symptoms are to be relieved, if the subtle patterns aren't restored they will continue to promote instability and imbalance, which manifests in the body, until we come to a necessary understanding in the search for a profound cure.

In André Luiz's book, *Missionários da Luz* (Missionaries of Light), instructor Alexandre states:

> Just like the physical body may ingest poisonous foods, that intoxicate its tissues, the perispiritual organism may absorb elements of degradation that corrode its force centers, with reflecting effects on the material cells. If the mind of the incarnated creature has not yet reached a discipline of emotions, if it fosters passions that are in disharmony with reality, it may, at any moment, become intoxicated with the mental emissions of those with whom it lives and that may find themselves in the same state of imbalance. Sometimes, such absorptions constitute simple phenomena of no great importance; however, in many cases, they are liable to bring on dangerous organic disasters. This mainly happens when those concerned have no habits of prayer, the benefic influence of which may avert countless ills. (Xavier 1995, p.325)

While it's true that our mental maladjustments are made more evident in the interference with physical harmony by the intensity with which they appear—the opposite is also true. Thoughts of optimism, fraternal and altruistic feelings, active faith, healthy joy, inner peace, and serenity are all elements that generate balance and health.

The will is the great agent that activates our positive animistic potential. It is the lever of thought, through which we drive our psychic forces to reach the desired objectives. It is a powerful resource, and should be cultivated and strengthened within for the moving of our mental field, for the disciplining of our emotions, and the overcoming of mental crystallizations that may affect our individuality. In all the events of this kind, one cannot do without the support of those directly interested in a cure, who are also seeking their own moral transformation.

In closing, I'd like to quote Calderaro: "It's indispensable to penetrate the soul, examine the core of the personality, improve the effects by helping the causes; therefore, we shall not restore sick bodies without the resources of the Divine Medical Doctor of Souls, who is Jesus Christ" (Xavier 1982, p.119).

Chapter 8

PSYCHOTHERAPY AND REINCARNATION
A Necessary and Fruitful Encounter

Julio Peres, PsyD, PhD

Introduction

Modern theories of human personality and the psychotherapies derived from them are based on people's life histories and their relationship with the environment. However, there is increasing recognition of the need to take into account the cultural environments of patients undergoing health care intervention (Bergner 2005). Methods used in recognized psychotherapeutic approaches such as Watson's behaviorism, Freud's psychoanalysis, or Beck's cognitive-behavioral therapy take no account of the belief in life after death held by most of the world's population.[1] These beliefs and values reflect basic assumptions about man's nature, and cognitive reference points used to cope with psychological difficulties. The growing experience of psychotherapy worldwide raises the question of the universality of the Western model's basic assumptions, and suggests that they arose in a specific cultural context over a certain period of time (Karasu 1999; Varma 1988). These reference points were and are transmitted in the academic world, which Thomas Kuhn (1962) described as an important propagator and upholder of paradigms in society. Fundamental milestones in the history of science were reached when researchers studied or revised phenomena not taken into account by the established paradigms of their times. Galileo and Darwin, for instance, collected substantial empirical evidence ignored by most scientists at the time. Their discoveries refuted long "established" concepts relating to astronomy and biology (Moreira-Almeida and Koenig 2007).

The concept of reincarnation, of the spirit returning to material form, is found throughout human history in different periods and cultures. The Western philosophical tradition posed the idea of survival of the soul after physical death, and its continuing journey evolving through reincarnation. This idea goes back to the ancient Greek Orphics, who influenced Pythagoras and Plato. In the culture of oriental peoples, the concept of reincarnation is also found in religions and philosophies such as Buddhism (from 525 BC) and Hinduism (from 1500 BC). The subject has given rise to much wild speculation, which may have kept scientific researchers away. However, it is now three decades since the reincarnation hypothesis moved from the religious and philosophical sphere to the field of scientific research.

Some disorders and maladaptive behaviors observed in medicine and psychology are difficult to explain through genetics and/or environmental influences alone. There may be specific phobias or symptoms of post-traumatic stress disorder not explained by events experienced in the present life. Beyond these symptoms, the reincarnation hypothesis may also help us understand phenomena such as unusual types of play or expressions of temperament in childhood, rare birthmarks related to supposed memories of death in a previous life, events in recurring nightmares, or traumatic memories from supposed previous lives related to maladaptive behaviors (Stevenson 2000a). Spontaneous memories (not induced or reinforced by family) from previous lives are sometimes reported by children in different cultures and countries. Investigation of these alleged memories, using rigorous methods, suggest that there may be an empirical basis for the reincarnation hypothesis (Stevenson 1983a). If this trend is confirmed, how would the paradigms of contemporary psychology be revised? How would this phenomenon be manifested in the human psyche and behavior? Could innate abilities, talents not learned in the present context, specific disorders, or unjustified fears be derived from unconscious reincarnation memories? Could environmental influences include other lives? This chapter will present and discuss the current data that poses these underlying questions that still await answers from contemporary psychology.

Research on Reincarnation

Several researchers argue that the hypothesis of reincarnation offers a possible explanation for unusual behaviors not produced by or imitated in the family context (Haraldsson 1991; Keil and Tucker 2000, 2005; Pasricha *et al.* 2005; Stevenson 1974a, 1987, 1993, 1997a, 2000b; Tucker 2005). For instance, a Sri Lankan boy called Sujith Jayaratne reported details of his supposed previous life as Sammy, a railway worker and liquor seller in the village of Gorakana. Prior to Sujith's birth, Sammy had quarreled violently with his wife Maggie, gotten drunk, gone for a walk, and been run over and killed by a truck. Sujith's mother paid no heed to the details of the story and had never been to Gorakana, but Stevenson (1977a) confirmed the truth of these and over 20 other statements. When the boy was taken to the village, he recognized several persons, places, and objects from Sammy's life, and showed strikingly similar psychological characteristics, including violent and aggressive behavior, and an unusually precocious interest in cigarettes and alcohol, which were characteristic of Sammy.

Children's spontaneous memories of their supposed previous lives have been studied, challenged, and in many cases confirmed for individuals from different cultures such as India (Stevenson 1975), Sri Lanka (Stevenson 1977a), Asia (Stevenson 1977b), Lebanon, Turkey (Stevenson 1980), Thailand, Burma (Stevenson 1983a), the US (Stevenson 1983a; Tucker 2005), Africa (Stevenson 1986), Brazil (Andrade 1990), Europe (Stevenson 2003), and Holland (Rivas 2003). Scientific approaches to the nature of memories of supposed previous lives pose certain questions. Are these memories brought on only in cultures that believe in reincarnation? Or is reincarnation a universal phenomenon, i.e. one that is manifested in different peoples despite cultural variations? The universal nature of the manifestation of this phenomenon strengthens the evidence for reincarnation. Thomas Kuhn (1962) noted that studies conducted from the viewpoint of certain theoretical reference points might neglect phenomena that would be observable using other more comprehensive paradigms. The body of evidence for reincarnation raises questions in relation to the mainstream paradigm of psychology, which fails to weigh influences of previous lives on present-life personality and psyche.

In addition to studies of children's spontaneous memories from their previous lives (Haraldsson 1991; Haraldsson and Stevenson 1975; Keil and Tucker 2005; Stevenson 1974a, 1987, 2000b; Tucker 2005), several other lines of research have found evidence suggesting life after death, including spontaneous memories of previous lives with corresponding birth marks (Keil and Tucker 2000; Pasricha et al. 2005; Stevenson 1993, 1997a, 1997b, 2000a), xenoglossia (knowing a language not learned in the present life) (Stevenson 1974b, 1984), therapeutic cases of regression to past lives with verifiable details (Wambach 1978), near-death experiences and out-of-body experiences with verifiable details (Athappilly, Greyson and Stevenson 2006; Greyson 2000, 2007; Morse and Neppe 1991; Stevenson and Greyson 1979; van Lommel et al. 2001), and messages received via mediums in the form of psychographic writing, with particular details not known to the spiritual medium writing the messages (Severino 1994).

Positive and False-Positive Cases

Stevenson and his team from the University of Virginia studied over 2500 cases of children aged four to ten who claimed to remember a previous life, and verbalized details such as proper names, relatives' names, names of cities, type of death in the previous life, and events leading up to that death (Stevenson 1974a, 1975, 1977a, 1980, 1983a, 1983b, 1987, 2000b). Not all memories from supposed previous lives can be checked, and a fair number have not been confirmed as true.

Reincarnation is not the only explanation for these memories, which these children seem to perceive as genuine memories, but is nevertheless a hypothesis to be taken seriously. Independent researchers—using the same method of investigation—have collected statements made by these children and observed by many witnesses. On challenging the information collected, they have verified them in many cases. Thus, independent investigators have obtained similar results (Andrade 1990; Haraldsson 1991; Haraldsson and Stevenson 1975; Keil and Tucker 2005; Mills, Haraldsson and Keil 1994; Tucker 2005). The children studied frequently (75–80%) remembered how they had died in their previous lives and provided details of their death. They often accurately described the areas where they had previously lived even though they were currently geographically distant and they had never been there in this life. The studies also reported a large number of unsolved cases (Stevenson 1983b). Haraldsson, Fowler and Periyannanpillai (2000) estimated that only one-third of the cases of children in Sri Lanka who claim to remember a past life provide evidence for reincarnation. Memories seemed to emerge spontaneously. In some cases, children who strongly identified with their previous lives insisted on being called by their previous name against the will of their present family. Stevenson noted that these spontaneous memories tended to diminish or disappear after some years, with the onset of adolescence (Stevenson 1977c, 2000a). Other cases studied revealed not only spontaneous assertive memories of past lives, but also unusual birthmarks corresponding to fatal wounds on the individual that had been identified as a potential previous personality (Keil and Tucker 2000; Pasricha *et al.* 2005; Stevenson 1993, 1997a, 1997b, 2000a). Stevenson (1997a, 1997b) showed that in some countries up to 35 percent of children claiming recall of previous lives had birthmarks and/or defects that they attributed to a traumatic death in a past life. In other countries, the percentage was much lower. The birth defects were usually of rare types, and, in 43 out of 49 cases in which medical records (usually postmortem reports) were obtained, the match between wounds and birthmarks or defects was confirmed. The research also showed a number of psychological characteristics—interests, personality traits, prejudices, specific phobias and cravings, behaviors quite unlike those of the present family but consistent with the supposed previous life—that were difficult to explain without the idea of reincarnation (Cadoret 2005).

The Riddle of Personality

Contemporary theories assume that personality is conditioned by a combination of unique genetic heritage and environmental influences in the course of one's life history. But genetic singularity and its interface with environment do not provide a full account of human individuality; if this were the case, two people with the same genome and the same life experiences would have identical personalities.

Dicephalic twins (two heads on the same body) and conjoined twins (two heads and two bodies) with identical life experiences and genetic constitutions would be expected to have the same personality traits, or at the very least similar ones. However, the American twins Abigail and Brittany Hensel, and the Iranian twins Laleh and Ladan Bijani, among others, have had very different personalities (tastes, temperaments, opinions, desires) since childhood (Thompson 2003; Wallis 1996). In addition to genetic and environmental factors, there must be more factors involved in the makeup of one's personality.

Having electrically stimulated the live brain to map cortical functions, Penfield (1978) postulated that neural networks alone would be incapable of producing consciousness, and stated that the mind had a distinct existence from the brain, although closely related to it. He added that there was no place in the cerebral cortex where electric stimulation would make a patient make a decision. Neurofunctional findings on psychotherapy, hypnosis, and the placebo effect, taken as a whole, challenge the hypothesis that the mind is a by-product of the brain (Beauregard 2007). Studies of cardiac-arrest survivors found that 11 to 20 percent of patients reported experiences that support the hypothesis that the mind can express itself independently of neural functioning (Parnia 2007). In line with these findings, some theories associate the brain with the role of mediating concepts such as spirit, which supposedly involves a repertoire of past experiences associated with personality.

Kelly and colleagues (2007) suggest that psychology needs to broaden its scientific horizons if it is to truly contribute to our understanding of the mind and its relationship with the body. Their *Irreducible Mind* discusses the implications of a wide range of important but neglected psychological phenomena, including psycho-physiological influences (psychosomosis, placebo, dissociative disorders, neurophysiologic changes induced by hypnosis, mental influence at a distance), memory, mental automatisms (identity, automatic writing/psychography, trance states, dissociative mediumship), near-death phenomena and similar experiences (near-death experience, out-of-body experience, death-bed apparitions, and lucid visions), genius (creative inspiration), and mystic experiences. After a detailed review, rather than an analysis limited to contemporary data from cognitive neuroscience, Kelly suggests that the main current theories of the mind–body complex are seriously flawed in light of the available evidence, and are unable to explain a wide range of human experiences. Following William James and Frederic Myers, the authors postulate that the brain may work as a filter for manifestations of the mind in our everyday life, instead of producing the mind. In other words, the brain may function as an organ that somehow confines, regulates, restricts, limits, enables, or allows expression of the mind.

Watersheds

Psychologists should not be dogmatic in taking an a priori monist or dualist approach based on as-yet embryonic neurofunctional research. For instance, the hasty theory of "the God spot," which postulated a point in the brain as responsible for experience of divinity, has been dismissed by recent neuroimaging studies (Azari *et al.* 2001; Beauregard and Paquette 2006; Newberg *et al.* 2003). Elucidating the neural circuits involved in subjective experiences such as prayer, contact with God, or mystic experience does not diminish or depreciate their significance or value. Crucially, contemporary psychology should also review the universality of its bases and theories so that it may understand and work with manifestations that are natural for human beings, and thus promote psychotherapy more efficaciously. Varma (1988) showed that contemporary psychotherapy's underlying premises, which do not consider reincarnation, fail to respond to the needs of most people in India and are not functional for them, since they believe in reincarnation.

Psychotherapists should contemplate the belief systems of the significant numbers of reincarnationists around the world. The World Values Survey found belief in reincarnation professed by 22.6 percent of the population in the Nordic countries, 20.2 percent in Eastern Europe, and 27 percent in Western Europe (Inglehart, Basanez and Morendo 1998; Inglehart *et al.* 2004); the numbers were 27 percent in the USA (Gallup 2003), and 37 percent in Brazil (Data Folha 2007). Psychotherapy must therefore take note of this significant group of people, regardless of the reasons that lead them to believe in reincarnation, such as vestiges of beliefs from the pre-Christian era, influences of Western and Asian scriptures/philosophies, finding a plausible explanation for issues not explained in other ways, experiences and personal memories of previous lives, or creating a cognitive framework for coping with the grief of the loss of loved ones. Like everybody else, reincarnationists want psychological treatment that takes their belief systems into account. Accepting patients' psychological realities and therapeutically working with their own reference points are predictors of satisfactory therapeutic results (Brune *et al.* 2002; Peres *et al.* 2007a). However, in opposition to the beliefs of most of the world's population, the dominant assumption made by science and psychology, as conveyed in the academic world, is that death marks the end of personal existence (Haraldsson 2006).

Growing experience in the psychological ambit points to the importance of non-dogmatic therapeutic approaches that take into account and appreciate the sociocultural realities of both large and small communities (Sayed 2003; Varma 1988). Many people think that their current difficulties may be related to traumatic occurrences in previous lives. Belief in reincarnation was associated with more severe traumatic experiences in some individuals with post-traumatic stress disorder (PTSD), including sexual abuse, rape, and loss of a family member through violent death (Davidson, Connor and Lee 2005). Studies of children who spontaneously recall past lives have shown that as a group they present the symptoms of PTSD, which may be best explained by the fact that 80 percent of them have alleged memories of violent deaths such as accidents, wars, or killings (Haraldsson 2003; Stevenson and Samararatne 1988).

Psychotherapy Considering Reincarnation

Even when the reincarnation hypothesis is not susceptible to scientific investigation, therapists must respect these subjective beliefs held by patients. Neurosciences have studied perception, which may be understood as the ability to associate sensory information with memory and cognition in order to build concepts about the world and ourselves, and guide our behavior. Perception and memory processes are directly related to the generation of adaptive behavior (Peres *et al.* 2007b). We do not perceive the world exactly as it is, but as we compute it is most likely to be, and these findings suggest that the richness of individual experience is hugely subjective (Ramachandran and Gregory 1991; Yarrow, Haggard and Heal 2001). Therefore the process of perception directing adaptive and maladaptive behaviors involves construction and inference. The implications of these studies are critical for psychology, since subjective assumptions about the world are among the pillars on which behaviors are erected (Creamer, McFarlane and Burgess 2005).

Emotional content configured as memory is a genuine representation of the individual's reference points. Psychological dynamics—or internal dialogues— will affect the way individuals relate to their difficulties (Peres, Mercante and Nasello 2005). For instance, belief in reincarnation considers a continuous cycle of learning and evolution through successive lives. From this point of view, difficulties are transitory and may be overcome when their lessons have been absorbed (Lee 2000). On the other hand, belief in the finite nature of life may amplify the dimension of present difficulty. We must remember that human psychological development is highly refined and self-correcting (Masten and Coatsworth 1998; Prochaska, DiClemente and Norcross 1992), and clients rather than therapists are the real healers (Bohart 2000). Therefore psychotherapy should turn towards clients and their respective belief systems, with the aim of boosting their ability to cope with problems. The type of service therapists provide comprises human self-healing processes that occur naturally, perhaps in a more refined and systematic way (Bergner 2005; Karasu 1986; Peres *et al.* 2007a; Sayed 2003).

Examples of Clinical Cases

The following two patient reports show how a therapist's respect for patients' beliefs in reincarnation may be helpful:

- *M.A. engineer, 38 years old*: I have three children but I was unable to relate well with one of them. I was unable to express affection, and I avoided contact with this child and was stricter with him. As a reincarnationist, I knew that we are a parent or a child in this life for a reason, and as a parent and adult, I had to change my behavior towards my son of six years of age. I sought psychotherapy to help me overcome this difficulty. After two unsuccessful attempts, with a third psychologist I felt comfortable talking about it, since my belief in reincarnation was accepted. As I responded to the psychologist's questions, lessons and details in relation to challenges I had to overcome became clearer. I exercised my insights and gradually managed to build a good relationship with my son. Professional help was very important for me to achieve what I could not do myself: Be in a good relationship with my beloved son!

- *P.L., musician, 23 years old*: Until the age of 22, I had a recurring nightmare: I would see a huge fierce wolf, drooling and sharp toothed, ready to attack me, but I awoke before he could bite me. I felt that this dream was related to a previous life, but I did not understand it. I sought psychotherapy to deal with another issue: a continuous state of arousal, anxiety, and feeling of helplessness that I could not explain. During psychotherapy I understood better what I was feeling on giving a detailed description of my symptoms to the therapist and in one of the sessions I talked about the nightmare and all that. It was like having a huge weight lifted off my shoulders... The psychologist asked me to go on talking about the nightmare, and then I saw myself as a child sleeping in a wooden shack in the snow. I awoke feeling cold and saw that huge wolf lunging at me through the open door. It was a traumatic death, I experienced terrible affliction through dying alone! I understood that the anxiety and helplessness belonged to the past and that now I am living in a different context, I am an adult, loved and supported by my family. I stopped having the nightmare, I managed to disconnect from trauma and live in the present, at peace.

Conclusion

William James talked of one single "white crow" that disproved the statement "all crows are black." We note that different lines of research and studies involving reincarnation suggest considerable evidence in favor of the reincarnation phenomenon. If the hypothesis of reincarnation is true, then current paradigms of human personality that do not take into account the influence of past lives over the present one will need to be revisited and rewritten. Therefore, the interest and pertinence of scientific investigations relating to reincarnation is justified, given the importance of their impact on people's quality of life through the answers obtained by science. As in any culture, when necessary, people may seek psychological treatments that take note of their belief systems. We postulate that psychotherapy must consider the client as potential self-healer. It would at least be salutary if psychotherapists asked clients themselves, in the therapeutic setting, about the roots/origins of their complaints and were open to working with the contents that naturally emerge, including supposed past lives. Professionals should be comfortable with clients raising existential and spiritual issues (Peres *et al.* 2007a; Shaw, Joseph and Linley 2005). There is a therapeutic need and an ethical duty to respect these opinions, and show empathy and respect for the reality a client poses, even though the therapist may not share the same beliefs (Shafranske 1996). Large numbers of people worldwide have been omitted from the contemporary psychotherapies accepted and taught in the academic world. Just as anybody may seek psychological treatment aligned with their values, reincarnation should be taken into account by psychologists, who should seek coherent and effective approaches to work with such content, particularly in cultures and countries where there is a widespread belief and acceptance of reincarnation (Peres *et al.* 2007c). Perhaps one of the greatest challenges for psychotherapy and health care in general is changing the paradigm of our view of man as a bio-psycho-social being that ignores the spiritual perspective and reincarnation. Research on the complex of factors involved in shaping personality must continue.

Note

1.   World Values Survey: www.worldvaluessurvey.org.

Chapter 9

THE GROUP FIELD

Emma Bragdon, PhD

At the Casa de Dom Inácio, a Spiritist healing center in Brazil, people coming
for healing are encouraged to sit in the "Current" (*Corrente*) room after meeting
John of God for a consultation (Bragdon 2006). Some would debate that these
rooms are not typical of Spiritist Centers—and they would be right, the rooms
for quiet meditation and prayer are unusual. There are 100–300 people sitting in
these large meditation rooms, all on chairs, eyes closed, feet and arms uncrossed
to better receive energy for their own healing and spiritual evolution—for one,
two, three, sometimes more than four hours at a time.

Why?

"Corrente" is a Portuguese word that is often translated into English as "current"
or "tide" but also literally means "metal chain." Thus, each person in the Current
room is becoming a link in a chain of consciousness. Linked together as people,
and linked with our sources of spiritual guidance, we create a powerful force
that is dedicated to healing all who sit, and all who walk through the Current
room on their way to see John of God in consultation. This chain also provides a
consistent energy to the healer, in this case the medium, John, as he works with
one person after the next, for hours at a time without a break. While being a link
to strengthen the energy, each of us is also receiving from the larger chain.

When you walk through the Current room you can feel the strength of
the group's energy field, and it often moves people to tears—as it is such a
concentration of the power of positive intention and prayer.

The group field not only has more energy than a single person, but can be
used to make energy manifest in more physical form. Think about the power
of ceremony. When a marriage or a baptism is sanctified by a group gathered
together in the name of God, it seals the positive intentions of the group and
those that are the center of focus—marriage partners, godparents, the child in
relationship to Christ, etc. Even in business and government, we gather people
together before signing important contracts or legislation. These agreements have
strength—we even call them "binding."

Cultures all across the globe have used a group field to both seal promises and
enhance healing. Indigenous Amer-Indians gather together for the Purification

Ceremony and Sun Dance Ceremony to empower the people and the elders endowed with leadership. In China acupuncture clinics are set up with banks of beds, one after the other, in one room, and the acupuncturist moves from one patient to the next, taking out needles here, inserting needles there. Each patient is humbly aware that he or she is one of many trying to find balance. In Slovenia today, Master BioEnergy Therapist Zdenko Domancic (Hochstätter and Coté 2005) sees 80 people in the morning and 80 in the afternoon. Patients waiting their turn sit in chairs in a circle witnessing the patient being treated in the center of the circle. The healing power of the healer and the healings performed continue to uplift those waiting, just as their positive intentions feed into those directly receiving the healing.

With so much energy available to speed healing within the group field, it is curious to consider how we in the USA and Europe feel entitled to—and expect— privacy when we interact with our health professionals. Our doctors divide their clinics into small rooms. We wait in such cubicles alone, often anxious, insistent on their undivided attention—if just for a few minutes. We have come to believe that the more undivided attention we get, the better it will be for our journey to health.

Are we missing something?

It is estimated that 70–80 percent of all illness stems from stress (Benson 1996). A symptom of stress is the feeling of not belonging in the web of life— being isolated and alone. One of the most effective therapies for prolonging longevity after a diagnosis of heart disease or cancer is participating in a support group.

When do we experience a positive group field dedicated to healing in the USA and Europe? If we don't attend prayer circles in church, then we might go to a large gathering when a noted spiritual teacher visits our city, such as Ammaji, the hugging saint, or John of God when he visits the Omega Institute in New York. However, these kinds of positive group fields are rare for us.

Recently, I watched the documentary film *Soul Masters: Dr. Guo and Dr. Sha* (Zeig 2008). It colorfully illustrates engaging group experiences in a hospital run by Dr. Guo in China. One sees lots of smiles and camaraderie in the common spaces used for the morning exercise program, evening dance program, sharing meals together, and massage rooms with several people being worked on at the same time. Dr. Guo and his loving family (his wife and five daughters) all live on a wing of the hospital. "So," says Daughter #5, "the hospital is more like a big family get-together than a place for 100 sick people." That could be one reason so many have been cured of advanced stages of cancer there.

At the Casa de Dom Inácio in Brazil some people experience spontaneous remission of cancer and other serious illnesses. It is believed that 95 percent of visitors have very strong spiritual experiences. We believe it is the love in the community (group field) that is one of the strongest forces at work in the healing. The sense of brotherhood and fellowship is vast, and yet touches people very personally. Yes, over a bowl of soup we can share where we are from: Brazil, USA, Malta, Greece, Germany, France, Russia, Sweden, Canada, etc. But, when it comes down to our true origins, we are links in one chain, working together to help each other, and that is both comforting and a source of immense strength and healing.

Chapter 10

SPIRITUAL COUNSELING AND FELLOWSHIP IN SPIRITIST CENTERS

Carlos Appel, MD, and Tania Appel, MA

Spiritist Healing Centers

There are approximately 13,000 Spiritist Houses, or Centers, called "Casas Éspiritas," in Brazil. Some are formal members of the Brazilian Spiritist Federation (FEB) and others are independent and do not follow all the regulations imposed on member organizations by the FEB. The FEB's largest center in São Paulo attends to 7000 people per day. Each person has the opportunity to receive laying-on of hands; attend classes, discussion groups, lectures, and artistic or cultural presentations; join others in charitable projects; train to become a medium and/or healer; or receive food for themselves and their families.

The role of the Spiritist Center transcends the simple goal of giving material assistance and is more than a mission of creating a solid community, although it includes both. It is truly a school where each Being (body, mind, and soul) can learn his reason for existence and for his suffering along this earthly journey, as well as take strides towards his own spiritual evolution. The notions are reinforced through Casa activities that the spirit is immortal and survives the grave, and that each spirit receives the grace of many opportunities for spiritual evolution through lifetimes in and out of the body.

Study

In order to receive the full benefit a Spiritist Center offers, each participant must commit him- or herself to study, discuss, and learn that Spiritism holds core beliefs such as reincarnation, and the possibility of communication with the dead (or disincarnated spirits). Mediums-in-training need to study for five years or more, observed and supervised by disincarnate mentors as well as incarnate teachers.

Some tasks at the Casa are carried out on the physical plane by incarnated individuals teaching classes and lectures through the inspiration of spiritual mentors, and other tasks, on the spiritual plane, are accomplished by the attending spirits with the collaboration of the incarnated. This is particularly true when mediums channel mentors to give counsel regarding the development of each center or how to help a particular person.

Reforma Intima/Personal Transformation

When a Spiritist Casa welcomes new people it receives them wholeheartedly and orients them with brotherly counsel so they may learn to acquire the knowledge essential for their recovery. Participants will also become aware that their full recovery, that is, becoming whole and balanced, depends entirely on their inner transformation ("reforma intima" in Portuguese). It is up to each person to make choices to enhance this inner transformation, to increasingly become more wise and compassionate.

Each Spiritist Casa offers a practical path to understand the truth written in the parables presented in the Gospels of the New Testament, teaching the Being to overcome his temporary limitations inherent in a bodily existence, enabling him to see himself as an immortal spirit journeying through time, inheriting his own past actions and shaping his future. One learns that one's actions need to be aimed at overcoming moral imperfections, like pride and selfishness.

The prophylaxis of the disease starts with an improvement in mental behavior (thoughts and attitudes become more positive) and will manifest in moral actions such as acts of kindness and compassion. Some primitive, deleterious energies must be fought by all those in need of help as well as those working at a Spiritist House. Energies such as pride, avarice, jealousy, vanity, envy, slander, hate, revenge, lust, anger, intolerance, hypocrisy, bitterness, sadness, fanaticism, illicit passions, pernicious vices, and lack of discipline or ill-meaning thoughts trigger vibrations in the perispirit which may seed diseases, which then manifest in the physical body.

Physical suffering is a call for awakening the need for inner moral reform. A significant example is evident in the life of a noble warrior wounded at the Battle of Pamplona, Spain, in the sixteenth century. After suffering a long, difficult convalescence in which he studied the life of saints, he underwent an intense process of inner transformation, from which he emerged as the great Ignatius of Loyola, founder of the Company of Jesus (Jesuits), active to this day all around the world.

Fellowship

It is now well recognized that support groups in which patients share deeply together with others in social and religious activities help increase longevity in patients with heart disease and cancer (Spiegel *et al.* 1989). James L. Spira, PhD, who chairs the Department of Health Psychology at the Naval Medical Center in San Diego, California, notes:

> Twenty years of research documents that psychosocial interventions impact a wide range of quality-of-life variables, including ability to sleep, fatigue reduction, improved mood, increased vitality, pain reduction and more general functional capacities like one's ability to exercise. (Spira and Reed 2002)

The fellowship one experiences among other participants at a Spiritist Casa offers empathic support in many ways: a listening ear, encouragement to successfully face personal issues, compassionate understanding for our challenges, a shoulder to lean on in tough times, and a group facilitator in discussion groups to help us focus on the important questions of life: Am I essentially a material body or a spirit exploring physical existence? Where am I going? What will happen to me at death? What is my mission in life?

Having the opportunity to speak to those who are well read or well versed in the Spiritist literature on the nature of karma, reincarnation, and spiritual evolution can be of immense value to those less aware of these universal laws and how they work. This form of fellowship acts as a gentle but pervasive support for consistent positivity in one's own life choices.

Those who have been raised in other religious traditions that do not believe in reincarnation, paranormal abilities such as mediumship, and spiritual evolution over lifetimes are relieved to find people, like themselves, with whom they can discuss and deeply explore these ideas. This is especially comforting when one personally faces end of life issues, or the death of one's child. Some qualified mediums at particular Spiritist Casas will hold group meetings in which they communicate messages from those who have passed on (died) and thus comfort the family members who are grieving. Simply acknowledging that the spirit is alive, and will greet other family members when they pass on, is also of great comfort.

In the classes and meetings, we also have the opportunity to practice being compassionate and wise—thus supporting our own inner transformation. For this reason, the word "Fraternidade" ("fellowship" in English) is often displayed on a wall of a Spiritist Casa. It is a reminder to all that we are not only exchanging concepts with each other, but we continually receive energy radiated from others just as we give them some of our energy. We are responsible for the quality of the energy we emit towards others; that's why we must watch what we feel and think about them.

Our own immunological system is affected by thoughts, feelings, and emotions (Spiegel *et al.* 1989). Certain attitudes (e.g. loving compassion) displayed by other participants may strengthen our state of mind, our faith, and even our immune system positively, and other attitudes (e.g. jealousy, envy, lust, prejudice, selfishness, hate) may influence us in a negative way—where we become more defensive, less hopeful, and our faith in God is challenged.

The Shadow in Fellowship

However pure our initial intent, fellowship at Spiritist Centers is not immune to the negative influences that beset people. In other words, the shadow exists in Spiritist Centers, just as it does in all other places. Participants drawn by the ideal of pure fellowship and unconditional love will find their human reactive emotions also arising as a stress response or "bad habit." These may include jealousies, the seduction of power, the fall into unnecessary competition, and the illusions of the ego.

These responses to emotional triggers can disturb all our relationships and must be dealt with and deliberately changed. The ideal is to become aware of the issue, and work on it to dissolve it—with help as needed. Only those who are able to reflect on the triggers, and work on them, will be able to put themselves on a path to spiritual evolution and an improvement in social interactions. When people have the perspective that this life emerges out of past lives and leads to a next life, they have more motivation to defuse their emotional triggers.

The principles of Spiritism, first collated and published by Allan Kardec in the 1860s (1986, 1996, 2004), consistently encourage us to embrace loving compassion and the wisdom available through evolved beings, such as Jesus Christ. Ways of going about this transformation are referred to repeatedly in classroom discussion and in the supervision of mediums and healers.

Discipline, Discipline, Discipline

In Spiritist Centers that are formal members of the FEB there are clear rules that must be followed. There tends to be more discipline and fewer interpersonal problems—less issues stemming from ego, and more of the feeling of a team of people working together in these centers. People put their own lives on hold in order to do the work, and they try to keep it simple.

Being a medium is simply this: Being here to serve.

- As you go deeply into the work, you realize you are a worker on the team engaging the consciousness of Christ, that is, you work together and focus on others in the name of what is the highest spiritual power for you… You need to accept the rules, be humble, and be prepared to be of service in any capacity.

- You work together in the same direction…you are in the same boat…to be of one mind… You share the attitude: we made the agreement before we were born that we would build a better world…to help people get the idea that through love we can make changes for the good. We have to solve problems we have brought from other lives…it's the way we get a better next life… Once people understand this…it changes everything…their relationship to themselves and others in home, work, and community.

- You are being of service through love. The physical body is your instrument… but most important is the connection you have with the Source.

- In a small community, when we work together, we can create a kind of energy that can change situations. Work flows when we pray together and for each other. We can minimize the negative and create something more positive. Concentration on the same thoughts also brings us closer… We feel we are the same, and each of us has the same importance. We accept the differences we have and who we are… Because of the love, we can also accept the frailties of others. If we refuse to continue to be at a center because we are disturbed by others, then we are not practicing fellowship. If we think just about ourselves, the chain of fellowship and fraternity will be broken.

Generally, if people don't like the Federation rules, they simply leave the center that abides by FEB rules. In those centers that are more independent and less disciplined there are less rigid rules and less discipline and relationship difficulties can emerge more easily. When each person does what they feel is right, as they tend to do in the independent centers, there can be more interpersonal problems.

Spiritual Healing Techniques

The Spiritist treatment of illnesses is complementary care. Spiritist Centers encourage people to attend to their medical issues through medically trained health providers. However, when illnesses arise from internal imbalances and stress, the Spiritist Centers make use of the following techniques for healing. All of these stimulate fellowship:

- "corrente" (current)
- spiritual counseling
- orientation
- study of the Gospel according to Spiritism
- prayer
- laying-on of hands

- "magnetized" water

- disobsession.

All of these protocols involve increasing compassionate connection to ourselves, and to others, including benevolent spirits who want to interact with us.

"Corrente"

The Portuguese word "corrente" is defined as both "current" and "chain." When the current of energy one experiences in fellowship to others is both loving and strong, one feels deeply connected as if everyone is a link in a strong steel chain which is not easily broken. In the best of times one feels this current so strongly that the notion of Oneness with all Beings is the only way to describe it.

At the Casa de Dom Inãcio (considered a very unusual Spiritist Center), where John of God works, there are three Current rooms, guided by prayer, to encourage each participant to move into higher states of consciousness, increasing his or her capacity for love and wisdom. Participants may be in "the current" for 3–9 hours a day, sitting quietly in the silence, eyes closed, in prayer and meditation—sitting until every person coming for healing has consulted John of God (Chapters 9 and 23 describe this in more detail). Less experienced people who participate find that their emotional and spiritual state is uplifted, their abilities to concentrate are enhanced, and they leave inspired and relieved. More experienced mediums and healers, connected to the disincarnate spiritual mentors of the Casa, anchor the Current rooms, infusing them with higher vibrations of spiritual peace, easing the way for the less experienced ones to reach higher states of consciousness. This is the manifestation of one of the ideals of fellowship within Spiritist Casas.

Spiritual Counseling

In a typical Spiritist Casa, an interviewer, who is a Spiritist "social worker" and likely a para-professional trained for the task at the Spiritist House, meets a newly arrived individual and initiates a form of spiritual counseling. The interviewer's job is to first make an evaluation based on asking questions of the interviewee, such as "How is your health? What health problems do you have? Do you get adequate sleep? Do you have adequate food and a clean place to live? When did you last see a doctor for a check-up? What are you seeking at this center?" Answers are briefly noted on a card to be kept on file at the center but may be coded by a number so as to protect the anonymity of the participant.

The person seeking help is subsequently advised by the interviewer to continue with his or her current medical treatment and other therapies of his or her choice while participating at the center.

Records at the center are never given to the public, or given to doctors so they could become part of the medical history of the participant. This is very important for people who feel that their engagement with Spiritism may be a reason for family or medical professionals to criticize or ostracize them. Some Catholic and Evangelical Churches in Brazil are highly judgmental of all spiritualist organizations, lumping all of them together as one, as if they are all doing the work of the Devil—without first truly understanding the work of the Spiritists who follow Kardec's principles and embrace a path of "practical Christianity," as opposed to those Spiritualists who practice black magic.

The new participant will subsequently be asked to follow a program of classes and meetings, including receiving laying-on of hands, before returning in 2–4 weeks to again speak to the interviewer. At that following meeting, the participant's needs are again assessed and a new program suggested.

Consistently checking in with a spiritual counselor, the participant establishes a more continuous relationship focused on re-establishing well-being: physical, psychological, and spiritual. This reinforces a good habit of periodically assessing his or her own well-being and pursuing a program to support health and personal growth. In the early stages of entry into Spiritism, or in crisis, the individual has an advocate, a witness, and source of support in the counselor, as needed. The individual must also be accountable, i.e. tell someone that he or she did or did not follow the suggested program, and what the results of these choices were.

As time goes on the participant can be assured of the stability of the ongoing relationship, as well as the positive intention of the counselor whose mission it is to help the individual find strength, will power, ability to make changes in life, and happiness.

Active participation is essential for anyone seeking to restore health and happiness. The subject's healing is a spiritual self-healing. He or she must avoid the repetition of conscious mistakes, for example giving in to an addiction that is self-destructive, the cause of his or her suffering, and the reason he or she has caused others to suffer. All this must also be used as a lesson for spiritual elevation. When this program is followed, it has been claimed that the Spiritist Centers are highly successful, for example 90 percent success in healing addictions (Bragdon 2008).

Healing practitioners and spiritual counselors within Spiritism do not seek any form of monetary reward or payment. This reinforces the Christian love that prevails as the ideal in all the centers' coordinated activities including spiritual counseling, and with the disincarnated benevolent mentors of the Casa, and all the work that happens through charitable giving.

Orientation

Orientation refers to an individual one-on-one meeting, or an orientation in a group where there is a leader. The leader bases his or her comments on *The Gospel According to Spiritism* (Kardec 2004) and the teaching of highly evolved spirits, such as those channeled by Chico Xavier or Divaldo Franco.

The coordinator of the orientation session listens compassionately to those with any kind of need, an offer of fellowship. This facilitator ideally fosters caring attention amongst all participants, developing consciousness of each spirit's eternity, studying the causes of disease or problems brought into focus, and counseling towards a shift in moral attitudes. The participant has the burden of committing to change and following the orientation.

The amount of time each participant spends in orientation depends on the agenda set by each Spiritist Center. Usually these orientation meetings are scheduled at a time of day when most people can attend, such as evenings, after work.

Further Study of *The Gospel According to Spiritism*

A very powerful treatment for the diseases of the soul is the repeated study of *The Gospel According to Spiritism* (Kardec 2004) together with *The Gospel at Home* (Payas and Romaquera 2003). The study of these books in the family or in a group at a center fosters and deepens fellowship. The foundation of the practice of mediumship is this same Gospel. It shows us that inner transformation is the most important goal and the source of a deep, quiet wisdom; the goal is not to manifest unusual phenomena, like incorporation of disincarnates.

Following are some words from Emmanuel, a spirit guide who wrote in the book *Leis de Amor* (Laws of Love) through the automatic writing of Francisco Xavier and Waldo Vieira (1981).

When Emmanuel was asked "Which are the medicines for the spirit?" he replied:

> In Spiritist activities we gather immediate sublime benefits from magnetism, be it in the form of the pass [laying-on of hands] under the influence of prayer, or in the systematic following of the Gospel at Home, in which benefactors and disincarnated friends rebalance our strength through elevated inspiration, calming our thoughts, or taking advantage of the available resources of mediumship in the group in order to provide aid to the afflicted soul or to exhausted energies.
>
> If you have embraced the Spiritist Principles, deepen your knowledge and you will understand that humility and benevolence, service and self-discipline, patience and hope, solidarity and optimism are medicine for the spirit, transforming conflicts into lessons and

hardship into blessings because at the bottom of each illumination and each consoling message flowing through your inspiration you will hear the words of Christ "Love each other as I love you."

Prayer[1]

A felt prayer is the time to speak with God, one's most intimate spiritual guide of any tradition, or with Christ. Prayer needs to be an intimate expansion of the soul in a loving dialogue, shaping the language according to circumstance, and avoiding clichés. There will always be a reply. If it is impossible to give what is asked, loving acceptance and spiritual protection will become available.

Prayer is a time of close connection to the sacred. It is encouraged so that one moves closer and closer to frequent practice of prayer and thus stays in close connection to the most benevolent good spirits.

Laying-On of Hands/Magnetic Passes[2]

Receiving an energy transfer through laying-on of hands stimulates vital centers in both the physical and spiritual bodies. The magnetic pass is performed by one or more spiritual workers (mediums), called *passista* (pass giver) in Brazil. To become a *passista* it is necessary to undergo a period of studies and training to become proficient in the appropriate technique. This powerful healing work increases the bonds of love within the centers.

The person receiving the laying-on of hands has to comply with the need for self-responsibility and inner discipline, such as the need to let go of resistance to change and accept the positive energy now being made available to them, in order to receive the intended benefit.

"Magnetized" Water[3]

Water naturally receives imprints from surrounding vibrations. Positive magnetic and fluidic energies may be transferred to water amplifying its therapeutic qualities. These energies especially arise through prayer from the feeling of love for others.

When one realizes that one's attitude and thoughts, as well as prayers, are being infused into water that will be used for healing purposes, one becomes more finely attuned to the importance of raising one's vibrations through inner transformation so as to increase one's ability to be a positive influence.

Disobsession[4]

Many symptoms of illness, such as negative attitudes, may be the result of influences from others, incarnate or disincarnate. Just as abusive verbal exchanges from parent to child can result in a lack of self-confidence in the child, lower disincarnate spirits may deeply affect anyone with their vibrations, helping form negative attitudes contributing to self-destructive tendencies. These influences may become manifest as *obsession*, *fascination*, or *subjugation*.

According to Dr. Lacerda de Azevedo (1997) in his book *Spirit and Matter*, obsession is the predominant contemporary disease. The number of cases labeled as mental illness or psychic dysfunction which in fact are obsessions is so great that we can safely say that, other than diseases caused by physical disturbances such as cranial trauma, infection, arteriosclerosis, and triggering traumatic issues from one's early life, *all* mental illness may be of a spiritual nature. The vast majority are from disincarnated spirits acting on the incarnated. Divaldo Franco wrote:

> The number of obsessed people on the earth plane is much larger than anyone might think. They are found alone, in groups, or in whole communities… These are critical times both for individuals and mankind as a whole. Spiritism has a giant task…to help science, encouraging it to look for the cause of diseases in the depths of the spiritual being rather than in the effects of its action. (Franco 1974)

The basic objective of the treatment of disobsession is to bring harmony to the obsessor–obsessed interaction by employing specific procedures and techniques, always with the help of God, Jesus Christ, and the good spirits.

The sensitivity to the reality of these relationships, and the conceptual framework which helps one understand the nature of these obsessions, is a source of support in the Casa Community, helping each person strengthen his or her inner sources to prevent or overcome obsession when it arises. Knowing that mediums are present to assist one with such difficulties is a tremendous source of support, increasing the bonding in the community.

Conclusion

Although Spiritist Centers emerged from a simple desire to help those in need, they developed an extraordinary path of fellowship and spiritual evolution. Emotional issues can be triggered and compassionately managed at these centers, so if one is willing to submit to self-discipline and study over a period of time, the goal of wisdom and unconditional love can be achieved.

Notes

1. Prayer is described more fully in Chapter 7.
2. Laying on of hands/magnetic passes are described more fully in Chapter 7.
3. "Magnetized" water is described more fully in Chapter 18.
4. Disobsession is described more fully in Chapter 3.

Chapter 11

JUNG, SPIRITS, AND MADNESS
Lessons for Cultural Psychiatry[1]

Joan Koss-Chioino, PhD

I tell you, one must have chaos in one, to give birth to a dancing star.

F. Nietzsche (1961, p.46)

There is ongoing discussion in psychiatry regarding the meaning and dynamics of phenomena labeled "dissociative states" and "altered states of consciousness," such as visions, trance, and possession by spirits (Hollan 2000). The unresolved problem of the nature and value of these states, in Western and other societies, ultimately turns on the meaning and definition of consciousness. Consciousness for Jung comprised both expressions and experiences under voluntary (ego) control *and* expressions/manifestations of the personal and the collective unconscious, the latter conceived as subterranean structures of the all-encompassing Self (as opposed to the personal self). "I define the unconscious as the totality of all psychic phenomena that lack the quality of consciousness." For Jung the personal unconscious is the "receptacle of all lost memories and of all contents too weak to become conscious…[and] all more or less intentional repressions of painful thoughts and feelings." Over and above this, the collective unconscious is comprised of "unconscious qualities that are not individually acquired but are inherited, e.g., instincts as impulses to carry out actions from necessity, without conscious motivation" (Jung 1960b, p.133).

Jung's special contribution to a discussion of behavior diagnosed as abnormal from a cultural and phenomenological perspective was his assertion—and conviction—that both neuroses and psychoses are potentially constructive, image-driven ways to deal with the intrusion of unconscious material into the ego. However, persons who suffer from psychotic episodes, in contrast to others, cannot maintain continuity of meaning when unconscious material inundates their ego and their everyday reality. "What the artist and the insane have in common is common also to every human being—a restless creative fantasy that is constantly engaged in smoothing away the hard edges of reality" (Jung 1960a, p.177). Jung also claimed that the "breakdown of ideas" characteristic of schizophrenia and the fragmentary and chaotic nature of dreams are analogous phenomena (Jung

1960a, p.258). Like dreams, schizophrenic expressions have meaning (Samuels 1985).

In this chapter I argue that one of Jung's potential contributions to a cultural psychiatry of mental illness is based on the recognition that even those who suffer psychosis share a creative relationship to the unconscious with all persons. Jung was explicit that the unconscious manifested not only in dreams but even more directly in belief in spirits and souls of the dead, as expressed by "primitive" persons, but also common to "highly civilized peoples," albeit "[currently] suppressed along with other metaphysical beliefs" (Jung 1960b, p.301). While we might question some of what Jung wrote about other cultures, since he was often operating within a paradigm set forth by Lévy-Bruhl (1926), who saw "primitives" as having different mental processes, Jung did recognize the similarities between psychological experiences that occupied European persons and the "non-civilized" others he met or observed in his travels. Through both external and intra-psychic explorations he concluded that all peoples shared a basic, human, unconscious world comprised of the archetypes and the collective unconscious, commonly manifested in the belief in spirits.[2] This is fundamental to his premise of a "plurality of relatively autonomous complexes that can behave like spirits" (Jung 1960b, p.309).

While recognizing a neurophysiological causality for schizophrenia (he favored a "toxic" etiology, especially in his later writings), for Jung the condition labeled schizophrenia or psychosis (he sometimes uses the terms interchangeably) was also a "complex" matter associated with "living units of the unconscious psyche" (Jung 1960b, p.101). Complexes are experienced by all persons, except that in schizophrenia the intrusion of the unconscious complex into ego consciousness has an unbalancing effect and brings "self-destruction…a disintegration of the means of expression and communication" (Jung 1960a, p.253).

This chapter first explores some early influences on Jung's ideas, particularly those that appeared to have led him to his theories about the nature of consciousness, the complexes, and the collective unconscious. Jung participated in Spiritualist séances led by his younger cousin, Hélène Preiswerk, which were attended by his mother and other family members (Ellenberger 1970; Hillman 1977). His interest in spirits extended into his years of medical training; his experiences with spiritual groups were the basis for the experiments reported in his doctoral dissertation. Since experiences of spirits and associated beliefs may be good candidates (in my opinion) for initiating the development of his theories of the collective unconscious and the archetypes, I explore relationships between some of Jung's early experiences and ideas, and his autobiographical reports of the experience of his own unconscious, particularly with regard to his period of "madness." I will not detail the influence of his travels in later years, which validated his ideas about the psychological role of spirits, which he then was able to perceive as widespread phenomena. Conceptual parallels and differences between current Spiritist views of consciousness (which I have studied and worked with over many years)3 and Jung's views are described, in an attempt to understand common ground relative to how he might have first perceived the world of spirits and the later confirmation of his formulations. This then leads to a brief discussion of Jung's theories on the psychogenesis of mental disease as compared to how some contemporary Spiritists conceptualize and work with persons considered "crazy" (in this case, diagnosed by mental health professionals as suffering psychotic episodes).4 Through an exploration of these topics I attempt to:

1. demonstrate how Jung's early formulation (and experience) of the notion of an overarching, universal, alternative "reality" (the collective unconscious) facilitates a somewhat different understanding of the experience of psychoses than we have inherited from the Kraepelinian model (Samuels 1985)

2. show how these views are paralleled by many of the notions of contemporary Spiritist healers, as only one among many groups who believe in and work with spirits.5

This exploration indirectly raises the question of the difference between "dissociation" as manifest by persons in psychotic states marked by hallucinations and delusions, and visions and fantasies experienced by persons who do not manifest psychoses. Both Jung and the Spiritists have explanations for this difference, related to their distinct but parallel views on consciousness and its relationship to psychoses, that readers might consider in the light of their own experiences.

Early Influences on Jung's Notions of the Unconscious

First we raise the question: Why did Jung become so interested in spirits? One part of the answer may lie in his apparently confused and paradoxical experience of religion. Homans (1979) devotes a chapter to the role of the early experience of religion in Jung's thought. Very early in his life Jung experienced religion in two very different ways: through his pastor-father's traditional Protestant Christianity, which was repudiated and feared, and through a modality that can be described as "personal-mystical-narcissistic," related to strong feelings of personal isolation (Homans 1979, p.116). Throughout his early life these modalities were sources of painful, personal conflict, both within and between them. He dealt with his distress mainly through personal imagery, fantasy, and rituals, such as making a manikin with top hat, black coat, and boots out of a ruler when he was 11 years old. This was an idealization of a male figure and a personal god, who served as a source of security when his feelings were hurt or he had done something wrong. With Jung's later repudiation of traditional Christianity, the personal-mystical-narcissistic mode of experiencing religion become the fulcrum of his critical years. Through reflection and self-analysis he assimilated these experiences into his core psyche. He also incorporated them into his concept of the individuation process, the goal of which was the formation of the Self and its relation to a god-image, which he called the "god within us," a "natural and spontaneous product of the human imagination" (Homans 1979, pp.130–131). It is of interest to this discussion that such experiences continued far beyond the critical years of his initial crisis and self-analysis. In his autobiography Jung remembers that in 1939 he awoke and saw a "marvellously beautiful golden image of Christ on the Cross" and he was "profoundly shaken by it." He states: "A vision is nothing unusual for me for I frequently see extremely vivid hypnagogic images" (Jung 1965, p.210). This was clear, though retrospective, testimony on the integration into his life of visionary experiences, which were shared at times with his family. On more than one occasion he heard spirits speak and held conversations with a spirit in a fantasy (see, for example, Jung 1965, p.191).

I have already mentioned influences from his mother's family, who were involved in Spiritualism. His maternal grandfather, a pastor and Hebrew scholar, is reported to have had visions and conversed with the spirit world (Ellenberger 1970). His mother Emilie was said to have had to sit behind her father when he wrote sermons to shield the writing from spirits. In his autobiography Jung (1965) recalls that he discovered a book on Spiritualist phenomena, written by a theologian, when he was a first-year university student. The phenomena the book described were the same as stories he had repeatedly heard as a child. This book established for him whether or not the "stories were physically true," that they occurred widely, and were reported over and over again (Jung 1965, p.99). In his words: "The observations of the Spiritualists…were the first accounts I had seen of objective psychic phenomena" (Jung 1965, p.99). These ideas were vigorously rejected when he spoke of them to his closest friends but his mother was sympathetic. Some years later, after mysterious happenings at his home (an old wooden table that suddenly cracked defied explanation, as did the spontaneous snapping into pieces of a steel bread knife inside a cabinet), he attended the meetings of a group of Spiritualists, relatives, who had a young girl, his cousin, as their medium. It was here that he gathered the materials for his doctoral thesis. However, he broke off his experiments after two years when he found the medium using tricks to produce phenomena. Despite some disillusionment he asserts that: "All in all this was the one great experience which wiped out my earlier philosophy and made it possible to achieve a psychological point of view" (Jung 1965, p.107).

It is well known that from 1912 to about 1919 Jung went through a period that he describes as a state of "disorientation" and "constant inner pressure" (Jung 1965, p.173). It was during this time that he reports his initial confrontation with the unconscious, the experience of elaborate images, fantasies, and dreams through which he followed the "laws of my inner personality" (Jung 1965, p.193). He considered these years the most important in his life; material "burst forth from the unconscious and at first swamped" him (Jung 1965, p.199). He came to two crucial conclusions: that the goal of psychic development is the Self and individuation, and that "the contents of psychic experience are real, and real not only as my own personal experiences, but as collective experiences that others also have" (Jung 1965, p.194).

For Jung, widespread belief in spirits in other cultures validated his formulations about the nature of the psyche, and particularly his formulations of autonomous complexes and the personal and collective unconscious. He comments somewhat later, when discussing the psychological foundation of belief in spirits, that one cannot believe in spirits without believing in souls; the former associated with the collective unconscious, the latter with the personal unconscious (Jung 1960b, p.305). He even briefly discusses whether spirits have an "independent existence" and concludes that, lacking proof, they are "exteriorizations," an "appendix of psychology" (Jung 1960b, p.318). However, he leaves the door open just a bit on the question of "Do spirits exist?" when he observes: "Feeling often arrives at convictions that are different from those of the intellect, and we cannot always prove that the convictions of feeling are necessarily inferior" (Jung 1960b, p.318).

Conceptual Parallels between Spiritists' and Jung's Views on Consciousness

Spiritists believe in spirits that manifest through visions as well as by visitations while possessing a medium. The reality of a parallel spirit world, comprised of the spirits of persons who have "passed over" from all times and places in the visible world, is virtually unquestioned. Although there are special factors in the selection of particular persons as mediums (i.e. severe or highly distressing illness that heralds development as a medium, for example), it is asserted that everyone has the capacity to "see into" the spirit world. Development as a medium implies that one can communicate with this world; in Latin American Spiritualism most communication is actually first through a bodily "knowing" what the spirits want to tell someone. The mediums both feel the distressing feelings of a client and see them through visions of the spirit world called *videncias*. As a prominent aspect of the healing ritual many mediums become a "vessel" (i.e. are possessed) for a spirit who wants to come through to the visible world and speak to the person to whom the spirit corresponds.

From Jung's perspective, spirit communications are manifestations of the collective unconscious. (From an anthropological perspective they are culturally constituted, and thus collective.) Jung defined the complex as a "feeling-toned image…of a certain psychic situation which is strongly accentuated emotionally and is, moreover, incompatible with the habitual attitude of consciousness" (Jung 1960b, p.96). Primordial images or archetypes, as Jung later called them, are usually represented by Jungians as Western culture (mainly Greek and Roman) mythological figures. In contrast, the description of spirits in Latin American Spiritism includes not only mythological, highly symbolic personages from their own cultural representations but also spirits of deceased persons from all times and places including famous physicians or wise men who are not named. The spirit world parallels the visible world of incarnated spirits, that of living human beings.

In a somewhat similar way, Jung was convinced that the structure of the collective unconscious was more or less built into the human psyche and asserted that the belief in spirits was proof of the "complex" structure of the psyche. There are obvious parallels between archetypes and spirits: they are both experienced as alien, and, at first, as intrusive, sometimes difficult, or fearsome. In Spiritism, spirits who come through to particular believers or sufferers are "tamed" and then accommodated as a part of the believer's self-description. This is possible when the spirit's true nature and relationship is discovered via communication through visions or possession-trance manifested by a practicing medium (Koss-Chioino 1992). Spirits of relatives or other associates from past lives are linked to believers' descriptions of their self; spirit presence becomes known when they manifest as troublesome, molesting influences in one's life. The goal of the healing ritual is to realize one's relationship to that spirit and come to terms with the spirit's demands upon the believer.

As I note in greater detail elsewhere (Koss 1986), there are differences in spirit influences on believers; some spirits, particularly deceased maternal relatives, come as potential guides to those who are in development of mediumistic faculties and are generally supportive and helpful, but may initially cause distress. Other, more threatening spirits come through because of a distorted relationship to a believer in the present or former life. This again somewhat parallels Jung's notion that there are complexes that intrude on the personal unconscious (because of repressed material) and complexes that are truly archetypal, comprised of basic human tendencies as part of the collective unconscious.

Spiritist parallels to Jung's description of the process of individuation are quite close. For Jung, complexes arise because of painful or distressing experiences that leave psychic wounds. Spiritist believers, in development as mediums, undergo serious and prolonged illness, and win through this distress through working with spirit intrusion conceived of as the cause of illness and distress. The process of "development" in Spiritism involves domesticating wayward and harmful spirits to become personal guides to the spirit world. Spirit guide/protectors are represented as personifications of universal human relationships (spouses, mothers, daughters from a former life, or famous persons with special abilities) and thus are archetypal.

Spiritual development is lifelong, as is the process of individuation described by Jung, and both processes are viewed as inexorable and beyond the control of those who are either elected to be healers or, in Jung's terms, affected by complexes. Should a medium decide to stop practicing and/or convert to another belief system, such as becoming a member of a Pentecostal church, illness or severe problems are inevitable. The health of mediums depends upon continuing to work with spirits, particularly focusing attention on relationships with personal guide protectors. Moreover, the guides demand or require certain types of moral behavior, as well as personal sacrifices. Jung's formulations of the dynamics of the psyche seem similar; he viewed neurosis as a call to deal with the unbalancing effect of material (autonomous complexes) arising out of the unconscious. To keep one's psychic balance individuals have to attend to and resolve the conflicts associated with the complexes until they are integrated within the psyche and become a part of the self. As illustrated by Jung, in the report of his own confrontation with the unconscious, both physical and mental health can suffer. Psychic balance, once achieved, must be maintained as a continuous effort.

Dissociative Experience

Before comparing views by Jung and Spiritists on madness/schizophrenia, a discussion of dissociation as defined by Jung is a necessary digression, since he and the Spiritists both point to differences between persons who "dissociate" in a "normal" way versus those who do not. For Spiritists, as described above, "dissociation" is equivalent to communication and/or working with spirits through visions, possession-trance, or, for the undeveloped, through discourse with a spirit whom the mediums bring to the session. The belief behind possession-trance is that the foreign spirit completely displaces one's own spirit; in other communications spirits merely impinge on a person's consciousness. The goal of the Spiritist ritual is to make the sufferer conscious of the spirit intruding in terms of its motives, gender, relationship to the client, and so on. Jung, in describing the structure and dynamics of the psyche, was very clear that the dissociability of the psyche is due to the "fact that the connecting link between psychic processes themselves is a very conditional one" (Jung 1960b, p.173). Dissociation occurs in neuroses (as described above) but the "potential unity of the personality" is maintained. Jung comments that, "Despite the fact that consciousness can be split up into several personal consciousnesses, the unity of the dissociated fragments is…visible to the professional eye." For those diagnosed with schizophrenia, however, "the dissociation is no longer fluid and changeable…it is more like a mirror broken up into splinters" (Jung 1960b, pp.234–235). For Spiritists, "development" as a medium involves learning how to control spirit intrusions and displacement (i.e. possession-trance) so that spirits come and go without undue distress; it also involves accommodating foreign spirits as self-related protector guides. Control over spirit presence is exactly what the "crazy" person cannot do.

Jung on Psychogenesis and Psychosis

Samuels (1985) observes that the first stage of Jung's formulation of archetypal theory arose not only from his self-analysis but also from his work with psychotic patients in Burghölzli Psychiatric Hospital, Zurich. Jung describes how (on autopsy) there were no regular brain lesions and so he followed "older clinicians" in fully investigating patients' psychological histories. He felt "rewarded" when he found that in each case "the illness broke out at a moment of great emotion which, in its turn, had arisen in a more or less normal manner" (Jung 1960a, p.161).

From these observations (and through association tests with patients) Jung developed the idea of the "feeling tone" or "affective state" accompanied by "somatic innervations" (Jung 1960a, p.40), the strongest of which (i.e. one that arises from a dangerous situation) can totally inhibit all other ideas that run counter to it. The ego or governing complex is "compelled to give way to other, stronger sensations connected to the new complex" (Jung 1960a, p.43), yet in most persons and instances it remains behind to reassert itself when the strong affect decreases. Strong complexes can become chronic and thus affect both health and psychic experience if they meet an already existing complex that acts as reinforcement. Obsessive complexes hinder the proper development of personality and are dealt with in most persons through defense mechanisms, such as displacement or repression. However, Jung emphasizes that "if the complex remains entirely unchanged," which happens "when there is very severe damage to the ego-complex and its functions," then one can identify dementia praecox (Jung 1960a, p.68). The psychotic person associates only with this very strong complex, and is unable to free himself from it psychologically. In this case, progressive degeneration follows.

In normal people, the "principal function of the unconscious is to effect a compensation and to produce a balance" (Jung 1960a, p.205). In the "insane," hallucinations and delusions arise out of unconscious processes that produce a disoriented and chaotic state, but their content is meaningful for understanding the cause and nature of the disease. This provided the basic position that Jung held, which opposed an explanation of insanity as primarily caused by "morbid processes of the brain cells" because "primitives may have visions and hear strange voices without their mental processes being disturbed" (Jung 1960a, pp.206–208). In normal persons, when the corrective compensation from the unconscious breaks through, there is the beginning of a healing process that corrects the psychically unbalanced attitude. In contrast, the mentally unbalanced person defends himself against his own unconscious, which results in a "condition of excitation" because the "unconscious corrective impulses" are perceived as unacceptable.

Puerto Rican Spiritists and Madness

There is general anxiety in Puerto Rico associated with becoming or being identified as "crazy" (*loco*) in the sense of "madness" (*locura*) comprised of extreme distress and out-of-control behavior. To be "crazy" is a deeply feared state, easily imagined. Fear springs in part from a general notion that the condition is hereditary and permanent (although this notion is changing); and is in part related to the stigma attached to erratic, uncontrolled behavior. What is being referred to as *locura* (madness) is more or less equivalent to a psychotic episode. The idiom "*nervios*" is often employed as a way to distinguish emotional problems from madness and links bodily distress with emotional disorder (Guarnaccia *et al.* 1992; Rogler and Hollingshead 1965). As a term of reference "nerves" does not carry the connotations of *locura* (madness) and tends to relieve family members of the guilt, shame, and hopelessness associated with the label. However, when people say that someone "has nerves" (*tener nervios*), this is often a oblique reference to what is labeled a psychotic episode in psychiatry. Even if the person manifesting out-of-control and bizarre behavior is identified as a "*loca tranquilo*" ("quiet crazy person," as opposed to someone who manifests extreme agitation or aggressive behavior), they may be brought to a Spiritist healing center, sometimes as a first resort, but more often when psychiatric services are not producing the desired effect.

Spiritist concepts regarding the nature and cause of madness focus on conditions of the mind or brain (*celebro*). A very frequent complaint is that the mind leaves or goes blank (*se le va la mente; la mente quedo en blanco*). The mind can also be "disturbed," "molested," "stalled," "turned over," "turned around," "running on," or "warped," most of which have bodily associations, but also describe cognitively abnormal behavior. All of these conditions are attributed by mediums to spirit influences on the way the mind/brain affects behavior. Spiritist healers say that "some spirit being is interlocked with, or hooked onto," the sufferer. The explanation of this state is that the client is "obsessed" by a spirit who perturbs the mind and causes it to malfunction. According to Spiritists, obsession by a "perennial thought" that invades the mind can also have this effect. Guarnaccia and colleagues (1992) report that Puerto Rican clients in a mental health clinic in New York use the term "*fallo mental*" (failure of the mind) for severe mental disorder.

Those affected in these ways have an impossibly large "emotional burden" or "tension" that renders them highly vulnerable to spirits who will become attached to them and cause problems. Fear is considered a major contributor to this state, yet symptoms of "nervousness" may not affect the mind for years until one day the person suffers a "nervous shock." (This parallels Jung's tracing the beginnings of the illness to an extreme emotional episode.) For example, Juana attributed her problems to her father's coming home drunk and knocking on her bedroom door; she was always unable to return to sleep. One night he was particularly insistent and she became extremely distressed and saw a "serpent." (She was later diagnosed as having schizophrenia.) However, this was not the worst type of obsession (the implication being that she feared or experienced sexual abuse, which was not openly discussed at the Spiritist healing session). "Persecution by an invisible enemy," sent by a living person or someone from a former existence who wishes a person mortal harm, can lead to homicide or suicide.

The above descriptions of madness were common to a majority of the approximately 100 Spiritist healers I interviewed over the course of 15 years; however, several Spiritists gave still another explanation, which they called "*locura espiritual*," distinguished from "physical madness." At a meeting of Spiritists and mental health professionals in the project I carried out in Puerto Rico (Koss 1980), where the case of a young girl with florid symptoms of schizophrenia was reviewed (she was diagnosed by psychiatrists), the Spiritists observed that the girl's own spirit was totally out of her body; she was "subjugated" by a foreign spirit. The result of this "obsession" by a spirit is that the person doesn't know herself or even who is behaving. She experiences great inner turmoil over not knowing the agent of her actions. Whether this explanation was influenced by contact with psychologists and psychiatrists in the project was impossible to establish, but it is clearly similar to theories of psychosis, beginning with Jung, that view the dynamics of schizophrenia as an overwhelming of the ego, defined as the control center of the psyche. It is worthwhile noting, however, that Spiritists did not condone the use of anti-psychotic medications because they claimed that to be drugged up (*endrogada*) with anything clouded the mind and prevented the return of the displaced personal spirit.

Spiritist mediums do not identify experiences that are labeled "hallucinations/ delusions" by psychiatric manuals. For them, a hidden, non-physical reality exists; it is populated by spirits who may manifest at any time. It is instructive that distortions of reality expressed by the young female patient were not attributed to her, but instead to the spirit-obsessors. These experiences were not perceived as "fixed false beliefs" or unreal perceptions, given the Spiritist concept of the self as one's own spirit, a central, observing entity. In other words, the girl's own spirit was not present in order for her to be credited as the agent of the disordered thoughts. In some cases, when visions of the spirit world do not conform to expectations (they have a limited pattern), then they are rejected as "true" experiences of the spirits and attributed to "mental confusion" introduced into the person's mind by molesting spirits.

Spiritists who worked with persons diagnosed with schizophrenia specifically recognize clients' emotional and cognitive limitations. For example, if clients appeared to be in a globally disordered state, with their minds "gone," they were *not* told that they were "in development" as a healer (which is a fairly common practice), nor were they asked to communicate with the possessing spirits brought to the session, in contrast to most clients.

Lessons for Cultural Psychiatry
Historical Perspectives

The prototype of Puerto Rican Spiritism I describe in this chapter is a Latin American synthesis of popular religious healing traditions and European Spiritualism, which had its beginnings before the middle of the nineteenth century. However, the movement really accelerated when the well-known Frenchman Allan Kardec (a pseudonym for Denizard Hippolyte Leon Rivail [1803–1869]) published his *Spirits' Book* in 1860 (1986), which was followed by six other books and a journal of ideas and reviews. Rivail was an educator and translator of scientific works but he was also both an atheist and avidly interested in Eastern religions. His own experiments consisted of exploring and describing the spirit world—the first truly spiritual ethnography. Kardec called his formulations "Spiritism" to distinguish them from the Spiritualism in England and the USA initiated by the table rappings of the famous Fox sisters. Both of these movements found congenial ground in Europe in the last decades of the nineteenth century among phrenologists, magnetists, and many other groups. What Ellenberger (1970) describes in the séances put on by Jung's cousin, Hélène Preiswerk, may have been related to either of the English or the French movements, but since the séances dealt with past lives, they seem more related to the Kardecian formulations.

It is perhaps futile to identify the actual direction of influence. Did his knowledge (and acceptance) of Spiritualist beliefs lead Jung directly (if not ultimately) to his central formulations about the unconscious, the complexes, and the archetypes? Ellenberger (1970, p.691) notes that when Jung entered Burghölzli Hospital in December 1900 he defined his work as the "scientific study of the human soul." However, since this discussion is about comparing recent Spiritist practices, it is possible (but not likely) that some contemporary Spiritists have read about Jung's ideas and adapted them, albeit to a limited extent. (The educated healers I knew were extremely eclectic and read all kinds of contemporary pop psychological and alternative religious literature.) It is also possible (although not documented) that the well-educated followers of Allan Kardec had some contact with Jung's writings. It is perhaps not coincidental that Kardec, a third of a century earlier, worked out the outlines of his system much as did Jung because they both were responding to the Zeitgeist of the times. They both incorporated some ideas from Hinduism, were both well read in the sciences but advocated a metaphysical approach, both carried out "experiments" to substantiate their ideas, and both rejected the institutionalized religions of their childhood which led to the development of basic notions of a personal deity who can be directly accessed.

Perhaps the actual direction of borrowing is unimportant because both "belief" systems—which considered themselves to be innovative "sciences" of the human condition at that time—were developing among intellectuals at the end of the nineteenth and the beginning decades of the twentieth century. This period witnessed both a reaction to the positivist scientific worldview beginning to assert itself with some force and popularity, and a reassertion that there are other realities—mysteries—that play an essential role in the affairs of all living human beings. As mentioned above, a number of social movements with more or less the same orientation competed for the attention of a growing intellectual class and for the role of interpreter of the "true" psychological nature of human beings. Spiritists in Puerto Rico during that period asserted that they were the "modern psychologists," just as did the followers of Jung somewhat later (Koss 1976).

Jung and Cultural Psychiatry

For more than six decades during the twentieth century, cultural psychiatrists, and anthropologists in synchrony with their views, have reported on and interpreted the spirit worlds of many peoples. They have examined conceptualizations and healing practices around spirit beings as related to mental disorders in general and schizophrenia in particular (see studies reviewed by Csordas and Lewton 1998). A recent example is the nicely detailed ethnographic description of a severe mental disorder in Indonesia by Broch (2001) and many more studies could be cited, including my own work (Koss-Chioino 1992). However, a majority of these studies begin with the premise that "schizophrenia" is a valid cross-cultural phenomenon, rather than leaving matters of recognition and definition related to spirit-filled realities as subjects to be studied (Hollan 2000).

Jung was a cultural psychiatrist in some sense, in his recognition of the ubiquitous role of spirits among non-European peoples as true psychological phenomena—even if he operated with what we currently consider uninformed— even naive—ideas about these people, given standard theories in anthropology.

His construction and elaboration of the personal and collective unconscious and their dynamics seem to have been validated by his cross-cultural experiences and observations, although I argue here that they seem to have been initiated by his early experiences with Spiritualism. Later, he attempted to penetrate and understand other cultural worlds even as he looked inwardly at patients and at himself, conflating the personal and the social and lacking a concept of "culture" (in the anthropological sense).

If we consult Jung on schizophrenia, we know that there were social dimensions to his ideas that affected his approach to treatment of persons diagnosed as schizophrenic. He certainly considered relationships with significant others: spouses, close relatives, and friends, and even the social milieu, the time and place, of his patients. However, he focused mainly on the internal workings of the psyche and in his last years unequivocally restated his earlier position that "the disease can be treated with psychotherapy" (though he qualified this assertion with "though only to a limited extent") (Jung 1960a, p.254). His main approach was through the recognition that those who appeared psychotic were overwhelmed by unconscious autonomous complexes and a resultant severe fragmentation of the personality. In his view this accounted for typical symptoms related to dissociation and depersonalization.

Conclusion

For those who believe, spirits exist on another plane, an alternate reality that interpenetrates the more readily visible world of everyday life. Spirits (in all the ethnographies that describe them) affect living humans, either to cause distress or enhance well-being; they bring forth and introduce salient aspects of individual history, but also human history, at one and the same time. This parallels Jung's formulations of the personal and collective unconscious. Spirits intrude upon, possess, or sometimes obsess persons; it is the individual's response that can lead to the special behavior and extreme disturbance of normal life labeled as "madness" or psychosis. Recent neuroscience research is determining why some persons are vulnerable to being overwhelmed by spirit intrusions or autonomous complexes in the ways Jung proposed. As part of this issue, Jung recognized the meaning and relevance of widespread experiences of spirits, framed by a theory that accounts for the sharing of psychological processes—between those who are "normal" and able to exert control over the disruptive effects of either spirit visitations or autonomous complexes, and those who cannot. Jung's formulations suggest that the mechanisms of madness (or of psychiatrically diagnosed psychosis— the equivalence is not established) are not alienated psychological conditions but rather shared, potentially creative, constructive attributes. They are the stuff that creates healers who work with spirits. It seems not fortuitous that submitting to and learning to control dissociative states of consciousness as the staging for healer development is found in folk theories in most of the world, as I have described for those Puerto Ricans who believe in spirits and Spiritism (Hollan 2000; Koss-Chioino 1992).

Notes

1. This chapter was first published in *Transcultural Psychiatry*. Reproduced by permission of Sage Publications, London, Los Angeles, New Dehli, and Singapore, from J.D. Koss-Chioino, "Jung, spirits and madness: lessons for cultural psychiatry," *Transcultural Psychiatry 40*, June 2003, pp.164–180 (© Sage, 2003).

2. In his essay "The Psychological Foundations of Belief in Spirits" Jung includes a footnote about his experience as a member of an expedition in East Africa when a young woman fell ill with a high fever and a *nganga* (medicine man) treated her for spirit intrusion by her dead parents, after the travelers' medical supplies proved inadequate. Although the travelers diagnosed the girl as suffering from a septic abortion, to their "astonishment" she recovered in two days (Jung 1960b, p.304). He uses this experience as a comment on the complex he describes as the "powerful psychological after-effects of the parents."

3. My discussion of Spiritism derives from data I collected in Puerto Rico over the years from 1968 to 1980, with follow-up during the decades of the 1980s and 1990s. I record my appreciation to the National Institute of Mental Health who supported four studies during the early years. Based on extensive review of the literature on Spiritualism and Spiritism, the observations I make here can be generalized to the practices and beliefs Jung was acquainted with in nineteenth-century Europe, which he refers to in his writings, since most Spiritist/Spiritualist practices stem from the same historic roots in Europe. However, there may be some differences due to cultural context, which I am not taking into account since I am constructing a general argument about belief in spirits and its ubiquity around the world. The reader who desires more details can refer to my book *Women as Healers, Women as Patients: Mental Health Care and Traditional Healing in Puerto Rico* (Koss-Chioino 1992) or the articles cited.

4. I collected details on 220 Spiritist cases to compare with over 1420 cases diagnosed and treated by mental health professionals. Using index cases in each major diagnostic category of the *Diagnostic and Statistical Manual of Mental Disorders*, revised third edition (DSM-III-R), based on case selections from case discussions attended by both therapists and Spiritist healers, as well as 15 cases receiving both types of intervention in a referral unit, I was able to diagnostically label most of the Spiritist cases using repeated pattern, discriminant function analysis (see Koss-Chioino 1992).

5. They are also similar to notions and clinical practices advocated by R.D. Laing and certain humanistic psychologists (Boyers and Orrill 1971).

Chapter 12

THE PRACTICE OF INTEGRATING SPIRITUALITY INTO PSYCHOTHERAPY

Mario Sergio Silveira, PhD

My Path of Learning

I will start by telling you about my path in life, as my current work is infused with this history. I was born in 1953 into a family that became Spiritist in the 1960s. Friends had suggested to my father that he should take my mother to a Spiritist Center to treat her depression, which had resisted all conventional treatments available at the time. Gradually, through the help she received at the Spiritist Center, she improved. Simultaneously, my father discovered that he possessed psychic ability. As he dedicated himself to study Spiritism, he found that he had the ability to channel spirits through automatic writing. After recovering from depression, my mother engaged herself in social work at the Spiritist Center, as well as studies. She was very grateful to learn new principles to guide her life. As a result of my parents' involvement in Spiritism, the whole family learned about a God of love and forgiveness, the survival of the soul after death of the physical body, its infinite evolution through multiple existences, and the possibility of communication with those who have left the physical body.

Until the time I entered university I was actively engaged in the Spiritist movement, deeply studying the basic works of Allan Kardec (1968) and associated books, especially the ones channeled by the Brazilian medium, Francisco Cândido Xavier.

At the time of my graduation in psychology in 1977, I was in inner turmoil: How could I reconcile the Spiritist philosophy and its worldview with the theories I had learned at university? How could I learn the new without trying to translate it always into the "old beliefs" with which I grew up?

Today I understand that one's perception of reality is influenced by one's formative beliefs, which may be unconscious. The way we are first taught to look at life usually acquires the status of "truth" and also forms the answers to the fundamental questions of each human being: "Who am I? Where do I come from? Why do I exist? Where am I going after death?" Each person's identity is constructed on these theories he or she has formulated about reality (Koenig 2005).

We further seek to unravel the conditions of our existence through the production of symbols and words, whether through scientific research, philosophical questioning, or through the search for the essence of being through spiritual paths.

In university I tried to set aside my previous knowledge tied to Spiritism, at least its formal and overt practices, so I could better grasp what the major masters of psychology had to teach me. After my graduation there were still vast holes in my knowledge. I wondered, "What is it 'to be' a psychologist?" I could not separate the "*to be* a psychologist" and "*to know* about psychology." My training in psychiatry, psychology, and psychotherapy for children, clinical psychodrama, as well as my studies in Freudian and Lacanian psychoanalysis, did not assuage my mental anguish. However, now I understand that questioning was the great compass that pointed me to what is Real, i.e. that which is primary and cannot be contained in symbols.

What cannot be put into words remains encrypted in the body, breaks through the containment of the unconscious, and is dramatized in dreams, emotional and psychological symptoms, and even physical illness. This is a natural way of the human mind to display and work out its conflicts. Neurotic symptoms represent the effort for resolution of conflict that failed, but they also reveal the way that psychic energy travels in search of satisfaction. My search was inspired by the "desire to know," that is, the desire to integrate knowledge of psychological theories, psychopathology, and the spiritual dimension of being.

A Fundamental Case

In Brazil, many psychiatric hospitals were built early in the twentieth century by the Spiritist movement to care for the "obsessed," victims of vindictive action of former enemies, who died in the recent or remote past. In the early 1990s a group of researchers, professionals, and volunteers gathered in the Psychiatric Hospital Bom Retiro in Curitiba, Brazil, in order to test the hypothesis that spiritual influences have a significant role in the genesis and triggering of what is called mental illnesses.

My first introduction to dealing with such obsession was in early 1991, when I was referred a six-year-old girl who needed a "Spiritist psychologist." She came to my office with her parents.

She was first evaluated by a pediatric neurologist, another clinical psychologist, and the family's psychotherapist. None of them could understand the cause of her "night terrors" in which the girl had crises of despair and could neither recognize her own identity nor her parents. During my evaluation session with the child, using some art materials, she had produced a mask describing to me: "This is what I see." It looked like a monster. After my first interview with the parents, I took the case. I told myself it was for purposes of "psychical research."

In light of the spiritual influences I felt were present, I understood that mediums were needed early in the course of therapy. Mediumship could provide an important "window" into other dimensions of the child's life. What a surprise I had when, after the start of the first disobsession meeting with the team of mediums enlisted to work on the case, I was immediately threatened by disembodied spirits who warned me not to interfere, as the young girl was not innocent just because she now appeared a child. Gradually, with the continued help of clairvoyant mediums who I invited to become involved, we were given access to a passionate drama that had taken place about two centuries ago, involving a woman and two men who now sought revenge.

During subsequent disobsession sessions, when the young girl was not present, we dialogued with the two characters of the girl's "past," helping them to understand that they could restart their lives, forgiving and forgetting. After these sessions, and their "leaving" the child, the child began to improve and today is a woman psychologically and emotionally well balanced.

The Paradigm of Consciousness

How was I to understand the girl's issues? How did I interpret the phenomenon of hallucination that had invaded the girl's nights, causing panic and depersonalization? How did I understand that this story, which took place in another era, could invade her mind today and take over her memory? It made me question again: Where is the memory? What was Real that was returning in the form of an image? Even assuming the hypothesis of reincarnation and obsession, how could I explain the action of another disembodied mind over this child's present life?

In order to describe how I answered these questions, I turned to the route that many scholars and explorers of the human mind have already taken through metaphysics, parapsychology, and modern consciousness research (Wallace 2009). Interested readers may already know that the greatest visionaries of modernity are physicists—among them are Fritjof Capra (1984, 2010) and Amit Goswami (2005). These readings brought me to a perspective that is the underpinning of my therapeutic practice.

> The objective world does not seem to exist outside of consciousness that determines its properties. The universe around us becomes increasingly less material; it is no longer comparable to a huge machine, but rather to a vast thought. (Guitton, Bogdanov and Bogdanov 1992, pp.4–5)

Currently, this same territory is being described by various hypotheses (Lazlo 2008; Moutinho and Melo 2010; Wilber 1991), such as the existence of multiple parallel universes. These hypotheses, inspired by discoveries of quantum physicists and their knowledge of the ancient wisdom traditions, are being brought into the practice of psychotherapy through Transpersonal Psychology and Humanistic Psychology. These psychologies work with a multidimensional model of the human mind in which the physical brain could be the transducer of other dimensions of consciousness and of other dimensions of the universe—so subtle they cannot be easily measured.

To put it another way: the complex mind–brain is like an energy system, organized in multiple fields that are in relationship with a vibrational, or subtle energy world. These have been likened to "informational fields" as they carry information not otherwise accessible.

In my clinical work I use the operational model of Roger Woolger, PhD's program "Deep Memory Process" (DMP) (Woolger 2007). It is a psychotherapy that uses a kind of regression process that perfectly integrates the transpersonal vision noted above. This training allowed me to integrate my understanding of spirituality into the psychotherapeutic process in which I was initially trained.

I understand that, at this point in humanity's evolution, we are immersed in the world of images that constitute our memory. These images are loaded with the energy (information) of feelings, emotions, and thoughts that we freeze at different points along our evolutionary trajectory through lifetimes. Each person's unique spirit, as part of the Divine Consciousness in the evolutionary process through time, stays connected to their multiple experiences. These memories are "saved in a file" labeled with space and time, as if our universe were a huge quantum computer. The human energy system, through the "chakras," as sensors, resonates with these memories from time to time and our ability to recall these files can be used for therapeutic effects.

Indeed, each thought we have acts as a kind of "carrier wave," carrying the informational frequency of our feelings and emotions. When we suffer an emotional shock (what Freudians term "trauma"), our system experiences a kind of overload, disorganizing the mind–brain system, allowing, through the phenomenon of resonance, the invasion of information from different files. This allows us to better understand the patient's psyche in times of crisis, such as when there are visual and/or auditory hallucinations, or the mind is in chaos.

Even though they are strange, the contents of these "files" delivered up from the unconscious mind must be acknowledged and investigated as part of the psychic reality of the patient.

The one-dimensional view of neuroscientific research reduces these phenomena to changes in the physical brain. We do not deny the potential for changes in the nervous system and in its complex system of information transmission, but we expand the understanding by studying the contents of these "altered" states of consciousness (Wallace 2009). Stanislav Grof's research (Grof 2007; Grof and Grof 1994, 1995) allows us to consider these phenomena "beyond the brain" as the cause of problems and not just as a consequence.

The same mind that meditates and can experience Oneness with the Divine in states of "expanded awareness," when disorganized, can live the states that psychiatry classifies as psychopathological: mental confusion, hallucinations, unusual physical sensations, disruptive changes in feelings and emotions, panic attacks, and behavior and mood changes. All these events can now be investigated in light of the resonance that Jung called "complexes" and Grof and Grof conceptualized (1995) as "systems of condensed experience."

Therapeutic Techniques

We look for trauma as the origin of problems for patients in crisis whom we attend in our psychiatric hospital. We believe what appear to be symptoms indicate the actual causes of the disease. Thus, the visions and voices or the elementary phenomena of psychosis would be the return of the material from other levels of perception. Usually we find patients are resonating with the biographical unconscious, somatic, archetypal, collective, or trans-existential levels of consciousness. In assessing the patient we need to identify the nature and origin of their experience. The resonances can occur in many different "files" of the cartography of consciousness.

In general, the symptoms that the patient reports when describing his or her crisis are "isomorphic" in relation to the original trauma, i.e. records of other space/time that manifest in the "here" and "now," producing effects with an intensity of feelings, sensations, and thoughts without needing the subject to identify their origin.

Sometimes in clinical practice we need to uncover the original stories or other unconscious material. The techniques we use are relatively simple. It is as if the therapist is guiding the patient in an internal psychodrama in an expanded state of consciousness. The therapist often focuses the consciousness of the patient to his or her feelings as one of the bridges to access the source of his or her symptoms. The therapist also uses the resources of body therapies, seeking a catharsis through the body to unlock the patterns of unconscious memory. These patterns constitute "programs" that we unconsciously repeat at the physical, emotional, and mental levels.

Another important link to the unconscious is through exploring dreams, which, as we have noted, are the natural way of working our unconscious conflicts. Once we access a memory, usually in the form of images, we work to bring the facts to awareness, but mainly the feelings, emotions, and physical sensations related to a traumatic situation.

The work of the psychotherapist is to help the patient connect to and derive meaning from these feelings, sensations, and thoughts and thus further his/her integration. As proposed by Jacob Levy Moreno in his book *Psychodrama* (1946), the goal of psychotherapy is transmuting and integrating the different levels of the psyche.

In the case of the child cited above, access to the cause of her symptoms was made with the help of mediums. Once the triggering cause of the night terrors was addressed, the symptoms ceased.

In the psychiatric hospital we usually find a correlation between depressive disorders and suicidal ideation, stimulated by "voices of command" (disembodied voices representing those seeking revenge from prior lives) and the trauma of sexual abuse in childhood. It is impressive how patients describe the "voices" in detail: their allure, their suggestions, and tips on how to achieve suicide. Patients engage in real inner debates trying to escape from these influences, called "obsessors," which they identify as "another consciousness" trying to convince them to say or do something they don't want to do. We also find the same phenomenon in schizophrenia.

When we treat adult patients who have the mental condition to directly access their memories, we proceed without mediums. The efficacy of therapy is greatest when the patient is working out his or her own experiences. The indirect access is justified in more serious cases, where the psyche is more compromised.

Unusual Capacities of the Mind

The study of mediumship, deeply investigated in the 1850s and 1860s by the French educator Allan Kardec (1968), has a place in the multidimensional view of the mind, as it is an intrinsic component of the mind. Formerly considered a symptom of mental illness, mediumship today is understood as a human potential and a fundamental key to understanding the human mind. It is true that this capacity of the mind to connect with other dimensions, if not trained properly or not utilized in a conscious way, can trigger the imbalance of the mind itself. But when mediumship is put in its proper place, the Self can take on a role as a kind of "psychic tool" able to observe and discriminate which reality is being seen and experienced.

The fundamental key is that the experience of reality is a function of the state of consciousness. According to the state of consciousness we are experiencing, we can access and experience different realities. For example, compared to conflicts from the present, while sleeping we experience the realities pertaining to dreams, which may have unusual origins. We come into contact with other dimensions of space–time with which we are in tune or possibly even bound up; we access the collective unconscious and its archetypal images in ways we cannot in waking consciousness.

Studies of "near-death experience" are already well known, as well as research on "out of body experiences." A new field is being investigated, "telepathic contact with patients in coma," through well-trained sensitives. We can obtain information about the mental state of these patients, including their feelings and thoughts about their situation. In addition to providing greater benefits to understanding the nature of human consciousness, this information can also be supportive to patients and their families.

Psychosis: A Great Challenge to Psychiatry

Psychotherapeutic methods of regression to access deeper levels of memory as a direct approach to uncovering the unconscious have allowed considerable progress in the broader understanding of psychopathology. Patients with psychic structures related to neurotic disorders are easily assisted by regressive therapies.

Patients with mood disorders, even with symptoms perceived as "psychotic" such as visual and auditory hallucinations, are perfectly treatable from the multidimensional view of being. Hallucinatory phenomena can be understood as a confusion in discerning the experience of reality due to the patient's altered state of consciousness.

We have the experience of patients returning to the "normal mode of consciousness" when using the "retrieval procedure of trance," as it is done in hypnosis. We understand that during the crisis, especially in neurotic structure, the patient is in an altered state of consciousness. In this state, the patient is in resonance with other dimensions of the psyche. It is possible, in some cases, to bring the focus of awareness to the here and now, to the body and the state of waking consciousness.

Patients hospitalized for more severe mental disorders are not as easy to work with using these techniques. The most difficult patient I work with is the paranoid schizophrenic who is certain of the reality of his or her delusion. According to Freud (1972) and Lacan (1988), psychosis stems from the failure of the paternal function, whose symbolic work is to unite the desire and the law.

A patient whom I attended at the hospital called my attention to the fact that she did not recognize her biological father as her father. Her explanation for this fact was superficial. Studying her biographical history I could not find any reasons for her to refuse her father. I then decided to investigate the hypothesis that her refusal could be caused by an unconscious process related to past lifetimes they had together. As access to the information through the patient herself was not possible due to her paranoid psychosis, I turned to a well-trained medium I work with. She focused on the patient in question, and was able to channel the "personality" of the patient's deceased biological mother. In great anger "the mother" said that she did not and that she would never allow her husband to approach their daughter (the patient). The mother did not see the patient as a daughter, but as a rival from a past existence who would have destroyed her marriage.

Certainly the "laws of life" put these souls together again, perhaps through what the Eastern traditions call "karma" or "law of cause and effect" as referred to in the Kardecist Spiritist movement and other theories of psychology.

In the above case, we can propose that the access to the father was barred by the unconscious intervention of the mother. In other cases of paranoid psychosis we have similar findings. When we investigated a case of sexual abuse of a patient in childhood by her own father, we found a passionate sexual relationship in a past life. In another serious case of continued abuse in childhood by the current father, the woman found an old slave master in a previous life who had taken "her" on when she was his slave as his mistress. This slave mistress had endured her master murdering her family, and then she had poisoned her master in their own "love" bed.

Since 1991, when our group began investigating relationships between mental disorders and spiritual influences, hundreds of cases have been investigated and generally the common denominator is continuity in the relationship as it relates to love, hate, and the need to take revenge.

What seems clear is that the dramas that unfold in our lives have continuity after the death of the physical body. The immortal consciousness transcends the limits of the physical brain and of the present personality. Until we can overcome these conflicts through forgiveness, and a choice to be compassionate to all others, we will continue to be prisoners of the "compulsion of repetition," repeating the passions born of love, hate, and the need for revenge. Unconsciously generated difficult relations between parents and children, presented to us first through Freud's Oedipus myth, may be better understood through this model of a "trans-existential" unconscious.

It may seem to the reader that we want to force the "spirit" hypothesis. This is not our intention; instead, we want the spiritual dimension of human beings to be definitively included in the practice of psychology as well as in psychological and psychiatric research (Nicolescu 1999).

Conclusion

According to the model described here, therapeutic action must occur at different levels of consciousness during the psychotherapy process and may include procedures taken from different schools of psychotherapy. It is important to expand the Freudian cartography of the psyche (Freud 1972) and use a multidimensional view of the self. Unlike psychoanalysis, the psychotherapist does not have to wait for the manifestation of the unconscious; instead, the psychotherapist can be more active and take the patient to a state similar to a conscious lucid dream in order to have access to deeper levels of consciousness for therapeutic purposes.

The psychotherapist can assist the patient to be conscious of the feelings, the emotions, the sensations, and the thoughts experienced in the scenes accessed, stimulating further integration of mental, emotional, and somatic levels. Patients with severe disturbances or those who cannot access their "files" can be helped by trained sensitives to serve this same purpose.

The process of spiritual psychotherapy as described is very efficient and certainly effective as a therapy. How far to go to enhance integration and self-knowledge with each patient will be the decision of each unique "being" and the resources of the clinic or hospital serving the patient.

Chapter 13

WHEN MEDICAL DOCTORS ARE MEDIUMS

Gilson Roberto, MD

Editor's Note

Gilson Roberto, MD, is one example among several whom I met in Brazil who are both maintaining clinical practice in a hospital or private office as a licensed health provider and very active as a medium and healer at a Spiritist Center. Those like Gilson are testaments to the fact that one can integrate one's psychic capacities and function very well as health care professionals—possibly even better.

The child of a materialist, atheist father and a non-practicing Catholic mother, I was raised without religious orientation, and separate from any values associated with spirituality. My father's influence was ever towards the denial of the spiritual reality, aiming towards the acquisition of material goods and professional success. At home we never spoke of God or religion, and we had no habit of praying. The focus was always study and work. Such was the legacy my father left me regarding what is most important in life, and which he strived for all of his own life.

My encounter with mediumship took place through some events that I witnessed over the course of my life, through faith-healers who lived in the region where I lived, and my maternal grandmother, who was a *benzedeira* (an umbrella term for women, generally elderly, who work as faith-healers and give blessings and spiritual healings). But at first I attributed no importance to these events, especially since my grandmother developed her *benzedeira* abilities spontaneously, acquiring her knowledge through dreams. She didn't possess any theoretical knowledge, or know anyone who could teach her about the mechanisms of her mediumship. My interest in the study of mediumship was only awakened through Spiritism, after I read a book containing messages from deceased people along with testimonies from their relatives. What called my attention was the precise information, to which the medium had had no possibility of access, contained in those messages. They consisted of personal details, known only by family members: a conversation that took place in private, an affectionate and particular nickname, names of ancestors, past facts accurately described. From then on, I started investigating and studying mediumship, eventually coming to exercise it alongside my medicine practice.

Mediumship and Intuition

Mediumship is the ability to feel, receive, and transmit the spirits' influence, making possible the exchange between the material and spiritual worlds. It's like a window that opens to another dimension, amplifying our perception of reality. It's an ability inherent to the human psyche, like intelligence and feeling. We are all endowed with some degree of mediumship, some of us possessing it in a more ostensible way. Its emergence does not depend on place, gender, social class, or religious affiliation. Although this ability is natural and spontaneous, it may be increased and improved through specific exercises and techniques, just as with any other activity that requires dedication, effort, and discipline.

Allan Kardec, codifier of Spiritism, named "mediums" the people endowed with "mediumship," which means mediator or intermediate, one who serves as an instrument for communication between the two planes of life. There are countless types of mediumship. In his work *The Book of Mediums* (1998), Allan Kardec classifies them, making clear the several existing types. I, however, will focus only on intuition, considered the most common and universal mediumship, as the base for these considerations.

Although intuition is more common among artists, probably all of us have had some kind of intuitive experience, even if we don't identify it as such. Intuition lies behind aspirations, be it through a new idea or an inner clarity; through perception of something that has happened or will happen in the future. It is very common in accidents or the passing away of family members, or even as an impulse for something we are led to accomplish. Since these phenomena take place in a psychological context, mixed up with our emotions, thoughts, and desires, we tend not to acknowledge or value them.

Intuition is a very common psychic phenomenon in certain cultures, and was very valued in the past as a way to apprehend reality and seek knowledge. In our post-modern society, the cognitive aspects, along with a materialist view, took a greater preponderance over the spiritual factors. Thus, great difficulty was posed for the sciences in understanding all that which is out of the ordinary, although there has always been research on these matters by its great scholars, which often ended up forgotten or opposed, victim of a pragmatic science that may sometimes be more fundamentalist than many religions.

These same prejudices can be found within the field of medicine, the result of a lack of knowledge or baseless fear of speaking about the subject, as though it was something prohibitive, in an attitude that goes against scientific argumentation itself, in denying something without a judicious analysis. Clearly, within the field of the imponderable noetic sciences, there is a wide margin for fantasy and quackery, but that must not be a reason for us to close our eyes to that reality. After all, in conventional science, the same knowledge used to heal may be used in the service of other interests. The atomic radiation used to destroy tumors is the same as that used in the making of bombs. What changes is the intelligence and intent behind it, directing it towards one end or another.

Intuition has always been the object of consideration and studies, demonstrating its great value. Many scholars, past and present, find an important path to knowledge in intuition.

Jung (1991) places intuition as being one of our possibilities of perceiving reality, being one of the four functions of consciousness. In Jung's view (von Franz and Hillman 1990), an individual's "psychological type" is determined by introversion or extroversion, and by the four conscious functions that the self usually employs, called the "psychological functions." He defined them as: sensing, thinking, feeling, and intuition. People utilize these four functions every day, establishing skills, aptitudes, and forms of relationships.

The psychological functions determine how a person reacts and relates to their internal and external world. *Sensation* and *intuition* are irrational functions, since the situation is apprehended directly, without the mediation of a judgment or evaluation. They are functions used to perceive things. The functions *thinking* and *feeling* are considered rational functions because they confer judgment, and are influenced by consideration, determining the way we make our decisions. These functions are also called "judgment functions," responsible for the conclusions regarding the subjects that consciousness deals with. If, in the perceiving functions, the word is apprehension, in the judgment functions the word is valuation (von Franz and Hillman 1990).

In intuition the perception takes place through the unconscious and the apprehension of the environment generally takes place through "presentiments," "hunches," or "inspirations." Dreams that are premonitions and telepathic communications that come to us unexpectedly are some of the manifestations of intuition. Intuition seeks the meanings and the future relations and possibilities of such received information. People of the intuitive type tend to see the whole and not the parts, and therefore can have difficulties in the perception of details (von Franz and Hillman 1990).

Jung (1991) discovered that one of the functions differs and becomes the dominant or main function, while the others develop with less intensity, becoming auxiliary to the former. The tertiary and inferior will not develop in consciousness, remaining thus unconscious. This preferential form of a person's acting in the world is due, among other reasons, to genetic heritage, family influences, and the experiences an individual has through the course of his or her life.

Philosopher Henri Bergson (1984), winner of the Nobel Prize for Literature in 1928, also developed a profound study of intuition and was among the first to reference the unconscious. His work, very relevant to this day, has influenced several fields of knowledge such as neuropsychology and bioethics, as well as literature and cinema. According to Bergson there were two ways of knowing an object, diverse and of unequal value: through concept and through intuition. The first is that of the way of the concepts of judgments, syllogisms, analysis and synthesis, and deduction and induction; the second is that of immediate intuition, which provides us intrinsic, concrete, absolute knowledge. For Bergson, an exponent of intuitionist philosophy, the true knowledge was not constituted by abstract knowledge, rationally by the intellect, but rather in the immediate apprehension, in intuition, as is evidenced by the inner experience. Although he considered that in the present day only rarely and with great effort may one reach intuition, he affirmed that there would come a day when mankind will develop intuition to a degree that it will be the faculty ordinarily used for knowing things.

Being an Intuitive MD

It was with this understanding that I sought to develop intuition and the other mediumistic activities I carry out, apply this resource in charitable work, and in improving my abilities as a medical physician.

I graduated in medicine in 1991 at the Pontifícia Universidade Católica (Pontifical Catholic University) in Porto Alegre, Rio Grande do Sul. My weekly medical routine consists in attending patients from Monday to Friday, morning and afternoon, in my private clinic. I reserve one morning to work in the Hospital Espírita de Porto Alegre (Spiritist Hospital of Porto Alegre) and on Friday afternoons I participate as a medium in a Spiritist Center giving lectures, *passés* (laying-on of hands), and spiritual orientation.

During the evenings I participate in the following spiritual activities: on Mondays I participate as a medium in the Instituição Espírita (a Spiritist Center), giving lectures, laying-on of hands, and free consultations with both medical and spiritual orientation; on Tuesdays, I lead a study group on the theme of Medicine and Spirituality; on Wednesdays, I work at the center as a medium again, giving lectures, and performing healing with the help of a team of mediums for those patients that were sent to us through spiritual consultation or by our associates who are medical doctors; on Thursdays I direct a group for the study and exercise of mediumship for those who apply for this task. All of these spiritual activities, as advocated by Spiritism, are voluntary and completely free of charge.

Furthermore, I engage in some academic activities as a guest professor in activities of Post-Graduation and Science Outreach. I am a coordinator and professor of the "Curso de Especialização em Saúde e Espiritualidade" (Specialization Course in Health and Spirituality) for health professionals. I participate in lectures, seminars, congresses, and study groups with fellow medical doctors about health and spirituality in Brazil and abroad through the Associação Médico-Espírita (Spiritist Medical Association).

It's important to stress that there is no antagonism between my academic training and discipline and my activities as a medium. On the contrary, they complement each other, since mediumship isn't something magical or supernatural, but rather something rational, a subject that can be both studied and subjected to analysis. My being a medical doctor helps me a great deal; besides allowing me a greater contact with human health it provides me with a solid basis of knowledge for the exercise of mediumship by providing elements to analyze the information accessed through mediumship and intuition.

When I have an intuition about or perception of an illness, I seek confirmation through medical examination, and only after this confirmation will I accept my intuition. Until then, my intuition is only an indicator. However, on several occasions it has been intuition that helped me find the correct diagnosis. On the other hand, mediumship, within the field of medicine, becomes a valuable tool, broadening my view of man and of the world. It's one more helpful instrument that adds to technical knowledge and to the use of investigative technology.

The use of intuition or the perception of some spiritual factor during medical consultations in my office is made in a silent manner, without any disclosure to the patient, avoiding sensationalism or offending the patient's sensibilities and beliefs. No mention of Spiritism or mediumship is made, nor any kind of explanation of related subjects, unless the patient spontaneously asks for my opinion in that specific context. When any spiritual factors involved in the illness are identified, I refer the patient to the Instituição Espírita for the proper treatment, as long as that is consistent with his or her beliefs.

Conclusion

For those colleagues that feel attracted to the expansion of their intuition, I suggest the practice of daily meditation and prayer. A reflective life favors access to intuition; and prayer prepares the mind for communion with the higher spheres, clearing the psychic channels used in mediumship.

Like Bergson, I believe medicine itself and patients alike would benefit greatly if doctors were to study mediumship with respect and seriousness, exploring intuition as a supplementary factor in the practice of their professional activity.

.

Part III

CURRENT SCIENCE, PSYCHOTHERAPY, AND SPIRITISM

Editor's Note

This part gives voice to researchers in consciousness, bio-physics, psychiatry, and neuro-anatomy whose work reflects on the value of Spiritism. Readers will recognize that Spiritist theory and practice is current with theories of soul-centered or spiritual psychiatry, quantum physics, the bio-physics of blessed water, and medical doctors studying dissociation. It's interesting to see parallels between what highly intelligent disincarnated spirits have said about such things as neuro-anatomy from their perspective 50 years ago vis-à-vis the findings of today's science.

Chapter 14

A SCIENCE OF UNDERSTANDING THE MIND
The Next Great Scientific Revolution[1]

Alan Wallace, PhD

Let's begin with a brief overview of three significant points in the history of modern science:

1. Galileo initiated the first great breakthrough in modern science, which took place in astronomy and physics. The central feature of his catalytic role was his rigorous observation of the phenomena he was seeking to understand. Nevertheless, medieval scholars of his time regarded his findings as impossible. Some refused to look through his telescope, saying that if they were to see something that was incompatible with their beliefs then what they would be seeing must be an hallucination, or a distortion, and therefore there was no reason to look. Galileo insisted that empirical observation must supersede metaphysical assumptions, even religious beliefs, and this was one of his great contributions to the scientific revolution—400 years ago.

2. One hundred and fifty years ago Darwin launched the next great revolution in the life sciences. This too was based on many years of careful observation of the phenomena he was seeking to understand.

3. By the late nineteenth century, the great pioneer of psychology, William James, proposed that a "science of mind" should be launched. (It's important to recognize that in the first 300 years of the life sciences there was no science of mind.) James proposed that this science of mind should be like every other successful branch of the life sciences: centrally moved by the direct observation of phenomena one is seeking to understand, in this case mental phenomena such as thoughts, mental images, memories, fantasies, emotions, etc. This proposed science of mind would be moved primarily by introspection, the rigorous observation of internal states. It was snuffed out. The potential of his revolution never took place in his lifetime.

Materialism was already dominating all branches of natural science at the beginning of the twentieth century. Thus, there was increasing interest in studying behavior and the brain. The world that scientists studied was to be objective, quantifiable, and physical. Non-physical causes and entities were not considered natural, or real. Subjective phenomena and consciousness itself were not considered real, from that perspective. This left us in the dark about the nature of consciousness and the role of consciousness in the natural world. Sadly, many of our scientists today have barely moved from this position.

At the end of the nineteenth century William James said, "Psychology today is hardly more than Physics was before Galileo." Before Galileo, all the sciences, like physics and astronomy, were based on naked-eye observation. Today one could call the astronomy of his time "folk-astronomy." All modern mind science, cognitive science, is based upon observations of behavior, which are very rigorous, observations of brain function, which are also very rigorous, and subjects' direct experience of their minds, which is, unfortunately, completely amateur.

How can this be so? In all of the modern sciences, including mainstream academic, cognitive science, there is no training whatsoever in directly observing mental processes and states of consciousness. So the mind sciences are unique among all the natural sciences. No way has been formulated to rigorously observe that which they are supposed to understand.

Consider mental processes engaged with inner images and recollections. Most likely, you can successfully imagine your home, recall what you had for breakfast, or recite a line of poetry. When you are dreaming, you can directly observe a wide range of phenomena that are happening in the dream, but what mode of perception are you using to do this? You are not using the eyes, ears, nose, tongue, or organs of touch. You do directly observe these mental processes concerned with inner imagery, but not with any of the five physical senses. Also, it is important to note that these mental processes are completely undetectable by all scientific systems of measurement.

Does this mean they are totally invisible? Of course not.

Right now, if you imagine a piece of fruit, you can directly observe if it is a pineapple, a banana, an orange, etc. This simple fact, which is so obvious, is hardly even acknowledged in modern mind science. They don't even have a word for it, nor do they even acknowledge that we can directly and accurately observe mental phenomena. The word "introspection" is more commonly used as thinking *about* the contents of one's own mind. The term "meta-cognition" likewise is thinking *about* one's own mind.

Recently, while attending a Mind and Life Institute conference, distinguished cognitive psychologist Ann Treisman made the comment that "Perception is a kind of externally guided hallucination" (Treisman 2009).

Cognitive psychologists commonly interrogate their research subjects about the content of their subjective experience and acknowledge it, but the same psychologist remarked, "Psychologists regard subjective reports as data, rather than as factual accounts" (Treisman 2009). This is remarkably similar to the dogmatism of medieval scholastics. They said people can have any kind of experience they like through their telescopes, but if they have any experience that is not compatible with scholastic beliefs, their experience is a hallucination.

Are all of our states of consciousness natural? How can they not be, for they are taking place in the natural world. But, are they physical? Subjective mental processes are undetectable by our instrumentation. This would indicate they are non-physical. But, scientists would say that the mind is the product of the brain, which is physical. Thus, the mind is physical…

One of the great keys for the scientific revolution is the use of "Occam's razor":[2] "It is vain to do with more assumptions, what can be done with fewer assumptions." So shave off all assumptions that are not necessary. Occam's razor has been in the drawer for 400 years, and I propose it is time to take it out and shave off the notion that everything natural must be physical. Shave off the notion that mental phenomena and states of consciousness must be physical. It's just an assumption. If you shave off those projections, what have you lost? Only an illusion of knowledge.

What might we gain by adding rigorous first-person inquiry to studying the mind? After 135 years of studying the mind, we have failed to do the necessary observation of the mind itself, as James suggested we do.

We could choose to follow the lead of Galileo, Darwin, and William James and observe the mental phenomena themselves. There is an instrument—we can call it "mental perception"—with which we can directly experience states of consciousness, diverse perceptions, dreams, and so forth. In fact, it may be our only immediate access to directly observing non-physical phenomena.

Consider, please, that technology, through telescopes and microscopes, x-rays, sonar, etc., advances and extends the capacities of the five senses allowing us to see and hear beyond our own limited physical capacities. These technologies enhance and extend our range of experiencing physical phenomena. The five physical senses are not very malleable through training. I don't know any exercises that can allow me to see or hear past my natural range. My eyes are getting old so I need glasses for reading. I don't know of any exercises that will allow me to recover the 20–20 vision I once enjoyed.

Refining Mental Perception

What about our mental perception? Can this mode of mental observation be refined through training and extend the normal range of perception? The contemplative traditions of the word, like Hinduism, Taoism, Buddhism, Christianity, and so forth, all respond with one voice: "Definitely, yes."

In this context, the existence of spirits is an issue that is of central interest, as is our relationship with spirits. Does anyone directly perceive spirits just as we directly perceive colors or sounds? Does anyone directly perceive types of sentient beings that are not physical? It appears that they cannot be detected with scientific instruments. But that should not trouble us too much, unless we are complete dogmatists, because what is going on in my emotions and in my mind right now is not detectable by the instruments of modern science. Does this mean that there are no thoughts in my mind because they cannot be measured scientifically? That's completely absurd.

Might it be that, through training, refining, and extending mental perception, in the direct observation of non-physical phenomena, one could increase the bandwidth, the spectrum, of phenomena, that one could directly observe? So, for example, with the naked eye we can see red and the other colors up to purple, but we can't directly perceive infrared, ultraviolet, or higher frequencies of light. However, we can extend the range of visual perception using technology, and see things that are otherwise invisible to the naked eye.

Might there be non-physical phenomena that can be directly perceived only by expanding the bandwidth, the spectrum, of what we can observe with mental perception? We can answer this question through experimentation, refining and extending mental perception.

William James' Radical Empiricism

The challenge here is to come back to experience, not just in the narrow bandwidth that conforms with materialism. To combat this habit, William James proposed a "radical empiricism":

> I say empiricism because it is content to regard its most assured conclusions concerning matters of fact as hypotheses liable to modification in the course of future experience. (James 1912, p.134)

In other words, James goes to the opposite of dogmatism, suggesting one should be willing to be skeptical of one's own assumptions, which is one of the hardest things to do. If we do this, we must treat the doctrine of materialism as a hypothesis, rather than a scientific truth or empirically validated conclusion. Unlike so much of the "halfway empiricism" that currently goes under the name of "scientism," this position does not dogmatically affirm materialism to which everything has to conform.

Perhaps it is time for William James to be brought back to life. As I said, he proposed that the primary mode of exploring the mind should be introspection. He wrote:

> Introspective observation is what we have to rely on first and foremost and always. The word introspection need hardly be defined—it means, of course, the looking into our own minds and reporting what we there discover. Everyone agrees that we there discover states of consciousness. (James 1950, p.185)

Refining Attention

Together with the cultivation and refinement of observation, there must be a cultivation and refinement of attention. Now this is something of universal importance. Not everybody is keenly interested in the nature of consciousness. Some people are simply trying to raise their families, or they want to play better football, or they want to be better in scientific inquiry, or business, and so forth. But for every meaningful human endeavor the ability to focus our attention with coherence, continuity, composure, clarity, acuity, and vividness is essential.

Galileo externalized the refinement of attention by developing and refining the telescope. He mounted his telescope on a very firm platform, so that when he was gazing at Jupiter, for example, his telescope didn't wander all over the sky because he could keep it focused with continuity. In this way he was able to observe the slow movement of the moons around Jupiter. Observing carefully over a sustained period of time, he could see the little white spots going around a larger white spot. You need continuity of attention and a stable platform for the telescope. Stability is not enough; you must have clarity: well-mounted, well-polished, sharply focused lenses that have high resolution. With these, Galileo could make his ground-breaking, revolutionary observations that really catalyzed the first great revolution in the natural sciences.

If we wish to direct our attention inwards to observe non-physical mental processes, we must have the same type of stability and vividness that Galileo achieved with his telescope for observing external, celestial phenomena. When we direct the attention inwards there must be stability, continuity, and coherence—sustained observation without distraction or agitation. The observation must be clear like a well-tooled telescope, so that you can make precise and accurate observations. Attention must be refined.

This was the great limitation, perhaps the debilitating limitation, of the crude attempts of introspection by psychologists in the late nineteenth century. They never learned how to develop or refine attention. So all of their introspective observations were quite primitive.

William James wrote about the potential of refining attention:

> The faculty of voluntarily bringing back a wandering attention, over and over again, is the very root of judgment, character and will. Education, which would improve this faculty, would be the education par excellence. But it is easier to define this ideal than to give practical instructions for bringing it about. (James 1950, p.424)

William James wrote brilliantly about the significance of attention, of the importance of refining attention, *but he had no idea how to do it*. He had very little access to the wisdom of the great contemplative traditions of Asia. He traveled extensively between North America and Europe but never to Asia.

Now, science has developed hardly any method at all for refining attention for any endeavor, be it athletics, business, mathematics, or music. Mainstream science has completely neglected the refinement of mental perception by means of which we might be able to directly observe a broad spectrum of non-physical events, perhaps spirits as well, the existence of which is acknowledged in all the religions of the world, including Spiritism and indigenous traditions of shamanism.

It seems that the only discipline that doesn't know about spirits is modern science. Why? Because they have limited their observations to the physical, the quantifiable, the objective. They are living in a tiny little box, a prison of their own construction.

Attention can be trained, and the great contemplative traditions of the world, such as Buddhism, have an enormous amount of experience over many, many centuries of devising effective means for refining attention and then using one's attention skills for probing not only into a wider bandwidth of perception but probing into the innermost depths of consciousness and discovering dimension upon dimension of consciousness…discovering that the space of the mind is every bit as vast as the external space of the universe.

The vastness of the external universe has become manifest only because wonderful scientists, engineers, and technologists have devised better and better telescopes for probing beyond the 3000 stars you can see with the naked eye, probing beyond the Milky Way, gradually discovering dozens of other galaxies, and now into the depths of space and time and discovering there are perhaps 50 or 100 billion galaxies, spaced billions of light years across. All because of the extraordinary advances of telescopes for observing external space.

What about developing telescopes for the mind and exploring the depths of the space of the mind? For probing beyond memories of this life, probing into and accurately revealing memories from countless past lives? Just as telescopes can penetrate way beyond the confines of a single solar system, as one looks into the deep space of the mind, one also looks into the deep history of the mind, going way beyond the confines of a single human life.

Mindfulness and Introspection

Therefore the refinement of attention is of universal relevance. It involves training two faculties:

1. One is mindfulness, the faculty of sustaining voluntary attention, continuously, upon a chosen object. Whether it's a planet, or your child engaging in conversation, a piece of music, a business negotiation, or directing it to your own mind and observing mental events, continuously, without forgetfulness or distraction. Mindfulness is an extraordinarily important faculty of the mind that can be refined…beyond anything that can be imagined by the scientific community.

2. Introspection is a faculty of monitoring the mind, direct observing states of consciousness, and other mental processes.

As one cultivates attention one can specifically recognize attentional imbalances: when the mind falls into excitation, recognize it swiftly, and bring the mind back to balance; when the mind falls into laxity or dullness, swiftly recognize it and bring it back to balance. In this way, we develop a telescope for observing the mind that is rigorous and gives rise to replicable and accurate observations.

The Goals of Training Attention

There are three goals of training attention:

1. To cultivate a deepening sense of ease and relaxation and looseness, of the body and mind…releasing stress, excess tension, feeling at ease in the present moment.

2. To cultivate stability: continuity and coherence of attention on an object, sustained continuously over time.

3. To cultivate a quality of vividness, which contains qualities of brightness, and focus of attention.

By cultivating them in sequence, and balancing and synergistically integrating these three qualities, you can apply refined attention to everything you do including: raising your children, music, art, business, athletics, science, and contemplative inquiry…even observing the depths of your own identity.

Integration with Science

How can we integrate this into scientific inquiry?

William James said introspection is difficult and fallible. Not everything we observe internally is accurate, and not everything we observe externally is accurate. There are optical and auditory illusions, but not all experiences are equally illusory. The difficulty is in all observation of whatever kind, including scientific observations, which are difficult and fallible. The only safeguard is in the final consensus of later knowledge of the thing in question, as later views can correct earlier, more fallible ones, until the harmony of a consistent view is finally reached…

Let communities of individuals trained rigorously in attention and introspection make their observations, and some of them will be incorrect, but by making further ones and more sophisticated ones, gradually the errors can be removed. Then, there can be a "science of mind" based primarily on introspection with the additional methods of behavioral psychology and cognitive neuroscience. William James was proposing that these two methods of studying the mind indirectly, by means of behavior and the brain, be integrated with our primary mode of observation, introspection. Again, that science has never occurred, but it could.

To return to empiricism in order to rescue science from the trap of scientific materialism is one of the great challenges of the day.

We need to bring science back to its truly broadly empirical roots…and encourage our scientists to be skeptical of their own assumptions. It is not truly empirical science to simply be skeptical of the assumptions of those who believe in spirits or believe in God, or believe in reincarnation. It is so easy…it is too easy to be skeptical of others' beliefs and not be skeptical of your own assumptions.

Richard Feynman, PhD, a Nobel Laureate in Physics, presents the ideal of scientific inquiry this way:

> It is only through refined measurements and careful experimentation that we can have a wider vision. And then we see unexpected things: we see things that are far from what we would guess—far from what we could have imagined… If science is to progress, what we need is the ability to experiment, honesty in reporting results—the results must be reported without somebody saying what they would like the results to have been… One of the ways of stopping science would be only to do experiments in the region where you know the law. But experimenters search most diligently, and with the greatest effort, in exactly those places where it seems most likely that we can prove our theories wrong. In other words we are trying to prove ourselves wrong as quickly as possible, because only in that way can we find progress. (Feynman 1965, pp.127, 148, 158)

An ideal beautifully stated…but hard to live up to.

I think we are poised now historically for the first true revolution in the mind sciences. This must include rigorous, sustained training in the direct observation of non-physical phenomena such as states of consciousness, mental processes, and all other non-physical phenomena to complement third-person, mainstream scientific methods of inquiry.

Such a true science of the mind must explore the broadest possible range of states of consciousness—not only states of consciousness of normal people, the mentally ill, and those with brain damage, which is where almost all scientific research on the mind is focused. Rather, it must also include first-person and third-person exploration of extraordinary states of consciousness—the consciousness of a medium, an advanced yogi, of a person who recalls past lives—and not reject such experiences simply because they are incompatible with what we assumed to be true. This is the attitude of medieval scholastics and closed-minded materialists. It is not worthy of science… It is shameful for science. It is the attitude of exactly what science was designed to overcome.

Who will rescue science from its own dogmatism? We must integrate the methods of psychology, neuroscience, and philosophy with first-person rigorous inquiry into states of consciousness by way of contemplative inquiry. I think that is the great challenge.

Notes

1.   This chapter was excerpted from the keynote address that Alan Wallace gave at the beginning of the Spiritist Medical Congress in Porto Alegre, in June 2009, titled "The Interface between Science and Spirituality."

2.   Occam's razor is a principle of adopting the hypothesis that makes the fewest new assumptions, when competing hypotheses are equal in other respects. For instance, they must both sufficiently explain available data in the first place.

Chapter 15

SPIRIT ATTACHMENT AND HEALTH

Alan Sanderson, MD

My Introduction to Spirit Release

How did a British psychiatrist, only recently returned to clinical practice after two decades of research, come to practice spirit release, a treatment strongly at variance with the concepts of conventional psychiatry? It was 1993. I was happy to again be treating patients in the National Health Service (NHS), but it was disappointing to find that, in my 20 years' absence, clinical practice had scarcely changed. Medication had failed to fulfill expectations and psychological therapies and social manipulation were often ineffective. There had to be a new way.

I heard of spirit release from a complete outsider. The idea appealed to me. I invited a demonstration and I was impressed by the response in some of my hospital patients. Through study, training, and practice I became proficient in spirit release and related therapies. Since then, I have used it on many hundreds of patients, initially in the NHS and now in private practice. Spirit release is a powerful but gentle way of helping patients to change. It has also changed me. I used to be a reluctant materialist, convinced by science that it was the only true system of belief. This new work gave me evidence of a spiritual dimension in which we are immersed as fully as fish in water.

Historical Perspective

Spirit release is practiced in many different forms. Familiarity with the subject requires some knowledge of how it developed.

In the West, for nearly two millennia following Christ's death, spirit release was a religious procedure, the Christian rite of exorcism. It was not until the mid-nineteenth century that Allan Kardec, intrigued by mediumship, entered upon his careful research into spirit manifestations. This led in 1860 to *The Spirits' Book* (Kardec 2003), purporting to contain the channeled wisdom from higher spirits, contacted through mediums. It constitutes the Spiritist doctrine, of which the most significant divergences from Christian teaching are the acknowledgment of reincarnation and the belief that angels and demons do not exist as such, but are human spirits at the extremes of moral development. It is obsession by the spirits of deceased humans which, Spiritists claim, is a common cause of psychological disturbance. Kardec's teaching was taken up strongly in Brazil where, 150 years on, Spiritist principles inspire the practice in many psychiatric hospitals and thousands of Spiritist Centers.

The twentieth century brought the influence of other major pioneers: Carl Wickland in the 1920s and Edith Fiore, William Baldwin, and Samuel Sagan in the 1980s and 1990s. Wickland, an American psychiatrist, describes in *Thirty Years Among the Dead* (1974, p.33) how static electricity was applied to the patient's head and back, in order to drive out possessing spirits. They entered his wife, Anna, who sat in a neighboring room, surrounded by a "concentration circle" of human helpers. Through Anna the spirits spoke with Carl, who engaged them in a lively dialogue and often persuaded them to leave. This was an effective but dangerous procedure. Mrs. Wickland ended her life in a mental hospital.

Sixty years passed before another professional, Edith Fiore, a psychologist specializing in past life regression by hypnosis, pioneered a new approach to spirit release. In *The Unquiet Dead* (1987) she describes conversing with spirits, through her clients, and releasing them, to the mutual benefit of host and spirit. Fiore had a great influence. Her work was developed with energy, dedication, and understanding by Baldwin, who extended it to non-human spirits and wrote the first textbook, *Spirit Releasement Therapy—A Technique Manual* (1992), still the best text of the new, interactive approach, for it is replete with technical descriptions and case histories.

Dr. Samuel Sagan, founder of Clairvision, though less influential generally, is a major voice in Australia and teaches in California. Sagan's approach (1997) to past life therapy and spirit release combines meditation and spoken guidance. He teaches that the great majority of attached entities come from fragmentation of the astral body at death. Other teachers include Ken Page (1999), a leader in intuitive therapy, Shakuntala Modi (1997), a psychiatrist in the USA who stresses the importance of demonic entities, and Sue Allen (2007), a leader in intuitive work. In the UK, the Spirit Release Foundation (SRF),[1] founded in 1999, teaches both intuitive and interactive approaches to release.

Spirit Attachment and the Cycle of Rebirth

Alternation between embodiment on earth and timeless, more or less blissful, existence in the spirit world, preparing for reincarnation, is the essential pattern. At death the spirit usually passes to the Light, the white brilliance seen in a near-death experience. However, it does not invariably reach the Light. It may be confused, even to the point of not knowing that the body has died. Ignorance or fear of punishment may cause it to be diverted. Some spirits remain earthbound in familiar places, where they may appear as ghosts, or they may attach to embodied humans. They may stay behind with the intention of attachment, perhaps out of concern for a relative, or to satisfy an addiction, even for revenge. Family sex abusers seem commonly to attach to their victims. Suicidal persons may have spirits with them which encourage suicide.

Phenomenology

The effects of spirit attachment may be so slight as to be imperceptible or so great as to cause incapacity. In the great majority of cases, attached spirits have no executive power. They may influence feelings and perceptions, but do not displace the host from environmental awareness or from control of bodily movement, except rarely, for brief periods, as during fugue states and in the "blackouts" experienced by alcoholics. Only a tiny minority show the switching of identity and memory gaps so characteristic of multiple personality. High levels of psychic sensitivity seem to predispose to spirit attachment. Attached spirits do not have the ability to help the host, except in rare instances; not infrequently they seem bent on causing trouble.

Most attached spirits are unable to leave without assistance, though occasionally they come and go at will. Sometimes a human spirit may be correct in saying that its body lives. Soul fragments of living people (described by Clairvision as cords; Sagan 1997, pp.128–139) may attach to others, usually relatives, and have a controlling effect. In addition, there are non-human entities, both positive and negative. People may also be subject to psychic attack, in the form of spells or curses, or they may be controlled by pacts, which they have made in this or in a previous life. These are real phenomena, which must be combated with appropriate measures.

Negative thought forms may cause difficulties. They may appear as images symbolizing fear, anger, and destructiveness, or they may have an identity and be sent by others to cause trouble. They may need healing and angelic help to move on. I find Ireland-Frey's approach to thought forms by negotiation particularly helpful (1999, pp.187–209).

Vulnerability to Spirit Attachment

Vulnerability to spirit attachment varies according to predisposition, health, and circumstances. Illness, injury, the misuse of drugs and alcohol, emotional disturbance, and the presence of attached spirits may all impair resistance. Attempts to invoke spirits, particularly by using the Ouija board, can be dangerous. Organ transplantation may be another risk factor (Sylvia and Novak 1997). Certain individuals seem to attract spirits, often from those who, during life, had a similar problem. For instance, those that have suffered sexual abuse may be drawn together.

Effects of Spirit Attachment

Spirit attachment can affect people in many ways, either mildly or profoundly. Here are some of the most common:

- unexplained fatigue

- unexplained depression

- sudden changes in mood

- hearing a voice

- addictions of all sorts

- uncharacteristic changes in personality or behavior

- anomalous sexual behavior

- unexplained bodily symptoms.

It is important to note that there are many other causes of the above symptoms. Hearing voices is a characteristic feature of schizophrenia and is often experienced in dissociative identity disorder (DID), previously called multiple personality disorder. However, voices may also be due to other factors, such as flashbacks of traumatic events or a more or less autonomous part of the personality, such as a child part. Wilson Van Dusen, a psychologist at a Californian mental hospital, described in detail the voices heard by chronically ill patients (1972, pp.143–160). He classed them as lower order and higher order. His book *The Natural Depth in Man* (1972) is of great interest.

Helpful voices, such as those reported by Gandhi, Martin Luther, Joan of Arc, and other famous figures, may be attributed to spirit guides or to a divine source. Angels and spirit guides are essential allies in guiding souls to the Light and in healing the effects of spirit attachment. They do not readily communicate during therapy, but may do so, when asked. Such cases have been well described by Petrak (1996).

Diagnosis of Spirit Attachment

Spirit attachment is not a recognized psychiatric diagnosis. For this there are two reasons:

1. Spirits have no place in the materialistic paradigm of contemporary science.

2. Current systems of psychiatric classification are chiefly concerned with symptoms, not cause. The term "spirit attachment" would not be consistent with such a classification.

Identifying and Typing the Attached Spirit

Two distinct approaches are available for identifying and typing attached entities. Therapists gifted with clairvoyance may be able to sense and communicate with attached spirits, the Intuitive Approach. This does not require the participation or even the awareness of the afflicted person. The outcome will depend upon the abilities of the therapist and the prevailing situation. Spiritists employ the Intuitive Approach. Their method combines two different procedures simultaneously. Patient and, where possible, relatives are counseled and encouraged to pray for Christ's intervention and support, and a medium, surrounded by human helpers, at a distance from the patient, but in cooperation with Spiritist colleagues, engages attached spirits, and encourages them to leave. This team approach gives continuous support to patient, relatives, and therapists. In Spiritist Hospitals such work is often undertaken for severely ill patients, to whose needs and situation it is particularly well suited.

The less gifted (I am one) can learn the Interactive Approach, comprising two distinct techniques, either of which can be used, as appropriate.

1. *Direct communication* between spirit and therapist, via the patient's voice. This is achieved with the patient in a hypnotic trance.

2. *Remote communication*, through a colleague. The facilitator helps a colleague, the scanner, into an altered state, and the scanner projects his/her conscious awareness to the patient, who may be at any distance and does not have to be aware of the procedure. Working closely together, the scanner responds to requests from the facilitator to relay words from any attached entities. In this way facilitator and entity communicate in much the same way as in the direct communication method, while the scanner is protected from the risk of channeling the entity. This technique may also be used during a direct communication session, should patient and therapist agree that it is appropriate to work on a relative. An important proviso when doing remote work is that the higher self of the target person should agree to the procedure.

Of the two methods described, direct work has the advantage that the patient is consciously engaged in the procedure, a desirable state of affairs when important changes are undertaken. However it depends upon the patient acting as his or her own scanner, a role for which he or she is not always well suited. The remote technique has obvious benefits in treating children, or adults who cannot enter an altered state, and it has the further advantage that an experienced scanner may discover things of which the patient is ignorant.

Uncovering Techniques

These techniques are necessary for interactive direct work.

1. *The use of finger signals.* These are set up in communication with the unconscious mind. They are a first step towards verbal communication with any attached entities.

2. *Engaging a voice.* If the patient (xxxx) hears a voice, it is usually appropriate to engage the voice directly. "What is your name? Are you part of xxxx, or someone else? Did you ever have a human, physical body of your own? What effect have you had on xxxx? Why are you here?" etc. The patient's voice may change markedly when an entity is communicating. Occasionally a patient will speak a language unlearned and not consciously known to the patient. This is known as xenoglossy, and has been described both in hypnosis and in normal consciousness (see Stevenson 1984).

3. *Body scan.* The patient, in an altered state, visualizes light filling the body and then focuses on any shadowy areas or abnormal sensations. The therapist encourages communication: "If that dark area were to make a sound, what would it be? What has the heavy sensation in the back got to say?"

4. *Mirror scan.* Have the patient imagine standing in front of a full-length mirror. Another figure or some unexplained bodily feature will give an indication of possible spirit attachment.

Treatment

Helping a spirit to move on can be a frustrating task. It may feel that its presence is necessary to the host, or it may aim to harm, even to kill, the host. The feelings of the host are also important, for without full commitment to being rid of the spirit the attempt is likely to fail. A harmful entity may gain acceptance in the guise of a guide, or by stimulating the patient sexually or by other enticements. Sometimes the entity does not see the Light, or the Light is only dim. In such cases there are several possibilities to consider. There may be fragmentation of the spirit, with a part attached to a relative or to a neighboring location. Or perhaps the reluctant spirit must itself be freed from spirit parasitism. A past life connection may need exploration. Once impediments have been cleared, the spirit of a loved one or a spirit guide from the Light is called for. It is necessary to check that these rescuers are in fact who they claim to be. This may be done by asking three times, "Are you from the Light?" Imposters leave when pressed on this point.

When the last entity appears to have left, one asks for healing spirits from the Light to remove any residue and to fill with light the spaces where the entities were. Finally the patient performs the Sealing Light meditation, filling the body with golden-white light, which extends an arm's length in every direction. Cleared patients are advised to regard themselves as convalescent, to lead a quiet life for a few days, and to be prepared for changes in behavior.

The environment, both human and physical, in which the affected person lives, also needs to be considered in the treatment plan.

It is important to mention here that not all cases respond to these methods. Those associated with physical movements or vocal utterances to the effect that the entity is determined to remain, and cases where voices give inconsistent replies or refuse to communicate, present particular difficulty.

The Effects of Treatment

While spirit release can bring dramatic benefit, it is only one aspect of the treatment process, and it is rarely sufficient in isolation.

To treat schizophrenia with this technique is a major undertaking, since the patient will almost certainly lack the ego strength and clear boundaries necessary to participate in *successful treatment.* Lack of trust is another problem. Shakuntala Modi, in *Remarkable Healings* (1997), reports a successful case in which treatment was first given remotely, through a relative who attended with the patient. Clearly, much depends on the expertise of the therapist. One must admire Dr. Modi's skill. If a schizophrenic patient consulted me I would hope to find an able Spiritist group to give assistance.

Spirit release has been used successfully in the treatment of gender identity disorder. Barlow, Abel and Blanchard (1977) reported the case of a 20-year-old male who underwent an exorcism, when about to have a sex change operation. He lost all his female behavioral characteristics, a change that was maintained two years later. Fiore has successfully treated a similar case (Fiore 2011). I have had some failures, especially in the severely mentally ill, but the great majority of my patients have improved. It is important to stress that even after spirit release there is often a need for other treatments, such as soul retrieval, regression, and counseling.

Before advising a release, the patient should be warned of three possibilities:

1. Other spirits may be found at a later check. The work is like peeling an onion.

2. Spirit release may be followed by exhaustion, even for days.

3. A sense of loss. For complications of this see the next section.

How can we prove that the beneficial effect of treatment comes from the release of spirits? There is no proof, nor can there be. Even detailed verification of information provided by spirits about their bodily lives will not convince the doubters. But because the treatment works, we can claim clinical validity.

It is necessary to enter a caveat here. There are two dangers that need to be considered before entering upon spirit release.

Dangers of Spirit Release

The first point to make is that spirit release is a very safe procedure and complications are exceptional. However, there are two important dangers that need to be considered before deciding on release work:

1. *Suicidal behavior.* This can follow a profound sense of loss in a patient who was dependent on a relative whose spirit attaches after death. Release should not be attempted unless the dependency has been effectively dealt with by psychotherapy.

2. *Excessive anxiety.* In considering the best action, it is important to distinguish between the fear of the patient, and the fear of an attached spirit, worried about being removed by the therapist. When a patient is unduly fearful about the possibility of a spirit being present, direct work is contraindicated. In such cases remote work or an intuitive approach may be preferable.

Assessing the Different Approaches to Spirit Attachment and Release

It is evident from the foregoing that there are many views on spirit attachment and many techniques of spirit release. Individuals and organizations have their own distinct outlook and methods of working. The subject resembles that of the elephant that was described differently by each observer depending upon whether trunk, ear, or foot was in focus. Church exorcists, mediums, psychiatrists, psychologists, and healers have all studied different population groups at different times and developed very different beliefs. Spiritism and Christian theology have different convictions and different methods of interaction with entities. Each has its own doctrine. While doctrine gives valuable coherence to an organization, it has the disadvantage that it limits openness to change, which is the essence of scientific exploration. This should be borne in mind when reading this chapter, since I write largely of my own beliefs and working practices, which are neither fixed nor certain.

Protection

The psyche has its own immune system—integrity. If you have integrity, wholeness of the psyche, and personal well-being, then all the little things which might attach to you don't grab hold, just as the physical body fends off attacks every day. Even so, it is wise for those who practice spiritual therapies to take precautions. Many protective techniques are in use (Matthews 2005). These include awareness of subtle energy, cleansing the aura, protective visualization, and grounding. Crystals, essences, and herbs are also widely used.

Some people are especially open to spirit interference and should avoid any psychic activity. Such people and all therapists would do well to arrange a regular scan by a psychic sensitive.

The Need for Research

In Western countries—Brazil is a wonderful exception—talk of attached spirits is likely to bring derision. We have far to go to reach a place of public and scientific credibility. I do not know of any research studies which use the accepted methodology of contemporary science. We have some good excuses—no time, no money, no academic support, no access to scientific journals. Even if these were overcome and impressive research confirmation was published, would anyone take notice? Eventually yes, but it will be a long journey.

I have two basic proposals:

1. *More case studies.* Outcome studies from individual cases are a first step. However, they need to be carefully recorded and have adequate follow-up information. Without this they have no research value. We need case studies in books, in journals, and on the Internet, our staunchest ally.

2. *Consistent belief.* We shall not gain respect if we speak with different voices. For instance, on the existence of demonic entities, there are profound unvoiced disagreements. Such a situation could not exist in science. Our views will not be seriously considered when there is such divergence. In a recent debate among Spirit Release Foundation members, concerning the existence of demonic entities, the two sides were balanced. The subject needs to be examined in case studies and discussed openly. Another debate might be centered on Clairvision's teaching that most entities are fragments of astral bodies.

How might one focus research, if the facilities for planned studies were to become available? We need clinical trials. It is necessary to study conditions of long standing, which do not respond to any other treatment. Persistent auditory hallucinations, gender identity disorder, and pedophilia are examples. To investigate spirit release for such conditions one needs good experimental design, time, money, and determination. We also need medical colleagues who will give access to cases.

Consideration of research deserves more than this brief summary. It is a major concern requiring persistent attention and funding.

The Future of Spirit Release

Things are moving. The increasing practice of spirit release and the appearance of books and journals on a wide range of spiritually based therapies augers well for the future. The related practices of past life and inter-life regression are also advancing strongly.

We must salute the Spiritists of Brazil, the only organization in the world to have therapy centers (12,000 plus!) and hospitals dedicated to spiritual work of this type, much of which is freely given. While there are active organizations in the UK, USA, Australia, and Germany, there is nothing to compare with Spiritism's 150 years of existence and considerable achievement.

In England a secular and evidence-based approach to spiritual work, under the name of Rational Spirituality, has recently been developed by Ian Lawton (2008), whose books focus particularly on past life and inter-life studies. This work seems likely to add to the acceptance of spirit attachment as a related phenomenon.

In addition to these developments there is tremendous energy under the heading of non-doctrinal spiritual activity and we seem to be moving on a tide of planetary change in human consciousness.

The time was not right when Allan Kardec made his optimistic predictions for change. Ahead of us now are opportunities that even he could not have dreamed of.

Note

1.   See www.spiritrelease.com.

Chapter 16

SOUL-CENTERED PSYCHOTHERAPY

Andrew Powell, MD[1]

Introduction

Spirituality can be described as the striving for a deep-seated sense of meaning and purpose in life, a wholeness that brings with it the feeling of belonging, harmony, and peace. It entails searching for answers about the infinite, and is particularly important in times of stress, illness, loss, bereavement, and death. For some people, but by no means all, this sense of oneness is found explicitly in relation to God as the ultimate source of love.

The spiritual longing for wholeness permeates body, soul, and spirit. Through the body we celebrate the gift of life in eating, drinking, making love, and bearing children—the primeval spiritual impulse that seeks to merge two into one. When we are attuned to Soul, we realize that we are mirrored in each other, indeed that ultimately there is no "other"—all humanity is therefore one. When we align with Spirit, we participate in the flux of the universe as it constantly creates form and dissolves back into energy, one such form being life here on Earth.

Trying to define terms like Spirit and Soul is fraught with difficulties. By Spirit I refer to the limitless and unbounded consciousness that energizes this universe (and doubtless others, too). I use the word Soul for the manifestation of Spirit through form. In this sense, a pebble on the beach has Soul—but it is at the level of a vibration of atoms. In the plant kingdom, Soul takes the form of a collective sentient field. In the animal kingdom, Soul has acquired awareness; dogs and cats are just as aware as you and me, and living as they do, entirely in the "now," their awareness is all the more keen. But in the human species, Soul has advanced to the stage of self-consciousness, the awareness of awareness; it is a privilege which opens the door to Heaven, but which, if abused, leads to Hell on Earth.

Self-consciousness bestows on us our sense of individuality. Whether individuality, once acquired, is forever preserved, or whether our ultimate destination is to merge with the source of All That Is, none of us can know for sure. However, I don't doubt that, for the time being, we exist in a multiplicity of virtual dimensions. It's just that I and you both happen to be here, in this one, right now. Even though I know this reality to be a sea of energy, of waves and particles, or, according to string theory, little vibrating loops of "string," it is, of course, entirely real, tangible, and solid to me, and to everyone who shares it with me.

The soul knows it is never alone, for there is a deep connection which goes back to our divine origination. Experiencing this life as a precious but ephemeral gift, the soul views the death of the body with absolute equanimity. On the other hand, the ego is separative. Formed from our individual personalities, it fears death, indeed tries to deny it, since it dreads the prospect of obliteration. Yet the ego is necessary to the outward journey, as it has been called, of the first half of life. This is when we desire to make our mark on life, an impression we may even think is going to last. The soul knows that any impression we make on the world is transient; instead, it takes us on the return journey, when we are obliged to harvest, for good or ill, what we sowed.

Soul and Ego must live together—for without Ego there would be nothing for Soul to learn from the classroom of life and without Soul we could not evolve beyond the most destructive life form on Earth. The human race killed more than 100 million of its own kind during the twentieth century. Never was the perspective of Soul more needed.

Despite this appalling statistic, I am an optimist, believing as I do that we are all here as spiritual beings on a human journey. The problem is that the human race is a very young species and we haven't yet learned how to stop acting on the impulse of Ego and listen more to Soul.

As a psychiatrist, I came to soul-centered therapy via a roundabout route that included psychoanalysis, group analysis, psychodrama, and the work of Carl Jung. Later I went on to study healing and other transpersonal approaches. But it was during my training in psychodrama that I first witnessed the power of Soul in action, and so this is where I shall begin with my case studies.

Soul Wisdom

During a psychodrama session, a woman who had been deeply embittered by the loss of her son years before returned to the roadside scene of the car crash in which he had been killed. Weeping in despair, she cried out, "God, why have you done this to me?" The psychodrama therapist immediately instructed her to reverse roles with God. At once this mother's face changed, becoming calm and composed, her sobbing ceased, and as God she exclaimed with immense dignity, "I have done nothing to you. Your son chose to die, so that he would not suffer anymore. Be happy for him and thankful for his life which brought you joy."

The woman was amazed by what had come out of her own mouth. She could see the meaning of it perfectly and for the first time since her son's death she could begin to heal.

What I had observed was a defining moment for me—I was amazed by the strength and wisdom of Soul. With hindsight, I might say that it was where my interest in healing began. Incidentally, the word "healing" comes from the same root as wholeness. Unlike the man-made concept of cure, wholeness is humankind's spiritual birthright, provided we don't mess it up.

Connecting with Soul

Christine was chronically depressed. Throughout childhood, she never felt valued for her own self. Academic success had temporarily bolstered her self-esteem. Later, it fell apart when a personal relationship failed. Her emotions froze over and she became profoundly withdrawn.

Christine had described her depression as a black cave, so I invited her to close her eyes, go inside, and report back with what she could find. After some minutes she found a pair of steel handcuffs, then a rope and an iron chain. I pressed her to go on looking. After what seemed an eternity, her expression changed to one of concern, so I asked her what she had found. It was a little puppy in a dark corner. I suggested she pick it up and hold it to her. With her eyes still closed, she cradled the puppy. What could she feel? She replied that she could feel the puppy's love for her. I urged her to let her own love flow to this puppy and she began to cry. I suggested she find an image for her emotion and she chose a heart made of gold.

The process can be understood psychologically, the puppy symbolizing the child Christine. She rediscovers and nurtures this child self, which she had lost touch with, and in doing so discovers that she still has the capacity for love. In terms of spiritual object relations, we can see Christine as reclaiming her soul, that had been buried in the wasteland of childhood.

Treasuring the Soul

Carol's story had been one of terrible abuse and for years she had taken refuge in alcohol. During the first interview, I encouraged her to look inside herself and tell me what she found there. What Carol saw was "her heart beating so hard it could burst." What did she want to do with it? She put it to rest in a silk-lined coffin, saying "only death will bring it peace." But then, after a moment, the heart transformed into a little whirligig of energy. It would not be trapped but flew about the room. So she released it and watched it fly away.

Images of the soul are incapable of death. But Carol was not ready or able to harness her soul for her own benefit and she did not take up the offer of therapy, which would have meant abstaining from alcohol.

Nearly four years later Carol came to see me again, in the meantime having faced up to her drinking. This time, when she went inside herself, she found a treasure chest. I asked if she could pick up the treasure chest. She put it under her arm and soon found an archway and went through. Now she found herself in a sandy desert, by a pool of water and some trees. She sat by the water, resting peacefully, and said with a sigh, "This is for me!" (All her life she has rushed around trying to please others.) Did she want a drink? She drank deeply of the cool fresh water. Now where did she need to go? She immediately found herself back home, still holding the treasure chest, studded with jewels and very beautiful. She placed it on the floor in the middle of the room. Following this session, therapy was offered and accepted.

A Soul Dream

My patient had been born into circumstances of great deprivation. Fortunately he was saved from a life in care by being taken in, aged four, by a neighbor, Bob, who from that time on was father in all but name.

The boy grew into a man and made good. He married, had a family, and moved south. But he often went back to see Bob, now ageing and alone but fiercely independent. Then the time came when Bob grew so frail, his neighbors had to come in and start washing and caring for him. Bob couldn't bear it. One day he got himself upstairs to the spare bedroom, lay down with his cap on his head as always, and swallowed a lot of tablets and died.

My patient was devastated at the news. He kept dreaming Bob was still alive only to wake up and find him gone. He fell into a severe depression.

He then told me that, just before attending this consultation, something had happened which had "knocked him for six." He had dreamed again of Bob but this was different.

In the dream, he knew for the first time that Bob was dead. Yet there was Bob, sitting across from him, large as life, cap on head, just the way he always sat. My patient asked him outright, "Bob, are you dead?" Bob answered him as direct as ever, "Yes!" His next question to Bob was, "Is there life after death?" Another emphatic "Yes" came right back. Then he challenged Bob head on. "Prove it to me!" Bob pulled out a book that looked like a Bible with detailed drawings in it and, sure enough, the proof was all there.

Then he awoke. All day he could intensely feel Bob's presence. He found his emotions welling up and, although it was very painful, he could say to me in that first meeting "I know I'm getting better."

Soul to Soul

Rosemary came to see me several years after her teenage daughter Tessa had attempted suicide, which had left her with severe brain damage. Rosemary felt deeply responsible and the torment of her grief was immense. She could no longer bring herself to visit her once lovely daughter, who now lay immobile, with severe contractures. "I cannot bear seeing what she has turned into," she raged, after a rare visit to the nursing home.

I had been struck by a comment Rosemary made, that she dreaded going to see Tessa because as soon as she approached the room, even on the other side of the door, Tessa who normally lay silent and motionless would start to make loud moaning noises. Could Tessa sense that this was her mother visiting?

It seemed to me there could be no healing until Rosemary was able to face her daughter. I advised her when going into the room immediately to fix her gaze only on Tessa's eyes, making sure not to look at her body while she drew near. We took time to rehearse this. When Rosemary came the next time, she said she had gone right up to Tessa, making sure to look only in her eyes. Tessa then stopped moaning and began to fixate on her mother's eyes. Rosemary found herself cradling her daughter and telling her that she loved her and would be coming again. One year later, Tessa was able to communicate a little with the help of a clock alphabet. She was now trying to crawl and surgery was being considered for treatment of her contractures.

It is no coincidence that the proverb "the eye is the mirror of the soul" is found throughout many cultures and countries.

Reunion of Souls

Joan came to see me about a year after the death of her husband, Ted, having nursed him through a long and debilitating illness. They had been together 40 years and her loss left her stricken with grief. She continually felt Ted's presence around the house, yet it brought only pain. I asked Joan if she thought there could be an afterlife. Yes, she thought there might be, but how could that help her now?

I asked her if she would like to try to make contact with Ted in a way that might bring her peace of mind. So at my suggestion Joan shut her eyes, relaxed, and was encouraged to see if she could "find" Ted wherever he might be. After a couple of minutes, a faint smile played on her lips. I asked Joan what she saw. She replied that she could see Ted in his cricket whites playing cricket and looking very fit and happy. I remarked that he seemed to be enjoying a game of celestial cricket. Joan's smile widened and she added that cricket had been Ted's great passion. Then a look of deep sadness passed across her face. I asked whether she would like to speak with Ted. She nodded, so I suggested she walk up to him and see what might happen. After a moment, Joan said that she was now standing next to him and that he had put his arm around her. What was he saying? He was saying, "Don't worry; everything is going to be all right." I asked Joan to look around her. Was anyone else present? Then she saw her deceased sister and parents there, smiling and waving to her. Being able to see death not as an ending but as a transition helped Joan to resume her life with hope and expectation.

A Soul That Never Got Born

Sometimes souls are together only a short time, as with children who die young, or who never reach their day of birth.

Gillian came with a depression that could be traced back to her earlier decision to have a termination of pregnancy. She has been a young single woman who found herself pregnant after a brief relationship. She felt sure at the time that it would be in everyone's best interests to end the pregnancy, so she sought medical advice and a planned surgical termination was carried out. Her physical recovery was uneventful, life moved on, and after some time she entered a new relationship which led to marriage. The couple tried for a child, but Gillian did not become pregnant. She became depressed, and found herself thinking back to the earlier termination of pregnancy, which she had kept secret. She started feeling that her current failure to conceive was a punishment for getting rid of her first baby.

In the session, as we explored her feelings about the termination, Gillian began to cry. I asked her if she had ever wanted to talk with her unborn baby and she nodded. I suggested that we might do that now, if she wished. Again she nodded, so I handed her a pillow and asked her to cradle it in her arms, close her eyes, and picture the baby she was holding. She began sobbing. "What do you need to say to your baby?" I urged her. Gillian burst out, "What have I done? I'm so sorry for what I did to you." "Now let the baby speak," I said, and, through her, I asked the baby, "What did Gillian do to you?" The baby answered, "It was a terrible shock, I was just lying there and then something came in and I was torn to pieces."

In a termination of pregnancy, the fetus, as it's referred to by doctors, is sucked out with a vacuum tube. What is not widely known is that, in the course of doing so, the tiny baby is literally torn limb from limb. Gillian was racked with remorse. "What else do you want Gillian to know?" I asked the baby. "Please stop crying," said the baby to her. "It was all over very quickly, and I'm fine now." I then said to the baby, "Do you know that Gillian cannot forgive herself for what she did?" The baby answered her, "You did the best you could at the time. And it was very nice being in you, even though I never got born. Don't blame yourself. I'm fine now, it's true." I asked Gillian if she wanted to say anything more to the baby. She said, "I'm so sorry, and I miss you and I think about you so much." The baby answered her, "It's only for now—we'll see each other again soon." I then asked Gillian to take some time in silence to be with her baby. As she sat rocking and holding the pillow, she gradually quieted. Then I asked her and the baby to say goodbye to each other for the present. Before she left, Gillian decided to tell her husband what had happened. I do not know if she subsequently became pregnant but I hope her chances will have improved.

Soul Retrieval

Sally, in her mid-fifties, was suffering from treatment-resistant depression. Her problems had begun in early childhood, which had been blighted with insecurity. When she was seven, she fell into the hands of a fundamentalist schoolteacher, Miss Edwards, who terrified the child with threats of hell and damnation. Sally had recurring visions of flames licking around her bed and the red face of the devil would appear at night and in her dreams.

In adulthood Sally seemed to overcome these fears but, following major surgery, which left her body scarred, she once again succumbed to these visions, living from day to day in a state of sheer panic.

First, Sally was encouraged to visualize her soul. She located it inside her chest but as a feeble thing, not much more than a glimmer of light. I asked her to look carefully to see if there were any strands or cords running out from it into the darkness. She found such a cord, so I urged her to follow it and see where it led. After a moment she looked up and said she could see Miss Edwards, looking very old but as fierce as ever, holding the end of the cord tightly in her hand.

I then had a frank discussion with Miss Edwards, speaking with her through the agency of Sally. Miss Edwards insisted that what she did what was right, the child had to be controlled and, if she instilled fear in her, it was for her own good. I pointed out that, instead of helping, it had only led to a lifetime of misery and torment. Is this what Miss Edwards as a Christian really intended? She faltered and I pressed home my advantage. She herself would now be nearing the end of her life and soon facing her Maker. How will she be judged? Then Miss Edwards became fearful. She hadn't intended harm and she hoped God would have pity on her. I put it to her that she could start making amends right now by letting go of Sally's soul and giving it back to her. Miss Edwards agreed and let go of the cord. I asked Sally to draw it back into herself, after which we spent some time on healing.

Following the session, Sally reported that the red devil had lost his power over her. The next step would be to help Sally find compassion for that child who had lived with so much fear.

A Soul Remembers

Peter, aged 27, came to see me with a water phobia. Having been a good swimmer and with no evident neurotic traits, he was traveling on a small ferry when he suffered a severe panic attack. He had been looking over the side of the boat at the time and the thought came to him that, if he were to fall overboard, he would be swept away and would drown. *No one would ever know what had happened to him.*

Going into Peter's personal history revealed no obvious cause for this acute episode. I asked him to close his eyes and re-live the scene, this time imagining falling into the water. Peter's body immediately began jerking and thrashing about. I said "What's happening?" and he cried out, "I can't get free, I'm drowning." I then instructed him to go back in time to just before this moment. He said despairingly, "We've been rammed and water's coming in the boat." "Why can't you get free?" "I'm chained to the boat!"

I took Peter forward again in time to the moment of drowning. His struggling movements became weaker and he went limp. What was happening now? "I'm leaving my body, I'm rising up through the water, and I'm going higher, up into the sky." "What can you see?" "There's a bright light, I want to go there." I said, "Before you leave, look back on this life you just lived and tell me about yourself and how old you are." "I'm 27," he said, and told the story of a young man fighting in the Greco-Persian wars, who had spent the last two years of his life as a slave oarsman on a Greek trireme. During a naval battle with the Persians, the ship had gone down with all on board. The young man's wife and children would *never know what had happened to him.*

By way of what is called an "affect bridge," Peter had slipped into a "past life." The process can be understood in various ways, from the psychological to the transpersonal. What is not in question is that resolving such soul dramas can have an immediate and lasting therapeutic effect.

Healing for Two Souls

Alice was a 43-year-old lady who came with a ten-year history of sarcoid, an auto-immune disease that was causing her to go blind. She was increasingly reliant on her husband, John, to care for her. Theirs was a loving marriage and she said of him with a smile, "He was a good catch!" Alice's loss of sight was challenging her to try to make sense of her misfortune. Recently she had heard about past life regression and wanted to see if it could provide any clue.

The sarcoid had begun with blinding headaches. In the session we went back to that time when she lay exhausted and crying, holding her head in her hands in a darkened room.

I asked Alice to find words for the terrible pain in her head. If her headache could speak what would it say? She cried out, "Let me alone. Let me be free." I suggested she give in to the longing and see where it took her. Her face relaxed and she lay with her eyes closed and a smile on her lips. At once, she found herself lazing in the warm, calm water of a tropical ocean. I asked her to look around. She could see the sandy shore some way off and, beyond that, dense vegetation covering the lower slopes of distant mountains. Next, I asked her to look down at her body. She said with astonishment, "I'm…like a fish." Then she exclaimed, "No, not a fish, I'm a dolphin!" Her expression was one of intense pleasure. I asked if there were any other dolphins nearby. It transpired that this young dolphin had disobeyed her parents and had swum off on her own.

I then asked her to go forward in time to the next important thing that happened. She found herself lying on the sand, unable to move. (Alice's body started making ineffectual jerking movements on the couch.) I asked her to check her body and she became aware of a large hole in her side. Now tears began to trickle down her cheeks. There was no pain but her strength was ebbing. She looked up and could see the prow of a boat a few feet away. Standing on it and staring at her was a fisherman with painted face and body, holding a spear in his hand. Then the boat slid away. As darkness fell, she grew calm. Suddenly she found herself rising up into the sky and looking down, without emotion or regret, at the lifeless body of the dolphin on the beach.

Did she need to face this fisherman who had killed her with his spear? At first she was reluctant, saying, "It wasn't his fault. He never killed another dolphin." Then she agreed that it could be important. So she waited there for a while until his turn came to die and he crossed over. Now she could see the fisherman coming closer. Involuntarily, she found herself going forward and embracing him. I asked her if she recognized him. "Of course, it's my husband John," she said, beginning to laugh and cry at the same time. "He caught me and this time I've caught him. We are together and he is here to take care of me!"

Release of an Earthbound Spirit

Pat had suffered from depression for many years. Since childhood, she had longed for approval but felt she could never please. Her mother would mock and belittle her and Pat was often full of anger that she never dared express.

When her mother died, Pat heaved a sigh of relief thinking she could now get on with her own life. But she found she could not, for Mother's presence was all around and she still seemed to hear her mother scorning her. Feeling possessed by her mother, as she put it, Pat had become suicidal.

I said to Pat that suicide would resolve nothing and that we needed to find a way to help the two of them separate. I invited her to confront her mother in death as she had not been able to in life. We did this by using an empty chair. Pat went right ahead; she was able to face her mother for the first time with a few home truths and told her it was time she got off her back.

I now asked Pat to sit in the empty chair and role reverse with Mother. Mother came straight through, saying she had no intention of stopping! She enjoyed hanging around Pat and in any case she had nowhere else to go.

I asked the mother, through Pat, about the life she had just lived and I learned that her own mother had rejected her from an early age. She resolved to escape from home and took the first man she could to help her get away. But getting pregnant with Pat when she was 17 ended her hopes of a career and tied her to a man she did not love. Her daughter became the life-long target of her resentment.

I explained to Mother the benefits to her of moving on and to see if there were any friends that could help take her on her way. To begin with, nobody appeared and so I urged her to look for just one person in her whole life that had shown her kindness. After a long pause, she recalled a Mrs. Cox, who had been a nurse staying with Mother's family for a time and who made a real fuss over the little girl. As Mother recalled her nurse, her face softened and I asked her to try to find her. Then she smiled and said she could now see Mrs. Cox, looking just the way she did all those years ago. I asked her to take her hand and walk towards the Light. There was no further protest and she left with her friend. When this was over, Pat looked emotionally drained but at peace. She went back to her own chair and said, "It feels that she has really gone, for the first time."

Suicide and Spirit Attachment

A young woman came to see me feeling unwell and "not herself." She had been told she was clinically depressed; anti-depressant medication had helped but she was still "not herself." I was struck by her use of the phrase.

Going into the background, I learned that, a few months before the symptoms began, this woman's friend had killed herself in the patient's home, having been staying there while my patient was away on holiday. By the time she got back, everything had been tidied up and the funeral had already taken place.

Remembering how she had twice said she was "not herself," I asked her if she had the feeling of someone else when she came back home. She replied that she hadn't wanted to mention it in case I thought she was mad, but every time she went into the house, she had the physical sensation that her friend was right there in the room with her.

Taking this at face value, I asked if she would like me to invite the spirit of her deceased friend to the consultation to see if we could get some further clues. She was willing, so I asked her to close her eyes, tune in to her friend, and try letting her friend speak through her.

Her friend came through and went on to express deep regret at having taken her life. Suicide had solved nothing. She remained unhappy and lonely and seeking comfort. I explained that staying on was having a bad effect on my patient, and was doing nothing for her either. She apologized. "If only I had known," she said, "what I know now. I was facing the biggest challenge of my life and I went and messed it up. I feel even worse than I did before." I said I was sure other opportunities would be given her. She was very relieved to hear this and we talked more about her hopes for another chance at life. When she said she was ready to move on, I asked her to look for the Light. She exclaimed with a smile "Yes, I can see it," and left at once. The moment she went, my patient felt the burden of oppression lift from her and it did not return.

Spirit Release from a Past Life

Barbara, my patient, had been visiting a well-known museum and wanted to look at the paintings on the first floor. There was a big central staircase with stairwells on both sides. Halfway up, she started feeling dizzy and could not proceed. Since that time, open spaces and heights triggered severe panic attacks.

I asked Barbara to close her eyes and imagine herself back at the bottom of the stairs. She became visibly tense and I asked her to focus on the sensation of fear and go with the feeling to the very first time it happened, wherever that might be.

With some surprise, Barbara reported that she was standing at the bottom of a stone pyramid with big steps leading upwards and a sheer drop on each side. She was wearing rough leather sandals and a long cotton skirt. I asked her what she was doing there. She replied that she was going to be sacrificed by the chief priest. She could see him waiting for her at the top of the pyramid, where he would cut her throat.

How had she come to be chosen? This took her back to a scene in the village the night before, when the elders had singled her out and said, "It might as well be her." She had no relatives to protect her and so she was dragged away. I asked her to go back further, to her childhood in that lifetime. She told me her name was Miria. By nature she was a solitary child, who liked to play alone in the forest. Later, being fiercely independent, she scared away her suitors, which left her with no husband to protect her and no status in village life.

As if in a trance she now climbed slowly up the pyramid steps. The height made her dizzy. At the top she was lifted onto the stone slab and the priest raised his sword. Suddenly it was over and she was free. There was no pain.

Miria floated away from the body but remained suspended in a shadowy, featureless world. I asked her to look around and tell me if she could see anyone. Looking down, Miria saw a five-year-old girl playing alone in the fields behind some houses. As she came closer, she could see that it was the child Barbara. Miria felt attracted to the little girl and so she stayed with her from that time on.

From the transpersonal perspective, Miria's spirit had remained earthbound, seeking solace in the company of another solitary child. The attachment only surfaced when the museum steps triggered a resurgence of fear in Miria, which had instantly and deeply affected my patient Barbara.

Once this was explained to Miria, she agreed to leave. I encouraged her to look for the Light, and after a short while, she found herself moving rapidly towards it and was gone.

"Demons" Have Souls Too

Janet, in her mid-twenties, had been depressed for many years. Her problems went back to an abusive relationship in her teens. Soon after, she developed chronic pelvic pain, for which she was now being told a hysterectomy might be needed.

I asked her to go within and "scan" her body and tell me what she saw there. Right away she described "a nasty dark red thing" attached to her womb. I invited it to speak and it explained, through Janet, that it had been there since Janet was 17. It was belligerent and boastful, saying it had made her ill and wasn't finished yet—it was going to give her cancer. When she heard this, Janet exclaimed, "It's a demon!"

She was anxious to free herself from this thing, so I suggested she visualize angels enclosing the "demon" in a bubble of light. At once it cried out in fear, "Stop, I'm going to burn." I pointed out to it that it was already trapped by the light, so it had better take refuge in the darkness within itself. I urged it to go deeper and deeper, and after a while it said with astonishment that it could see a light. The next moment it cried out in wonder, saying, "This feels so good, I feel so warm and nice!" Then it went on to say with great remorse, "What have I done? I have caused such pain and misery!" I said that only by going into the Light would it find forgiveness and the opportunity for redemption. It couldn't wait to leave!

This transformation of "negative" energy is an important aspect of spirit release work. We can see the "demon" as being just that, an attached entity, or we could regard it as a split-off complex of pathological object relations. From the clinical standpoint, the important thing is to decide when to work for integration and when to go for removal. In this case, the energetic complex was treated as a spirit attachment and released into the Light. However, further therapy would be helpful for Janet to understand why she had been vulnerable in the first place, and to stay well.

Psychotherapy for Soul Trauma

Helen, a woman in her forties, had become suddenly aware of feeling deeply emotionally burdened. There was nothing she could identify to account for it. All she could say was that she sensed the presence of a woman calling out to her in distress.

Helen wanted to understand more about this voice speaking to her from within. Through hypnotic induction I was able to make direct contact with the woman, Marianne, as she called herself, and below is the story that she told.

Marianne had lived several centuries ago. Her mother had died in childbirth and she had been brought up by her father who was an impoverished crofter. As a small child she fell ill, and the father, at his wit's end, left her close to death on the doorstep of a convent. Mother Superior found the child there and took her in. Marianne was nursed back to health, and although deeply affected by the loss of her father, she grew to love Mother Superior, who showed her great kindness. The convent became her home.

When she was little more than a child, there was a civil uprising and a band of drunken militia broke into the convent. Mother Superior insisted that Marianne hide herself and then went out with the other nuns to face the militia. The nuns were all raped and killed. Marianne could hear what was happening and was terrified. Later, she crept out to find bodies everywhere. Weeping, she ran into the nearby woods and there, overwhelmed with guilt at not saving her beloved Mother Superior, she hanged herself. Immediately she found herself, in spirit, back at the convent, unable to leave the scene of the massacre. From that time on, she wandered alone in a state of shock and deeply burdened by guilt, until she found herself attracted to Helen and "moved in."

The therapeutic task was to take this traumatized soul back to her suicide and help her complete the transition to the afterlife. As soon as she crossed over, the first person to greet her was Mother Superior. Marianne wept and asked for forgiveness. Mother Superior embraced her, saying, "You have nothing to blame yourself for." Marianne answered, "But how can I repay all you did for me?" Mother Superior replied, "I have waited a long time for you to come and you are repaying me now by enabling me to be the first person to greet you."

Then Marianne looked round and saw her father. He had died a few years after leaving his child at the door of the convent. Still in anguish as to whether he had done the right thing, he asked her to forgive him. Finally, Marianne's mother, who she had never known, appeared and lovingly greeted her. For the first time this family was complete and reunited.

Marianne never troubled Helen again. The therapeutic effect on Helen was profound, for it also addressed a life-long concern of her own, the feeling that it was dangerous to love without reservation, for fear of abandonment.

In a letter from Helen some months later, she explained how she and Marianne had both been released from what she called "the trap of abandonment." Through witnessing Marianne's reunion with Mother Superior and her parents, Helen could see that no one in Marianne's family had wished to cause hurt and rejection; on the contrary, their love for Marianne was profound. In the light of this experience,

Helen could now see that her own family, imperfect though it may have been, had done its best for her.

Conclusion

What is required when working with Soul? First, a willingness to consider spiritual reality to be as "real" as any aspect of life; second, a readiness to work beyond the bounds of consensus reality; and third, to trust that our patients already hold the key to their own healing, if only helped to make use of it.

I am not advocating soul-centered therapy as a catch-all. Many human problems can be explored and resolved psychodynamically without recourse to Spirit. Indeed, for some patients, too much "spirituality" can be a defense against confronting painful emotion, while other patients simply prefer to stay firmly grounded in the affairs of daily life. However, in the examples given here, the chosen field of action has been psycho-spiritual, unconstrained by the limits of physical reality, especially birth and death. Yet the aim is always to throw light on the complex challenges of human life, mindful that each scene in the play is essential to the working out of the greater whole. And when the depth and wisdom of the human soul is harnessed, it is plain to see that there is far more to life and death than, as some would claim, random mutations of "the selfish gene."

Note

1. Dr. Andrew Powell's publications on spirituality and health are available from the publications archive at www.rcpsych.ac.uk/spirit.

Chapter 17

CURRENT RESEARCH ON SURVIVAL OF CONSCIOUSNESS AND MEDIUMSHIP

Linda Russek, PhD

The mechanistic worldview has existed for three centuries. Scientists who held a mechanistic worldview sought results that were materially observable, localized, and could be correlated with hypothesized cause–effect interactions. These same scientists had the erroneous belief that they could remain separate and apart from their experiments, and thus maintain objectivity and not affect the outcome of their research. Through the application of the scientific method and experimental designs, consciousness was viewed as an emergent property of brain function, a mere by-product of the brain that ends with physical death.

There was no place for a wider view of consciousness in a deterministic universe where inviolable laws, reductionism, and local actions and their measurable effects on physical matter ordered the physical landscape of all there is. The non-local, non-material aspects of consciousness were simply left out.

Against this backdrop, in 1882, the Society for Psychical Research (SPR) was born and during more than 125 years of research they have explored avenues of human consciousness that have been disenfranchised by the scientific community. The two main lines of research that still dominate their proceedings are: Do human beings possess psychic abilities? Does personality survive physical death?

The seriousness with which this task was undertaken was stated by William James:

> Were I asked to point to a scientific journal where hardheadedness and never-sleeping suspicion of sources of error might be seen in their full bloom, I think I should have to fall back on the Proceedings of the Society for Psychical Research. The common run of papers, say on physiological subjects, which one finds in other professional organs, are apt to show far lower level of critical consciousness. (James 1956, pp.303–304)

Other serious researchers have now joined the search, and share this same rigor modeled by the SPR. During the initial 50 years of research on "trance" and "mental" mediumship, a significant amount of evidence was accumulated that suggested to almost everyone involved that qualified mediums were receiving information through some super-normal means but there was substantial disagreement about what this process was (Braude 2003; Fontana 2005; Gauld 1982).

In Braude's opinion (2003) we can confidently affirm that human beings possess psychic abilities. What remains to be decided, however, is how all-encompassing, extensive, and refined psychic abilities might be. This apparent predicament greatly complicates efforts to determine whether we survive death, for we must scrutinize the evidence suggesting postmortem survival to determine whether it is actually veiled psychic functioning among the living.

Mediums: A Valuable Resource

Mediumship can be regarded as a talent that develops spontaneously in a few gifted individuals. Information gleaned from the minds of some of the most outstanding mediums of the last century, most notably Mrs. Leonora Piper (1857–1950) and Mrs. Gladys Leonard (1882–1968), inspired and intrigued such open-minded scientists as E. Dodds (1934), R. Hodgson (1898), William James (2009), Oliver Lodge (1935), F.W.H. Myers (1903), and others to rigorously explore uncharted territory—to discover whether memories are stored in the brain, whether consciousness and brain function are identical, and what may survive death.

The study of consciousness and mediumship, in particular, can be credited with igniting scientific advances in neuropsychology, psycho-neuroimmunology, biology, psychology, sociology, and physics, and in advancing our understanding of dissociation pathologies, exceptional mnemonic gifts, extreme or unique forms of savantism, or equally rare latent creative capacities.

The Importance of Current Research on Mediumship

The study of near-death experiences, mediumship, and reincarnation hold influential positions in psychical research as they are phenomena in which researchers can use the experimental method and combine aspects of field studies, spontaneous case studies, the study of special individuals, and survival research. So far, mediumship appears to be the only phenomenon directly related to the survival issue that can be produced and observed under experimentally controlled conditions.

Mediumship encourages the manifestation of powerful emotional and psychological concerns that often lead to strong psychic effects, seen in spontaneous experiences, without losing the ability to control the conditions. Hence, it reduces the uncertainties that too often accompany spontaneous cases where there are possibilities for other explanations or sources of information.

Psychical research is a field where there is the tendency to separate different kinds of studies, like spontaneous case studies, survival research, and experimental research, one from the other. Since mediumship is a phenomenon that embraces all these elements together, it is advantageous for broadening the scope of psychical research.

In addition, the study of mediumship may help us to tease apart and address the fundamental question at the root of psychical research and parapsychology: Who is the source of the psi experience or event? Is it primarily emanating from the living (the sitters or the medium) or the discarnate communicators (spirits)?

Current Challenges in Research on Mediumship and the Survival Hypothesis

When evaluating mediumistic material we must follow this sequence:

1. Rule out those with mental pathologies through appropriate testing procedures.

2. Determine whether the statements of the medium might have come from some "normal" process.

3. Determine whether the most likely explanation is that they are derived from some "super-normal" process.

"Normal" explanations would include fraud, fishing for information (known as cold-reading), cryptonesia (a hidden memory experienced as new), and trying to obtain information and direction during a reading by using statements that sitters respond to with "yes" and "no" answers. The last normal explanation to be watched for is the medium's use of vague or general statements that could apply to any person. It is only after we have ruled out such normal explanations, such as these, that we can consider a "super-normal" hypothesis.

The third step attempts to account for what the "super-normal" process is and whether it includes:

- the collaboration of a discarnate communicator (a spirit without a physical body)—giving evidence to the survival hypothesis

- telepathy with others (called "super-psi" or "super-ESP")

- information psychically extracted from a reservoir of information (Beischel and Rock 2009). The "psychic reservoir hypothesis" assumes that since the beginning of time all information has been stored in the universe and some mediums access it rather than communicating with the deceased.

Since the late nineteenth century mediumship researchers recognized that telepathy between living persons could seriously challenge the discarnate communicator hypothesis even though heroic efforts had been made to identify and study mediumistic communications that were difficult to account for by a super-psi hypothesis.

In order to increase discernment so that researchers could begin to recognize cases in which the survival hypothesis seemed the most reasonable, they put more focus on:

1. the motivation for communicating

2. deliberation in the selection of the sitters experiencing the medium's communication.

Researchers defined three kinds of mediumistic communications: cross-correspondences, drop-in communicators, and proxy sittings. In cross-correspondences and drop-in cases, the motivation for communicating is perceived as coming most strongly from the discarnate communicators rather than from any living persons and therefore provides good evidence of survival (Kelly 2010). In proxy sittings, there is no person present who knows the deceased so it appears less likely that a telepathic connection had been established between the medium and living people who knew the information contained in the communications.

As knowledge about psychic phenomena expanded, it was suggested that the intent of the medium to provide evidence of survival of consciousness was all that was necessary to produce information about the departed, but this still did not explain the means of obtaining the information. After 50 years of amassing research on mediumship, an apparent impasse was reached when it came to evaluating the opposing explanations (Cook 1987; Gauld 1961) of how mediums obtain information. Qualified researchers (Rock, Beischel and Cott 2009) are now trying to make these distinctions.

Although there is a resurgence of interest in mediumship among the general public today perhaps due to television shows, movies, and books from several celebrated mediums, few serious scientists are pursuing the field. Kelly (2010) argues:

> Simply because the theoretical impasse seemed so difficult to surmount, was, in my view, a serious self-inflicted wound on psychical research. It will only be by the accumulation of more evidence that we may eventually begin to see our way beyond the impasse... (p.251)

Laboratory Research

Mediumship studies undertaken primarily in naturalistic settings have long played a pivotal role in parapsychology's exploration of consciousness and in researching the main questions concerning psychic abilities and the survival hypothesis. A few field studies of extraordinary findings that tip the scales toward the survival hypothesis have also been reported, as in the case concerning a medium who provided key information that helped lead to the conviction of a murderer (Playfair and Keen 2004).

The two most predominant lines of mediumship research being conducted today include laboratory-based proxy-sitting experiments on the one hand, and qualitative phenomenological studies of the medium's unique experiences during mediumship readings, on the other. Whereas some researchers are using one or the other of these two approaches, the Windbridge Institute for Applied Research in Human Potential[1] has developed and uses a specific two-prong research focus with both.

Mediumship research today at the Windbridge Institute takes place in the regulated environment of the laboratory that permits the controlled and repetitive assessment of anomalous information reception by mediums (Beischel 2007). The Windbridge Institute's laboratory setting seeks to optimize the mediumship process for both the medium and the discarnate as well as to utilize research methods that increasingly magnify the experimental blinding of the medium, the rater, and the experimenter. Julie Beischel, the Research Director at the Windbridge Institute, has also managed to build a powerful quintuple-blind protocol different to the protocols of Roy and Robertson (2001, 2004), and previous researchers who used protocols that were single, double, or triple-blind controlled.

In this manner researchers can eliminate all conventional explanations for the information and safeguard its accuracy and specificity. Building upon earlier (Schwartz and Russek 2001; Schwartz, Russek and Barentsen 2002; Schwartz *et al.* 1999, 2001) as well as modern (O'Keeffe and Wiseman 2005) mediumship research, several methods are now used at the Windbridge Institute which include the thorough screening of all research subjects (mediums, sitters/raters, and discarnates), the pairing and formatting of readings, experimental blinding, and the scoring of readings by raters. Would-be mediums at the Windbridge Institute are run through a battery of psychological tests, interviewed, evaluated for talent in mediumship, and trained in research methods and grief prior to being certified as research mediums and participating in research studies.

It is hoped that one of the aforementioned researchers will, in time, find a way to prove the survival of individual consciousness after death. For now, we can analyze cases that appear to do so.

An Extraordinary Case

Following is a single case study of a chess game purportedly played between two leading grandmasters, one living and one dead, in the hope that the reader may get a sense of the intense commitment and care required to advance the field.

This special circumstance was staged by Dr. Eisenbeiss of Switzerland, an asset manager and amateur chess player, and publicized in the 1980s in the popular media. After reviewing the case and sorting through material not previously published, Hassler determined that a deeper analysis before a scientific audience was warranted (Eisenbeiss and Hassler 2006).

This game was played over the course of 7 years and 8 months, where the alleged moves of the discarnate grandmaster, Géza Maróczy, were transmitted through an automatic handwriting medium, Robert Rollans (1914–1993). Rollans claimed no knowledge of chess or chess history, was not cheating through secret communication with a living chess expert, and was not paid for his participation. Dr. Eisenbeiss knew and worked with Rollans for eight years and attested to these facts. Rollans's motive for participation was to support the survival hypothesis, believing from his experiences as a medium that physical death was not the end of personal life. His widow signed a written declaration attesting to her husband's belief.

To set up the event, Dr. Eisenbeiss gave Rollans a list of deceased grandmasters in the hope that he could encourage one of them to participate. On June 15, 1985, Hungarian Master Géza Maróczy (1870–1951), ranked second in the world around 1905, purportedly responded, assisted by Rollans's control. At the beginning of the game, Rollans received the words of Maróczy: "And you, dear Robert, will convey the game to its end." At the time, none of the participants anticipated that the game would take so long and therefore didn't realize the possible meaning behind Maróczy's comment, which looking back might have appeared prescient of Rollans's own death on March 2, 1993, just 19 days after Maróczy finally resigned at move 48.

Eisenbeiss was able to persuade living grandmaster and, at one time, number two rated chess player in the world, Viktor Korchnoi, to take on the match. Grandmaster Korchnoi knew that his opponent could be either the physical medium himself, or the mind of a deceased chess player, depending on the explanation attributed to what would follow. Subsequently, the chess moves were given from Maróczy to Rollans, purportedly forwarded from Rollans to Eisenbeiss, who, in turn, sent the move onto Korchnoi. Korchnoi's replies were communicated in the opposite direction. At no time did Rollans and Korchnoi have direct communication with each other (except for a handshake when they met in the SAT1 TV show four and a half months before the end of the match at the end of September 1992). This procedure remained consistent, always with

Eisenbeiss as the intermediary. The match ended on February 11, 1993, when Maróczy resigned.

Approximately a year into the match, Eisenbeiss judged the communication stable enough to request further identification from Maróczy that he was the true communicator. Some days before move 27 was received, he asked Maróczy (with no prior notice) via the medium, Rollans, to communicate a report about his life with special focus on his chess playing on earth. On July 31, 1986, from 11:04 am to 1:50 am the next day (interrupted by long breaks) Rollans received a lengthy text of 38 handwritten pages with an abundance of information on Maróczy's life, and also producing move 27.

In order to properly assess the veracity of the information that had come through, Eisenbeiss devised 39 questions in three basic areas that resulted in 91 question points:

1. Questions about "Maróczy's personal sphere."

2. General questions pertaining to "Maróczy's chess-playing."

3. Questions concerning "Maróczy's tournament successes."

Korchnoi was asked by Eisenbeiss if he could verify Maróczy's alleged statements about his chess tournaments, but Korchnoi stated that he didn't know the answers nor could he dedicate the time to finding out. Next, Eisenbeiss contacted the Hungarian Chess Club and was fortunate enough to make contact with historian and chess expert, Mr. Laszlo Sebestyén, in September 1986, who agreed to provide the answers. Sebestyén was not given any background information concerning the questions, had never met Korchnoi or Rollans, and was led to believe that he was contributing to a publication on Maróczy's chess life. He worked for over 70 hours consulting several libraries, Maróczy's two children (both over 80), and a cousin, managing to find the answers to almost all the questions. Sebestyén was reimbursed for his contribution by Eisenbeiss on September 17, 1986.

The percentage of overall correct statements Rollans had transmitted from Maróczy is 87.9 percent (for 80 responses), which is remarkable. Even more amazing is the percentage of correct responses given to the most difficult questions. Using a scale ranked in difficulty from low (1) to high (6), those in the category of 5 were perceived as "needing expert knowledge, difficult to investigate (hidden resources)." Those in the category of 6 were held as "private knowledge (known by few persons only, not known to be written down)." Thirty-three (36%) of the total of 91 question points fall into these higher categories (5 or 6).

Effectively, after careful and detailed re-analysis, 31 of the 31 esoteric questions to which an answer was known were correct. Neppe (2007), an accomplished chess player himself, re-analyzed the data initially presented above and increased the level of overall correctness to 97.5 percent (31/31 of the most difficult correct:

100%) as previously missing information was authenticated and included. Only 2.3 percent were then incorrect—of these, even incorrect data were very minor, like exact positions of others in tournaments. In two more items, the answers remain unknown.

One of the exceptional elements in the case was Maróczy's response to Eisenbeiss's question relayed through Rollans about a specific match against a relatively unknown player that he thought might still be remembered by Maróczy because of an important move he made at the end that won Maróczy the game. It was a match against a certain "Romi," played in San Remo, Italy, in 1930.

Maróczy's insistence on the correct spelling of Romi with an "h" is described below:

> But now it's time to answer your question whether I played a game with a certain Romi, I am sorry to say that I never knew a chess-player named Romi. But I think you are wrong with the name. I had a friend in my youth, who defeated me when I was young, but he was called Romih—with an "h" at the end. I then never again saw the friend whom I so admired. In 1930 at the tournament of San Remo—who is also present?... And so it came about that I played against him one of the most thrilling matches I ever played. (Eisenbeiss and Hassler 2006, p.74)

After consulting multiple source documents with conflicting spelling, Sebestyén and Eisenbeiss finally settled on the Slavonic origin of Romih because Maróczy claimed to have known Romih from his youth and they both came from the Habsburg Austro-Hungarian dual monarchy. For the super-ESP hypothesis to succeed, the controlling mind, on perceiving the differing references to Romih or Romi, would have to be able to retrieve the correct one from Maróczy's perspective, choose to address the situation, devise a response to the conflict, and perform it in the context of a teasing exchange with Eisenbeiss/Rollans about the correct spelling.

Two other fascinating examples where information was spontaneously provided in lieu of the requested and expected responses occurred. These suggest a possible window into the psychological motivations and personality of Maróczy that could tip the balance of probability in the direction of one hypothesis over the other (psi or survival).

In the first, the rationale Maróczy gives for forgetting the name of the founder of the Vera Menchik Club, he refers to as a "pointless joke." He then continues with an unrelated and unprompted story about a woman whose beauty impressed him. In the same transcript of August 21, 1988, he describes the following story:

> I have been talking about the embarrassing situation of the world champion Capablanca in Karlsbad. He was playing a chess match

with Samisch when his wife unexpectedly showed up from Cuba. He was a quite a "lady's man" and had hugely neglected his wife. He was not only busy enjoying triumphs in his chess matches but also in love-matches with the ladies, which ended with many conquests. He was accompanied by his Russian mistress, who was even more striking than his wife, having black hair and deep dark eyes, into which some colleagues dreamily gazed. I myself was also impressed by her femininity and beauty and that is why I can remember the incident very well.

The moment when Capablanca caught sight of his wife, his face turned white and then red. I was there. He said nothing, as if nothing unexpected had happened, but his behavior changed, which until then had been relaxed and even happy, because in fact he was better than his opponent, and also because his mistress continually flattered him. [He was] happy with her adoring glances. His mistress could not grasp what had happened because she probably had never seen his wife. She did not know who she was and thought her to be one of his many lady friends. When she realized what was afoot she didn't know where to flee and eventually left the hall... I can imagine what was said because, shortly after, Capablanca left his wife and married the striking Russian lady. But this also spelled the end of his amorous conquests, as the new lady never gave him a chance for an affair: she was with him at all tournaments. (Eisenbeiss and Hassler 2006, p.76)

Maróczy relates that, in all the excitement, Capablanca made a poor move that lost him the game.

The second example, a 1924 New York tournament, is inherently similar to the first. But here the anticipated—yet missing—information about how Maróczy ranked in the tournament is replaced by other disclosures about himself.

I had a thrilling game against Alekhin there, ending in a draw. You certainly have observed my trick in saying, "I no longer know which of us won the game." In doing so I want to bury a failure in order not to have to write so much, because failures are rather common among all chess players. This is a joke only, my dear friends: in fact it is true for me that I am not able to remember everything, most of all whenever winning eluded me. (Eisenbeiss and Hassler 2006, p.77)

The above serves to illustrate how scrupulously detailed Rollans's transcripts could be and how striking it is that he did not recount important highlights of the New York tournament which were readily available and existing in the public domain. Instead, if we examine the character of Maróczy, it is clear he was quite ambitious and he would not be prone to remembering his failures. However, for Rollans to censor information concerning Maróczy's failures would contradict his main purpose—to provide convincing evidence to support the survival hypothesis.

Neppe (2007) also concluded that the level of chess-playing by Maróczy had major stylistic differences that a chess computer of the 1980s and even today could not simulate, and many living chess players could not play at this high a level. This level could not have been achieved by the medium, Rollans, even after great training, assuming the medium was not a chess genius, which he was not. Neppe performed a simulated computer analysis using an appropriate-level computer and both Maróczy's and Korchnoi's play were superior to that of the computer. Effectively, Korchnoi's play acted as an exceptional comparator for Maróczy's. This then becomes far more than just a data analysis but also the first case of skills plus data, an extended case motivating survival, and the first use of computer simulation in survival research.

Discussion and Conclusion

Was a weakness of the case the fact that there was no independent witness consistent throughout? According to Neppe (2007), this is minor. Eisenbeiss performed a similar role to Hodgson in much earlier research in the case of medium Leonora Piper. Dr. Eisenbeiss (Eisenbeiss and Hassler 2006) attests to the faithfulness of this account and the integrity of the "players" involved. The press had investigated this case halfway through and Korchnoi has also attested to this case, plus it was independently analyzed by a Swiss chess champion at that time.

Neppe (2007) analyzed in detail the alternative possible explanations and, given the skill components, these fail:

- Cryptomnesia cannot explain the skills.

- Rollans did not have access to all the information and skills needed to engage in a grandmaster chess match and narrate details of an obscure life in the early twentieth century. This proved extremely difficult (if not impossible) even for a paid historian.

- The same holds for Eisenbeiss who had no prior access to most of the sources (books and witnesses). Even the expert, Korchnoi, when asked by Dr. Eisenbeiss, saw himself unable to answer the 39 questions and said it would require too much effort to find out.

The most probable alternative explanation to the survival theory would interpret the case as a perception by Rollans of existing knowledge and abilities through telepathy and clairvoyance in its highest form: the super-ESP or super-psi hypothesis.

Eisenbeiss and Hassler (2006) rejected super-psi since it has not been established under controlled laboratory conditions. However, Braude (2003, pp. 15 and 19) argues that one should not rule out spontaneous cases of psi where the phenomenon is particularly strong. At present there is insufficient understanding of alleged super-ESP and its limits. The authors argue that, apart from this, they are not convinced, like Braude and others, that the events attributed to psi cannot be explained by the survival hypothesis (when we lack in-depth understanding of what causes psi). Braude (2003, p.91) concedes that "Super-psi explanations have trouble handling both multiple sources of obscure information and also the consistency of mediumistic achievements." Most psychic researchers agree on the assumption (not fact) that intellectual (and practical) faculties are not communicated via extra-sensory perception. For a more comprehensive debate of the super-psi versus survival hypotheses refer to Almeder (1992), Braude (2003), Gauld (1982), Griffin (1997), Grosso (1999), and Schiebeler (1988).

Neppe (2007) points out that super-ESP in this form has never occurred and the consistent requirement of skills and transmission of 48 moves by ESP over seven-plus years has never been shown even in super-ESP. This case involves far more than just an example of objective knowledge acquisition which even if extending the super-ESP hypothesis order of magnitude beyond what was demonstrated before still fails the super-ESP hypothesis. What is so fascinating is the blend of acquired skill (playing chess) and objective knowledge (confirmed diffuse hidden information) over an extended period (7 years, 8 months) enhanced by an unexpected disclosure about a small (previously unknown) detail about the spelling of a name (Romi(h)). Furthermore, Rollans's skill at chess cannot be taken as an expansion of a skill he already possessed. Braude (2003, p.122) uses this argument to raise doubt on the survival hypothesis as an explanation for cases of spontaneous fluency in an unlearned language (xenoglossy).

Neither Rollans nor those around him were aware of the many details about Maróczy's life in advance. For Rollans to have been able to extract the information appearing in the transcripts from diverse domains would have required extraordinary psi ability. He also would be up against a huge amount of background "noise" from other sources (Braude 2003). When he was fully engaged in giving a voice to a discarnate spirit he would have had to simultaneously access the personal memories of living people to get facts (that had not been previously written down) at a time when those living people were likely not thinking about the subject he was wanting to understand.

Furthermore, Rollans's psi ability would have had to extend to pondering all the conceivable moves of the chess pieces and choosing the right one or tuning into the faculties of a chess-master who unconsciously assisted play. This feat then would have had to continue at a constantly high level over many years (one of the elements of Braude's "Argument from Crippling Complexity" [2003, pp.86–95]).

Neppe's (2007) analysis of the chess game itself judges this possibility as next to impossible.

If one searches for a psychological motive, Eisenbeiss and Hassler (2006) postulate that Rollans did not have one. However, Maróczy, who knew Romih in his youth, may have stuck with the spelling of "Romih" as he knew it, and may have rejoiced in deflating Eisenbeiss's seeming omniscience as interrogator. In addition, I feel that it is justified to draw conclusions from information spontaneously provided in lieu of the requested and anticipated responses to take into account psychological motivation. In this case, it seems to tip the scales in favor of Maróczy's unique personality.

This author is pulled in the direction of Ducasse (1969):

> When Occam's razor is alleged to shave off survival as a superfluous hypothesis, and to leave ESP as sufficient to account for all the facts in evidence, it turns out that ESP cannot do it without being arbitrarily endowed with an ad hoc "beard" consisting not of capacity for more far-reaching perception but of capacity for reasoning, inventing, constructing, understanding, judging, i.e. for active thinking; and more specifically for the particular modes of such thinking which only the particular mind whose survival is in question is known to have been equipped with. (Ducasse 1969, quoted in Kelly *et al.* 2006, p.41)

The Maróczy versus Korchnoi chess game may currently be the most remarkable case in demonstrating survival after bodily death.

Note
1.   See www.windbridge.org.

Chapter 18

THE POWER OF "MAGNETIZED" WATER

Beverly Rubik, PhD

Introduction

Spiritist Centers and Hospitals create and use what they call "magnetized" or "fluidified" water to facilitate healing, which is water informed through prayer and energy directed from healers' hands. It must be clarified that, in science, "magnetism" refers to conventional magnetic fields and their influence on matter. Here, the more popular use of the word "magnetic" is intended—of human beings purportedly affecting water energetically through intention and/or subtle energies. Indeed, there is a long history of "blessed" waters thought to have special healing properties, from the springs of Lourdes in France to the Hunza water of Pakistan. Recently Masaru Emoto (2004) popularized the notion that water can be programmed with specific "vibrations" associated with thoughts and feelings such as love, and that these result in different morphologies of ice crystals upon freezing. This notion has a basis in the frontiers of science, both from experimental findings and new theory. In this chapter we examine aspects of this new science that demonstrate that water is not a simple chemical substance, as was previously thought, but rather a complex liquid that interacts dynamically with signals from its environment and even with information from conscious intent. The evidence also suggests that water imbued with life-positive information can be especially beneficial to life. These results fit together like pieces of a puzzle toward a scientific basis for the "magnetized" water used in Brazil by Spiritists as well as its healing potential as a treatment.

Studies and Observations on Energized Drinking Water, Health, and the Biological Terrain[1]

Water is involved in virtually every function of the body, which consists of more than 70 percent water. Yet water is far more than just a constituent of life. Increasing evidence points to the efficient *flow* of water throughout the body as key to health and healing (Batmanghelidj 1995). Other evidence shows that certain "functional" waters treated with electromagnetic and possibly other forms of energy improve health in various ways. Thus certain waters may have much more subtle effects on life than previously thought.

The hydrating, cleansing, and restorative effects of various types of drinking water can be observed using live blood analysis, a holistic health assessment of the biological terrain or "soil" of the body. Figure 18.1 is a photograph of normal, healthy blood as seen under a dark-field microscope, showing the blood of a person who has been fasting.

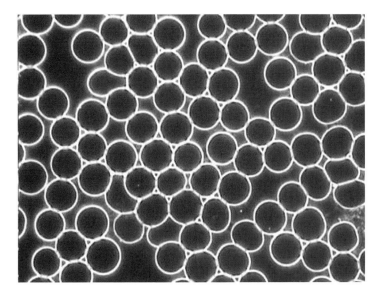

Figure 18.1: Dark-field microphotograph from live blood analysis of a normal healthy person's blood sample. The circular cells are red blood cells

After examining the effects of different kinds of drinking water on blood for years, we found that drinking alkaline water from an ionizer appears to be among the best drinking waters for health. An ionizer is a device connected to a water faucet that filters the water and then exposes it to an electric field and does partial electrolysis. The drinking water collected from the cathode is alkaline, rich in electrons, and has antioxidant properties, all of which are properties of water from a mountain stream, considered ideal drinking water. Like water flowing in a natural stream and exposed to earth fields, the molecules of ionized water are present in much smaller clusters (5 to 6 molecules) compared to tap or bottled water, due to the electrical energy treatment. We discovered that drinking ionized water over time slowly clears up congestion in the blood and improves the biological terrain. For example, Figure 18.2 shows the initial congestion in the blood of a 55-year-old person before drinking this water. The red blood cells are stuck together and barely recognizable.

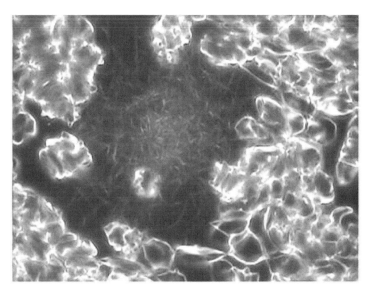

Figure 18.2: Dark-field microphotograph of the initial live blood analysis of a 55-year-old man that shows considerable blood congestion. The red blood cells are stuck together, and fibrin, a fibrous clotting protein, is also seen

After drinking ionized water for six months, the congestion is reduced and the blood improved, as shown in Figure 18.3.

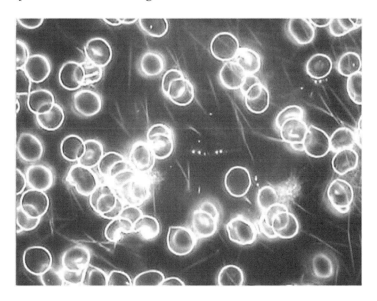

Figure 18.3: Dark-field microphotograph from live blood analysis of the same 55-year-old man (see Figure 18.2) after six months of drinking alkaline water from an ionizer, showing that the blood is less congested

There is less red blood cell stickiness and aggregation (which is indicative of a higher zeta potential, the electrical charge on the red blood cell surface), with less fibrin, the fibrous protein in clots, seen as white threads in the photo. The medical literature shows a number of beneficial effects from drinking ionized water, including protective effects on the pancreas in diabetic mice (Kim, Kyung and Uhm 2007); fewer medical complications from dialysis in kidney patients (Huang, Yang and Hsu 2006); protection of DNA from oxidative damage (Shirahata, Kabayama and Nakano 1997); and thwarting cancer by inhibiting the formation of new blood vessels linked to tumor growth (Ye, Li and Hanasaki 2008). Evidence is mounting that certain energized drinking waters such as ionized water have greater health benefits than untreated water. It is thought that the electrical treatment of ionized water erases the "memory" of water, of its past encounter with water treatment chemicals, agrochemicals, and drugs, and possibly also revitalizes it. By contrast, tap and bottled water are stagnant, low energy waters.

To further explore the influence of energized water, we conducted a limited study to look for an effect from drinking water energized with 7.83 Hertz (oscillations per second) on four middle-aged adults. This frequency corresponds to a key natural earth energy, called the Schumann resonance, known to be beneficial to life. Life has been resonating with this frequency throughout evolutionary time. This same frequency also corresponds to the alpha rhythm of the brain when a person is relaxed with closed eyes. Bottled water was treated overnight with an electromagnetic field of 7.83 Hertz in a resonant chamber. When participants drank this water, within an hour we found less red blood cell stickiness and aggregation, with reduced blood clotting, compared to their drinking untreated water (Rubik 2010).

The pilot study results of drinking water over the short term imprinted with the key energy frequency of the earth were quite similar to the long-term effects of drinking ionized water. Both of these energized waters reduced red blood cell stickiness, aggregation, and clotting. Since these factors are related to inflammation, these findings suggest that certain energized waters may be useful for combating the effects of inflammation. Because chronic inflammation has been identified as a key factor underlying virtually all chronic degenerative diseases including cancer and heart disease, drinking water imbued with certain energies may be particularly beneficial to health.

Basic Science Studies on Water Imbued with Frequencies

Can we measure changes directly in waters imprinted with certain energies? Can we assess any changes in waters imbued with intent or subtle energy associated with healers? Any changes in the structure of these waters, if present, are often so subtle that they cannot be recorded by conventional scientific instruments.

One method that we found to record changes in water imprinted by these means utilizes the GDV (Gas Discharge Visualization) Camera Pro (Korotkov 2002). This camera performs digital electrophotography, using high voltage electricity to stimulate water droplets to emit a pattern of light that can be analyzed quantitatively. This method is known and used worldwide for its capability of showing subtle energetic changes in substances, for example homeopathic remedies (Bell, Lewis and Brooks 2003). A GDV photo of ordinary tap water is shown in Figure 18.4a. It is seen to be smaller and less complex than the GDV photo shown in Figure 18.4b, which is that of water from a mountain stream. Figure 18.4c shows the GDV photo of water energized by an ionizer, which looks quite similar to Figure 18.4b. In short, mathematical image analysis of the GDV photographs of energized water droplets show that they emit larger, brighter patterns of light with certain changes in geometry compared to un-energized water. Thus the GDV camera appears to depict certain features of energized water.

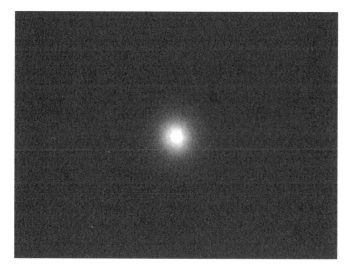

Figure 18.4a: GDV photo of induced light emitted from a tap water droplet

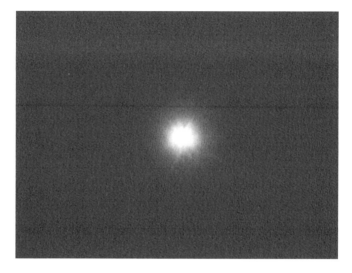

Figure 18.4b: GDV photo of induced light emitted from a droplet of water from a stream in the High Sierra Mountains of California

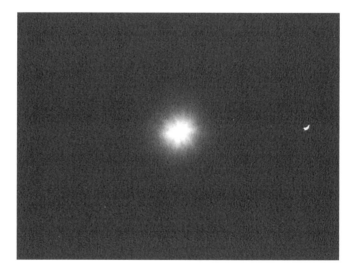

Figure 18.4c: GDV photo of induced light emitted from a droplet of water from an ionizer. The same tap water whose GDV emission pattern is shown in Figure 18.4a was sent through the ionizer

Few controlled experiments have demonstrated effects of energized water upon biological systems in the laboratory. In one blinded study in which alfalfa seeds were germinated using energized water compared to control water, the final dry weight of the sprouts watered with energized water was measurably greater (Rubik 2007), indicating a faster growth rate leading to more biomass.

In bio-electromagnetics, it is now well established that biological systems can respond to extremely low-level, non-ionizing energy fields, in some cases even less than thermal noise. Thus, an extremely low-level energy field may only be a carrier of key information, "electromagnetic bio-information" (Popp *et al.* 1989), which living organisms decode and utilize. Water imbued with energy, such as electromagnetic frequencies, that has beneficial effects on life, apparently conveys such information that is central to life. The author has proposed a unifying concept of bio-information as a holistic perspective underlying all types of biological effects at various levels of order, from the atomic and molecular levels through higher levels of organization, including interactions with mental intent and prayer (Rubik 1997).

Water with Sentience

In several field experiments, we have worked with groups of people who believe in a collective power to energize water through intent and/or "sending energy." We assess changes in the water using the GDV camera. Figure 18.5a shows an induced light pattern from tap water just before treatment, and 18.5b shows another after the group projected "healing love" onto the water sample. In three out of four blinded controlled experiments in the laboratory, we found measurable changes in water treated with "healing energy" by a spiritual healing group located 500 miles away. Apparently water shows sentience in being able to respond energetically to specific information directed to it from humans across large distances. These changes that we observed in the water are also reminiscent of local and distant healing effects of healers on people or organisms in the laboratory (Rubik, Brooks and Schwartz 2006).

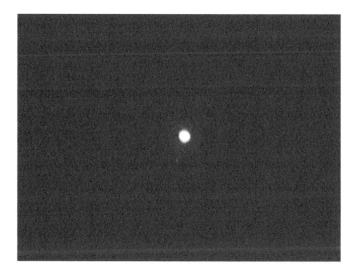

Figure 18.5a: GDV photo of induced light emitted from a tap water droplet

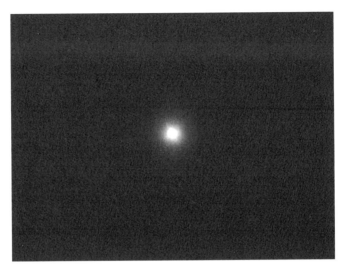

Figure 18.5b: GDV photo of the same tap water as in Figure 18.5a after a group of six people project "healing love" to the water

A New Science of Water

Previously water was regarded as only the "stage" on which the biomolecules of life acted. But recent discoveries support the notion that life is a collection of biomolecules "dancing to the tune" of water. Water is the "matrix of life" (Szent-Gyorgyi 1979). We are now in the midst of a paradigm shift in which liquid water is seen as an active substance rather than a passive constituent, exquisitely sensitive to signals from its environment, and as responsive as a living being (Ball 2008). For example, in physics, water and living systems are equally sensitive to a single quantum of magnetic flux (Smith 2004). Water shows long-range ordering around surfaces such as living cells, biomembranes, and biomolecules, where it is more akin to a liquid crystal with distinct properties in those regions that radically distinguish it from bulk water (Zheng and Pollack 2006).

The late physicist Giuliano Preparata (1995) made the first systematic attempt to develop a quantum electrodynamic theory of the structure of liquids and solids. Long-range forces acting over larger distances in the liquid phase gave rise to spatial domains wherein all the molecules oscillate in phase, like a stage full of ballerinas dancing pirouettes in unison, simultaneously, again and again. These are called coherent domains. Furthermore, Del Giudice and Preparata (1998) theorized that a certain proportion of liquid water contains collections of coherent domains of water molecules that are fluctuating and resonating with fields in the environment. The water molecules within those coherent domains vibrate in unison, because they are in a state of coherent excitation in which photons (quanta of light) are trapped in resonant states. These coherent domains of structured water provide order over long distances and can also act as "antennae" for external fields, such as extremely low-level electromagnetic fields from the environment. Employing this concept, the quantum structure of water with its intrinsic, vibratory, coherent domains exquisitely sensitive to externally applied fields may underlie the organization of life itself. Due to this dynamic substructure that is in constant interaction with the environment, water can register extremely subtle aspects of its environment, even across distances, through rapid changes in its internal properties. Decades ago, in climatology, Piccardi (1962) found that the stability of aqueous colloids, for example of milk mixed with water, was connected to extremely small changes in the earth's magnetic field. Today, the quantum electrodynamical theory of water can explain these extremely subtle interactions of water and its environment.

Preparata and Del Giudice's quantum electrodynamical model of liquids offers new insights into the *modus operandi* for many well-known phenomena in physics, such as superconductivity and magnetism. Moreover, it is the only physical model that correctly predicts and calculates from first principles many of the physical properties of water, most of which had previously been considered anomalies. Their model is also the best physical model of water that explains its "memory."

The Memory of Water

The observation that water can hold a "memory" of its past exposure to energies or substances is gaining support from several fields—material science, physics, climatology, and energy medicine—and in particular, homeopathy (Roy *et al.* 2005). Imprinting information from an electromagnetic frequency into water appears to be encoded as a frequency of alternating magnetic vector potential (Smith 1994a). There are techniques for embedding frequencies in water, for analyzing them using dowsing techniques, and for erasing them using high-energy fields or heat (Smith 1994b). Moreover, natural water with dissolved minerals appears to retain information longer than ultrapure water. Thus, minerals dissolved in water may play a role in its memory properties.

Homeopathy is an alternative medical practice founded around 1790 by Samuel Hahnemann, which involves prescribing remedies made from very high dilutions of medicinal substances in water. The most potent homeopathic remedies are, in fact, the ones with the highest dilutions, in some cases so dilute that there are no molecules of the original medicinal substance left. The fact that homeopathy persists over centuries is evidence for an enduring "memory" of water, which is the basis of these remedies that have been found to have beneficial effects on various disorders and illnesses. Numerous controlled clinical trials on homeopathic medicine as well as basic science studies on homeopathic remedies exist (Endler and Schulte 1994; Schiff 1995). GDV camera studies on homeopathic remedies that are infinitesimally dilute, whereby no molecules of the original substance could be measured, shows these ultradilutions to be distinctly different from ordinary water, demonstrating a "memory" of past exposure to the substances (Bell *et al.* 2003). In 1988 French immunologist Jacques Benveniste, in collaboration with 12 scientists in four countries, conducted basic research on solutions of antibodies so dilute that they no longer contained a single molecule of antibody. Nonetheless these ultradilute-aqueous solutions produced a response from immune cells (Davenas *et al.* 1988), which at the time rocked the scientific establishment. In recent explorations by Luc Montagnier (2010), who won the Nobel Prize for discovering the HIV virus, certain DNA sequences were observed to organize water,[2] and, at very high dilutions, that water emits low frequency waves that can communicate information about the DNA sequence.

Healer Interactions with Water

Still others have conducted research that goes beyond imprinting water with the memory of substances or conventional electric, magnetic, and electromagnetic fields. However, this area of inquiry is in its infancy, as there are very few published studies showing the influence of healers directly on water. One controlled study on Therapeutic Touch-energized water that was given to guinea pigs to drink, compared to control water samples, demonstrated positive effects from healer-treated water on wound healing (Savieto and da Silva 2004). Tiller, a retired Stanford professor of material science, has conducted research on imprinting of water by healing and intention (Tiller 1997) as well as electronic devices storing intent and conveying information to water (Tiller 2001).

The human body radiates energy, which is comprised of conventional (Hertzian), albeit extremely low-level, electromagnetic fields that may impact water. It has been found in basic science studies on water dynamics that, in the presence of such radiant energy, the organized liquid-crystal type structure of water expands extensively and is dependent on this incident electromagnetic energy (Chai, Yoo and Pollack 2009). Moreover, we must also consider the role of intent in spiritual healing, including the possibility that other putative subtle energies (non-Hertzian) may be involved, too. Therefore, a complex interplay of these various modes may interact with the water to change its dynamic structure. In Brazil, the mediums that "magnetize" water engage in prayer and place the palms of their hands facing the water, which may bring together this interplay of information from intent plus human energy fields. The water thus imprinted through intent and biofield[3] is then given to the people for drinking to enhance health and wellness, conveying the information imprinted in the blessed water to their bodies.

Spiritual healing is a challenging area for scientific research because the dominant scientific paradigm has no role for conscious intent in the physical world. A new epistemology for a science-with-consciousness, along with appropriate research strategies, would deepen our understanding of spiritual healer interactions with water and life.

Conclusion

As we explore the interface of science and spirituality, especially the power of intent and prayer, we find apparent paradoxes, seeming impossibilities, and wonders such as blessed waters that can heal. That intent or prayer can somehow alter the structure of water to increase vitality, improve health, and even cure disease seems to be in the realm of the miraculous. However, as shown in this chapter, there are several lines of evidence from frontier science that fit together like pieces of a puzzle to spell out a new dynamic view of water and its intimacy with life, energy, and consciousness. We have brought together some strands of evidence from observations, theory, and experiment that provide support for "magnetized" water. This is the start of a scientific basis for understanding how "magnetized" water may heal, beyond a placebo effect.

What presently exists are various studies from mostly isolated scientists, but what is needed to move this field forward is a concerted scientific effort. We need more studies to lead to a generally accepted scientific explanation for the phenomena of "magnetized" water, water with memory, and water with sentience. Besides further basic science studies on energized water, it is also recommended that controlled studies on patients who drink "magnetized" water be conducted, especially studies that would assess outcomes measured in suitable parameters as well as qualitative dimensions of the healing experience.

Research in this realm of subtle energies and intent requires an entirely new perspective. A new paradigm, on the verge of developing, will blossom when humanity embraces more of its full potential and resolves to bootstrap itself into a new phase of existence. In order to develop a science ready to encompass spirit and consciousness, we first need to change ourselves. We need to recognize the primacy of consciousness in the world and become more self-aware in directing our will and intent. Then we can work at a more causal level of creation, both in our science and beyond.

Notes

1. The biological terrain is the ground or "soil" of the body, which is the aqueous material between the cells of the body, and all of its properties (pH, relative cleanliness, etc.), that is an important measure of health and wellness. It is assessed by many holistic health practitioners through examining the fluids taken from the body (i.e. blood, urine, and saliva).

2. DNA is a large polymer molecule that has a sequence of genes, which involves a sequence of base-pairs attached to the double-helical backbone that spell out the arrangement of amino acids in proteins.

3. The biofield is the complex dynamic organizing field of the organism, which is within and all around it, which I hypothesize is intimately involved in biocommunication, bioregulation, and healing.

Chapter 19

THE POSITIVE POTENTIAL OF DISSOCIATIVE STATES OF CONSCIOUSNESS

Melvin Morse, MD

Introduction

This chapter will discuss the dissociative states of consciousness and emphasize their protective, healing, transformative, and restorative functions (see Table 19.1).

The Current View of Dissociation

The term "dissociation" was first used by Janet in the late nineteenth century, to understand and describe hysterical personalities. He described a life of "psychological misery" because of, in his view, the resultant segmented and dissociated life of the hysteric (Janet 1901).

This viewpoint persists to this day. The American Psychiatric Association's (1994) *Diagnostic and Statistical Manual of Mental Disorders* (DSM-IV), while stating that dissociation should not be considered inherently pathological, offers no diagnostic category for non-pathological dissociation. Near-death experiences, simply because of the out-of-body component and detachment from the physical body, have been categorized as dissociative events and are discussed in that context (Krippner and Powers 1997).

Other theorists, however, have pointed out that dissociation in general and the near-death experience in particular may well serve to connect consciousness to other realities (Evan 1989). It has become increasingly appreciated that the majority of dissociative clinical conditions do not represent pathology. As a result, there has been a call for a reclassification of dissociation based on function and clinical situations, not simply the phenomenon itself (Spitzer *et al.* 2006).

Table 19.1: The spectrum of dissociation as seen in healing, health, and mental dysfunction

Dissociation as a healing tool	Dissociation as a therapeutic tool	Dissociation for spiritual improvement	Spontaneous dissociation	Dissociation with mild functional disturbances	Severe dissociation with independently functioning personalities
Well-trained Spiritist mediums and healers; NDE	1. EMDR 2. TRVP (Past Life Regression Therapy)	Controlled remote viewing or astral projection	Simple out-of-body experiences (OBE)	PTSD with anxiety and mild DID	Severe DID (formerly known as multiple personality disorder)
Persons enjoy excellent mental health and are using dissociation to interact with spirits and other realities, and to help others	Experienced therapists guide the patient through protocols which involve dissociation and non-local perceptions	Techniques and protocols used by individuals which promote non-local perceptions and dissociation	About 3% of population will have sudden OBE for no reason; it just happens	Patients are fairly functional and have anxiety and brief dissociative episodes	Ordinary seamless stream of consciousness is significantly disrupted as various personalities struggle for control of the self

Even in severe situations such as Dissociation Identity Disorder (DID), it is not clear that it is dissociation that is the root cause of the pathology. Dysfunctional dissociation is often the result of severe and chronic childhood traumatic experiences where the dissociative barriers are developed to aid the child in his or her psychological survival. However, this type of response later in life can inhibit a person's natural development and may contribute to the debilitating symptoms of post-traumatic stress disorder (PTSD), depression, and anxiety. It appears that the very thing the child used to survive, *dissociating*, can later help to heal them when used in the context of therapy.

We All Dissociate: It Is a Normal State of Consciousness

It has been known since the mid-nineteenth century that there are two independent streams of consciousness operating in the human mind (Crabtree 1993). There is the "internal narrator" or ordinary consciousness, which recently has become associated with left hemispheric function. There is also the unconscious stream of sensory input and memory, associated with right brain functions but in fact found in multiple areas of the brain (Binet 1890; Crabtree 2006). Normal healthy well-functioning adults can even have as many as three or more independently functioning streams of consciousness (Beahrs 1982; Crabtree 1985; Hilgard 1977).

Although consciousness in the brain is far more complex than simple "left brain" versus "right brain," split brain research documents that the two hemispheres of the brain process information differently (Gazzaniga 1989; Sperry 1974, 1993). Understanding the strengths and weaknesses of each consciousness can clarify the need for integration of the two major streams of consciousness.

The "left brain" is analytic, verbal, and creates our ongoing sense of reality. It is our normal personality. One important function it has is to make sense of the ordinary world and facilitate our daily lives. It creates our sense of meaning of life, and the myths and belief systems by which we live.

The "right brain" is conscious of the left brain's mental activities and although considered "unconscious" actually contains the entire conscious record and memories of the person. It is relatively non-verbal, communicates with symbols, and sorts and organizes data and information but rarely tries to judge it or make sense of it (Gazzaniga 2008). It is this arena of consciousness that is associated with automatic writing, vivid perceptions of deceased persons, remote viewing or otherwise accessing information through non-ordinary means, and mediumship (Braude 1995; Myers 1885). It is this same stream of consciousness that I have speculated is connected to a timeless space-less source of all knowledge. I have theorized that the right temporal lobe and hippocampus is our "god spot" (Morse

2002). Others feel this is simplistic as the entire brain is connected to the Divine (Beauregard and O'Leary 2007).

Case Report

Dissociative experiences in the context of dying (near-death experiences; NDEs) can have powerful transformative effects independent of the psychological aspects of coming close to death and surviving (Morse 1994a). This case report comes from the experimental model for near-death experiences inadvertently developed by the US military when studying the effects of high acceleration forces on the human brain. James Whinnery, MD, the lead investigator, found that dissociative experiences occurred to the test pilots when they were at the point of maximal accelerations in a centrifuge. They did not occur at lesser accelerations. These dissociative experiences included a full return to consciousness (after first suffering seizures and coma), a perception of being transcendent with the Universe and merging with a spiritual white light or "god" (Whinnery 1989; Whinnery and Whinnery 1990).

Jeff Smith was a warrior. He was a flight officer in the US Marine Corps. Now he is one of a hundred approved consultants in EMDR (Eye Movement Desensitization and Reprocessing) therapy and an advocate for the homeless. He is dedicated to treating veterans with PTSD. As part of his military experience, he was part of Whinnery's research on G forces and consciousness. He had the typical NDE seen in clinical studies of children and adults who describe near-death experiences, especially merging with a spiritual white light. The experience had a transformative effect on him. He altered his career path and trained as a family therapist and then specialized in EMDR. He integrates his spiritual understandings gained from his near-death experience with traditional EMDR therapy.

Dissociative Experiences and Non-local Perceptions

Dr. Whinnery; Pim van Lommel, a Dutch adult cardiologist; and myself, a former pediatric intensivist, have done prospective studies of NDEs. Our research and conclusions are well accepted by the mainstream scientific and medical mainstream literature (Morse 1994b; Morse, Castillo and Venecia 1986; van Lommel *et al.* 2001).

All three of us concluded that NDEs:

- occur in dysfunctional or (briefly) dead brains

- involve a sense of expanded awareness and consciousness implying that consciousness does not depend entirely on brain function

- involve out-of-body perceptions, merging with a transcendent reality or "god," speaking with deceased persons, encountering spirits, etc.

- are not caused by coma or trauma, a lack of oxygen, or medications, and are not a psychological reaction to the fear of nearly dying

- are associated with positive personality transformations

- seem to imply that memories can be stored outside the brain and that consciousness exists independent of brain function.

(Morse and Whinnery, personal communication 1996–1998; Morse and van Lommel, personal communication, October 26, 2008)

This last point is not as controversial as it seems. In fact, there is no current modern theory of how memory can be stored in the brain. Allan Gauld, in reviewing the subject, states that the idea that memory must be stored within the brain is a neuroscientific myth, unsupported by the evidence, and now hardened into dogma (Gauld 2006, p.281). In the same text, Bruce Greyson, MD, states: "the central challenge of NDEs lies in asking how these complex states of consciousness can occur under conditions…[which neuroscience now] deems impossible. This conflict between neuroscientific orthodoxy is head on, profound, and inescapable" (Greyson 2006, p.421).

Near-death research clearly supports the concept that dissociation can involve contacting spiritual realities and a "god" that exist independent of us, and may not be pathological at all. The need for more neutral terminology led van Lommel (2010) to propose the term "non-local perceptions." Non-local perceptions include spirits, deceased relatives, a god, past life memories, remote viewing, angels, and spiritual realities which cannot be perceived with the ordinary senses and yet seem completely real.

Dr. van Lommel's "non-local perceptions" reinforce my theory that we have a "god spot" or "spiritual brain" which allows us to interact with the theoretical physicists' current concept of reality, a timeless space-less conscious informational universe (Stapp 2007). At the very least, this new research suggests that we are designed with the hardware in the brain to connect to an altered or "unconscious" consciousness for a positive purpose of healing and growth. Regardless of the objective reality of these non-local experiences, it is clearly beneficial to have them. For example, dissociative experiences have been associated with genius and creativity (Braude 2002).

Using Dissociative Experiences to Transform and Heal the Mind

Simply being in a non-verbal unconscious mental "dissociative" state, without any specific reference to spirits or encounters with a "god," has been shown to be protective against severe psychological trauma. Researchers have shown that PTSD can benefit from patients being immersed in what those researchers called "the separate sensory stream of consciousness" by playing a video game that involves sorting shapes (Holmes *et al.* 2010).

There are specific therapies and protocols that facilitate healthy dissociation, which typically involve non-local perceptions.

Controlled Remote Viewing (CRV) or Controlled Out-of-Body Perceptions

Protocols for the controlled ability to dissociate and/or access information by non-ordinary means were developed independently by the US military and "projectiologists" in Brazil and Portugal. Their protocols are strikingly similar. They involve a "viewer" who first accesses the sensory stream of consciousness and then creates a "virtual reality" within the mind. While in this virtual reality, the viewer obtains information otherwise not accessible through memory or the ordinary senses. Automatic writing and dissociation are key elements of the experience. There is a monitor of the sessions to guide and direct the viewer in the process and help the viewer remain within the structured protocol.

The Brazilian group uses the experience to develop good mental health and have a body of research documenting this (*Journal of Conscientiology*). Although the US program was developed for military intelligence gathering, the same result occurred. Most of the originally trained military remote viewers have written books with titles such as *Captain of My Soul, Master of My Ship* to describe the positive transformational effect their training had on them (Atwater 2001). Lyn Buchanan (2003), for example, states that high quality viewings correspond to creativity, happiness, and excellent mental health in the viewer. He has moved beyond the military targets he was trained for and frequently monitors and assists persons during their own dying process.

Eye Movement Desensitization and Reprocessing

EMDR is one of the few evidence-based therapies documented to heal PTSD. It is approved as a first-line treatment intervention for PTSD by the American Psychiatric Association, the US Department of Veterans Affairs, and the US Department of Defense. EMDR is an eight-phase, integrative psychotherapy approach that uses specific protocols and procedures (Shapiro 2001) to access the unconscious. There is bilateral activation of both hemispheres of the brain using eye movements or the other forms of bilateral stimulation. In EMDR a client's sensory stream of consciousness is engaged while they are asked to talk about their experiences. At the onset of EMDR treatment a virtual "safe place" is created as a mental construct to ensure a place for the client to return to for self-regulation. The process of creating this safe place is strikingly similar to the mental processes of controlled remote viewing.

The specific details and memories (auditory, somatic, visual) of the traumatic events are accessed, and otherwise linked trigger memories are reprocessed, resulting in positive thoughts and feelings which were unavailable prior to the processing. At times in treatment, other "virtual" persons can also be engaged, such as healthy adult parts of the person, fallen comrades of a soldier in war, dead family members, abusers, and spirit helpers to assist in the healing process. This often catalyzes a profound healing response where clients report a sense of deeper healing, even a spiritual experience, while new material comes forward of forgiveness, compassion, and love for the self and others. This healing process occurs much more efficiently compared to traditional talk therapies. Clearly EMDR involves healthy dissociation and creative use of non-local perceptions.

Experiential Regression Therapy de Peres (TRVP)

This is a seven-stage experiential treatment of PTSD. This technique was developed by Julio Peres, PhD, a neuroscientist and psychologist in Brazil. The entire therapy typically takes six months. Patients were hypnotically regressed to past life memories and experiences. Cognitive behavioral therapy was then done. Peres studied 610 patients between 1996 and 2002. Two-thirds of the patients had complete resolution of PTSD. Facilitating dissociation and non-local perceptions is a key part of the therapy (Peres 2009).

Mediumship in Psychotherapy

When we understand communicating with the human second consciousness as a linkage with a timeless, space-less, all-knowledge domain, much of the confusion in this arena disappears. Whether it is a medium contacting a "dead person," or an EMDR therapist helping the client to interact with an abuser or a fallen comrade in battle, all of these experiences really involve interactions with the body of information that represents a given situation or person. They all are simply mental experiences involving the accessing and processing of non-local information.

Examples of Mediumship in Psychotherapy
The Author and His Wife's Experience[1]

We have treated over 30 patients with severe DID, all within a spiritual context. Early in therapy, we seek to find as an ally the "artist within" and/or the "being of light" that is typically present. We engage the various consciousnesses as if they are completely real, with respect, dignity, and unconditional love.

For example, one conscious state I refer to as "the monster soul" usually has the most complete memories of the childhood trauma. They have voluntarily taken on horrific trauma to allow the core personality to live a happy and uncontaminated life. I explain that their anger and fury is to be expected and respected. As the therapeutic process continues, I ask them what the best resolution of their anger would be for them. One "monster soul" told me that she wanted to be sealed in a stainless steel museum in a graveyard that everyone could admire, but never enter. Rapid resolution of disabling anger then occurred.

To facilitate healing, with my wife as monitor, I openly enter into a spiritual and/or dissociative state with the patient. I have had consciousnesses "talk" through me as if I am channeling their words. My therapeutic model is entirely one of love, respect, and wonder. The patient has his or her own healing solutions which I could never anticipate. For example, with one patient, I realized that the core or central personality was frightened and perceived herself as a seven-year-old girl and a "frozen sausage." There was in fact no adult personality to take charge. She had been misdiagnosed as a "schizoid" or "borderline personality." The previously hidden "artist within" stepped forward and "thawed out" the core personality. Over many years, she gradually matured and healed. I cannot think of a single patient I have helped in any way other than by being a witness to their healing by being willing to believe in the unbelievable (Cline 1997).

A Psychotherapist Medium

At least one well-trained and highly successful psychotherapist has written about his clinical practice which straightforwardly involves, at times, communication with spirits who have therapeutic information and suggestions for the client (GoForth and Gray 2009).

Mediums as Psychotherapists

Conversely, it has recently been proposed that mediums may play an important role in grief therapy, and should be studied in that context (Mosher, Beischel and Boccuzzi 2010).

This immediately raises legitimate concerns about untrained and undisciplined mediums actively practicing psychotherapy with the potential for significant harm. The above examples involve well-trained, highly skilled physicians and psychologists who add the element of mediumship to their other skills and training. Clearly it is appropriate to begin a dialogue on what are the proper standards of care for such integration of mediumship into therapy (GoForth 2011). Until this is better understood, in my opinion only persons already skilled and licensed to practice psychology and medicine should attempt to integrate "interactions with the all-knowledge domain" or mediumship into their clinical practice.

Conclusion

Dissociation is best understood as a spectrum state of consciousness. At one end of the spectrum are the mediumistic experiences of the best-trained and supervised mediums of the Spiritist movement who lead a well-disciplined and balanced way of life. They may be highly educated professionals or not, but all of them do group mediumship for the purpose of helping people who are suffering as well as purported disincarnated spirits. They do not charge for this practice (Spiritist Medical Association of the USA 2010). The spontaneous dissociation of the near-death experience is also at this end of the spectrum.

Next is dissociation in the context of positive therapeutic experiences discussed above. These therapies depend on the healing power of shifting to what is loosely called "right brain" consciousness, and then creating a loving and safe place for healing to occur.

Controlled remote viewing and astral projection are at this part of the spectrum. They are skills that can be learned and clearly can enhance spirituality and ordinary consciousness. It is one non-local perception validated as objectively real by considerable scientific research (Dunne and Jahne 1982; Targ and Puthoff 1974).

In the middle of the spectrum is the simple out-of-body experience. These occur to 3 percent of the normal mentally healthy population, spontaneously. They typically have no secondary meaning or transformative effects (Gabbard and Twemlow 1985).

Towards the pathological end of the spectrum would be PTSD. Such patients often have entwined clusters of memories, and seemingly unrelated non-traumatic experiences can suddenly trigger traumatic memories resulting in panic attacks and momentary dissociation. Many patients with DID fall in this mild category. They may well have many dissociative experiences in a given day but have learned how to cope and manage them in a functional way. Finally at the end of this spectrum is severe DID disorder and PTSD where the patient experiences major and disabling dissociative events out of conscious control. It is not the dissociation that is disabling; it is the lack of conscious control.

Modern research and therapies have the potential of creating a new healthy holistic approach to dissociation. This has enormous potential to enhance our ordinary state of consciousness as well as help disorders such as PTSD and DID, when directed and guided within a therapeutic context.

Note

1. The author and his wife are an experienced controlled remote viewing team. They have adapted the structure, protocol, and discipline of controlled remote viewing for working as a team with DID patients.

Chapter 20

COMPASSIONATE INTENTION AS A THERAPEUTIC INTERVENTION BY PARTNERS OF CANCER PATIENTS
Effects of Distant Intention on the Patients' Autonomic Nervous System

Dean Radin, PhD, Jerome Stone, MA, RN, Ellen Levine, PhD, Shahram Eskandarnejad, MD, Marilyn Schlitz, PhD, Leila Kozak, PhD, Dorothy Mandel, PhD, and Gail Hayssen

Introduction

A 2004 government survey of adult Americans, conducted by the US National Center for Health Statistics, showed that, of the top ten complementary and alternative medicine (CAM) healing practices, the most popular was prayer for self and the second was prayer for others (Barnes *et al.* 2004). From a psychological perspective, the former may be thought of as a coping mechanism in the face of uncertainty or dire need. The possibility that prayer for self may promote one's own healing is not considered controversial because of the growing literature on the salutary effects of meditation and placebo and the plausibility of psychoneuroimmunological models of self-regulation (Kiecolt-Glaser *et al.* 2002).

Prayer for others is likewise understandable as a practical coping mechanism, but the idea that it might be efficacious for another person remains contentious. To avoid unnecessary religious connotations, the descriptive phrase "distant healing intention" (DHI) is sometimes used in the scientific and medical literature to refer to this practice (Schlitz *et al.* 2003). DHI effects are considered scientifically doubtful by some because the "distant" in DHI means shielded from all known causal interactions (Sloan and Ramakrishnan 2005; Wallis 1996). Science is beginning to reconcile with the concept of "spooky action at a distance" within fundamental physics, but so far the idea that non-local effects might also exist in living systems (Walach 2005), and be pragmatically useful in some way, evokes as much contempt as it does serious interest.

Because the mechanisms underlying postulated DHI effects are unknown, most DHI experiments have focused on the straightforward empirical question: Does it work? Can DHI affect medical symptoms and outcomes? Some clinical studies of hospital inpatients and medical outpatients suggest that DHI might be medically efficacious (Astin, Harkness and Ernst 2000; Krucoff *et al.* 2001), but as a whole the clinical evidence remains uncertain (Benson *et al.* 2006; Krucoff *et al.* 2005).

In contrast, when DHI is tested under controlled laboratory conditions, the evidence is less ambiguous. Meta-analyses indicate that DHI produces repeatable effects in the human autonomic nervous system, detected typically by monitoring fluctuations in one person's electrodermal activity while a distant person mentally attempts to influence the target person's emotions or attention (Schlitz and Braud 1997; Schmidt *et al.* 2004). The literature also indicates that DHI effects can be detected in the central nervous system, as measured in brain electrical activity (Duane and Behrendt 1965; Grinberg-Zylberbaum *et al.* 1994; Radin 2004a; Standish *et al.* 2004; Wackermann *et al.* 2003) and hemodynamics (Achterberg *et al.* 2005; Richards *et al.* 2005), and also in the enteric nervous system (Radin and Schlitz 2005).

The laboratory evidence may be clearer than the clinical evidence because there are no "competing" intentions to interfere with the test results, such as the prayers of clinical patients' loved ones, and also because physiological fluctuations can be objectively monitored in real-time, whereas healing responses in the clinic may progress over days or weeks. The context of laboratory studies is also quite different from that of clinical studies. In the lab, the person assigned to "send" DHI (hereafter called the *sender*) is typically a volunteer who is not especially motivated or trained to provide DHI, and the person assigned to receive DHI (the *receiver*) is often just curious to see what will happen.[1] Given these low motivational factors, it should not be surprising that the magnitude of effects observed in such studies is rather small; for example, the meta-analytic effect size estimate reported by Schmidt *et al.* (2004) is Rosenthal's $d = 0.11$ ($p = 0.001$) (Rosenthal 1994).

The goal of the present study was to see what would happen when the powerful, real-life motivations associated with clinical trials of DHI were combined with the controlled context and objective measures offered by laboratory protocols. In addition, most previous DHI studies assigned the sender's role to a laboratory staff member, so the sender and receiver were often strangers. The present study sought to enhance the ecological validity of postulated DHI-type connections between couples by recruiting long-term, bonded pairs, and by exploring the role of training and motivation in potentially modulating DHI effects. Given the laboratory context we did not test for distant *healing* per se, but rather the physiological effects of distant intention. With this caveat in mind, the term DHI will be used hereafter for ease of exposition.

Method

Participants

Pairs of friends, long-term partners, married couples, and mother–child pairs were recruited to participate in one of three groups. Two of the groups were comprised of adult couples, one of whom was healthy and the other undergoing treatment for cancer. The cancer patients and their partners were recruited throughout the San Francisco Bay Area by health care provider referrals and newspaper advertisements. The study design was explained to interested parties, including the random assignment to different conditions, the data collection procedures, potential risks and benefits, and their rights as voluntary participants, including informed consent. Couples were excluded if they were participating in family therapy, were receiving any form of "energy healing," if the partner was enrolled in a cancer support group, or if they chose at any time to leave the study.

The healthy partner was assigned the role of the sender of DHI and the patient the role of the receiver. In the "trained group," the sender attended a program involving discussion and practice of a DHI technique based on the cultivation of compassionate intention, defined as the act of directing selfless love and care towards another person, with the intention to relieve their suffering and enhance their well-being.

The training program, developed and provided by the second author, consisted of a day-long, eight-hour, group workshop, followed by a daily half-hour practice at home for three months. The program included a lecture on the healing potential of compassionate intention, discussion of common resistances to positive expectations about DHI, guided instruction in several meditation and mental focusing practices, and guided exercises in breath-based techniques for enhancing compassion, as variously practiced in Tibetan Buddhism (the practice known as Tonglen meditation) (Chodron 1996; Rinpoche 1994; Rosenthal 1994), Judeo-Christian meditation (Davis 1997; Lerner 1995), and Therapeutic Touch (Krieger 1993).

After attending the training session and practicing the DHI meditation daily for three months (healthy partners were asked to keep a daily log to verify their practice), these couples were tested in the laboratory. In the "wait group," the couple was tested before the healthy partner attended the training program. A third group consisted of healthy couples who received no training (the "control" group). Of those recruited for the trained and wait groups, ten couples eventually dropped out. Reasons provided included time constraints, dissolution of the couple's relationship, the couple was in search of a "quick fix," death of a patient, spouse was not available, complications of cancer, or because one or more concepts in the training program clashed with the couple's belief system.

When a couple arrived at the lab, they signed informed consents and then the experimenters attached electrodes to each person to monitor five physiological variables. The principal measurement was electrodermal activity (EDA), specifically skin conductance level (SCL), as this is the variable most frequently employed in similar, previous studies. Electrodermal activity was monitored with two electrodes, each filled with an isotonic electrode gel,[2] and attached to the left palm using double-sided adhesive collars.[3] These electrodes were attached to a Biopac GSR–100C EDA amplifier, set to the 0–2μS range.[4]

For exploratory purposes, we also monitored one channel of electro-encephalogram at C_z, fingertip blood volume on the left thumb, electrocardiogram, and abdominal respiration. Results of those measurements will be reported in other publications. All signals were recorded at either 500 or 1000 samples per second, and each person was monitored by a separate physiological recording system.[5] To assist in the computational process, all raw physiological data were downsampled to 100 samples per second before analysis.

The couple was asked to maintain a "feeling of connectedness" with each other. To assist with this intentional focus, each person was asked to exchange a personal item, like a ring or watch, and to hold that object in his or her free right hand for the duration of the session. In the control group, couples were asked to decide which of the two might be more receptive, and that person was assigned the role of the receiver. In the trained and wait groups, the cancer patient was always the receiver.

Environment

The receiver (R) was asked to relax in a reclining chair inside a double steel-walled, electromagnetically and acoustically shielded chamber, as illustrated in Figure 20.1.[6] R was informed that the sender (S) would be viewing his or her live video image at random times from a distant location, and that during those periods S would try to make a special intentional effort to mentally connect with him or her. No one involved in the experiment knew exactly when those random periods would occur, as they were selected by a computer (described below).

A low-light video camera was focused on R's face, and the interior of the shielded room was illuminated with a 25 watt incandescent bulb. The physiology and video signals were routed outside the shielded room via optical fiber to two computers,[7] one dedicated to recording R's physiological signals and the other used to automatically run the experimental session, including switching the video image to S's location at random times.

To test for possible sensory cues between the S and R locations, audio tests were conducted to check whether tones as loud as 110 dB at 1000 Hz sounded in

S's room could be detected inside R's shielded chamber. Subjective hearing tests along with quantitative audio tests using a digital sound level meter confirmed that the test tones were indistinguishable from background noise inside the chamber.[8] To further isolate the shielded room from potential infrasound cues, the chamber rested upon a vibration-dampening vinyl mat in the basement of a building.

After R was settled in the shielded room, S was led through two closed doors to a dimly lit room 20 meters away and asked to sit in a chair about a half-meter in front of a video monitor. An experimenter explained that, when the video monitor showed R's image, S was to try to mentally "connect" with R with as much intensity as possible. The principal experimenter (first author) was blind to whether a couple was in the trained or wait group, but was aware of the condition for the control group participants, the majority of whom were recruited by and guided through the experimental sessions by the last three authors.

S's electrodes were connected to the same model Biopac system as R's, using the same type of amplifiers, settings, and data sampling rates. The digitized outputs from both Biopac systems were transmitted over a local area network and streamed to two Windows-based PCs, each running Biopac's Acknowledge 3.7.1 data collection software (Figure 20.1).

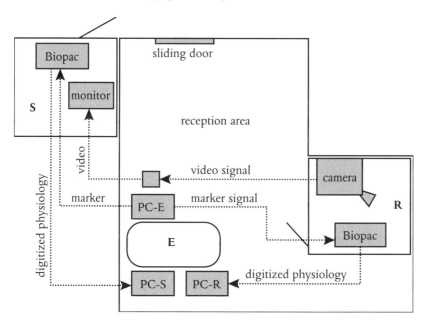

Figure 20.1: Laboratory layout. The experimenter's workstation (E) consisted of three computers: Two recorded the physiological data from the S (PC-S) and R (PC-R) Biopac systems; the third (PC-E) controlled the random timing of the stimuli and a video switch. The receiver was in an electromagnetically and acoustically shielded room; the sender was in a distant room behind two doors and a double wall

Stimulus Procedure

The timing of the viewing periods was controlled by a Windows PC running a program written by the first author in Microsoft Visual Basic 6.0. When that program was launched, it created a random timing schedule for either 25 (control group) or 36 (motivated groups) 10-second visual stimulus epochs. Epochs were separated from one another by a randomly determined 5 to 40 second inter-epoch interval (Figure 20.2).[9] To synchronize the S and R physiological signals, at the beginning of each stimulus epoch the computer switched the video signal from R's chamber to the video monitor in front of S and simultaneously sent onset marker signals to both the S and R Biopac systems (using signals generated by an analog to digital circuit[10]). At the end of each stimulus epoch, the computer switched the video signal off and sent offset markers to the two Biopac systems. After both participants were secured in their respective rooms, the experimenter checked to see if the physiological recordings, marker signals, and video switch were operating properly. When everything was in order an experimenter started the controlling program and attended to other tasks while waiting for the session to end.

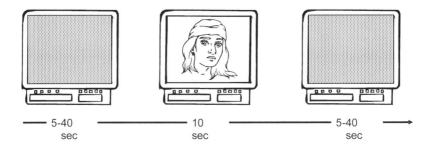

Figure 20.2: Protocol for sender stimulus. Random inter-epoch intervals ranged from 5 to 40 seconds separated by 10-second distant healing intention periods. The receiver's live video image appeared on the monitor during the sending periods, otherwise the monitor was black

Hypotheses and Analyses

The principal hypothesis was that S's DHI directed towards the distant, isolated R would cause R's autonomic nervous system to become activated. A secondary analysis explored whether the factors of motivation and training modulated the postulated effect.

In the following description, the term "epoch" refers to the 20-second period from 5 seconds before stimulus onset to 5 seconds after stimulus offset (this range was used to examine the physiological responses in a temporal context), and "stimulus epoch" refers to the 10-second DHI period between stimulus onset and offset. The analysis examined changes in skin conductance levels (SCL) averaged across epochs ("ensemble average") to see how S and R responded to DHI in time-synchrony.

To determine the statistical significance of the observed results, the following procedures were independently applied to the R and S SCL data. This "bootstrap" analysis, a common method within the larger domain of computational statistics, is a non-parametric way of analyzing physiological data because it makes no assumptions about the underlying structure of the data, and because it answers precisely what we wish to know: Did SCL change in an unexpected way during the actual stimulus epochs, as compared to other, randomly selected times? All SCL data were smoothed using a one-second sliding average window ($\pm$ 500 msec), then a sequence of steps was applied as follows:

1. For each SCL sample in a given session, subtract the SCL value at stimulus onset to form a measure of change in SCL during that epoch.

2. Calculate the ensemble mean of the baseline-subtracted epochs in step 1 for each session.

3. Calculate the grand ensemble mean across all sessions of interest (e.g. trained group sessions).

4. Select random starting points in each session, one for each epoch in the original session, and from those create new, 20-second random epochs. Subtract the baseline from each of these random epochs as in step 1.

5. Form the ensemble mean of the random epochs.

6. Do the same for the other sessions, then calculate a grand ensemble random epoch mean.

7. Repeat steps 4–6 10,000 times to build up a "bootstrap" distribution of ensemble random epochs that *could have occurred* in the experiment if the original epochs had occurred at different times than they did in the actual experiment (Blair and Karniski 1993).

8. Normalize each sample in the original ensemble average curve (20 seconds $\times$ 100 samples/second = 2000 samples) using the mean and standard deviation of the bootstrap distribution formed in step 7, as $z_i = (x_i - \mu_i) / \sigma_i$, where i ranges from 1 to 2000 samples, x_i is sample i from the original ensemble mean, and μ_i is the mean and σ_i the standard deviation of the associated sample from the bootstrap distribution. This step essentially creates a z-score for each sample in the original ensemble epoch. Basing the results on normalized scores weights each epoch equally.

Under the null hypothesis the precise timing of the epochs should not matter because R was thoroughly isolated from S. Thus, if at stimulus offset the normalized ensemble epoch for R significantly deviated from chance (as determined by the bootstrap process), it would suggest that R had responded to, or more generally was correlated with, S's DHI. To avoid multiple testing problems, the preplanned hypothesis examined the normalized deviation only at stimulus offset.

Results

Participants

A total of 72 people participated in the study (Table 20.1), including two minors (a mother–son and mother–daughter pair). They consisted of 36 couples who together conducted a total of 40 sessions, 38 of which were usable (two control sessions could not be analyzed because S's physiological data failed to record properly). Ideally, the three groups of participants would have been matched by gender and age, but in practice this was difficult to achieve as the clinical groups mostly involved women with breast cancer, and this tended to skew the age and gender of those groups. In addition, two couples in the control group switched roles as S and R, and all individuals in the control dyads were healthy.

All participants in the trained and wait groups filled out demographics questionnaires upon beginning the study, then before and after the training periods they filled out questionnaires on mood (McNair, Lorr and Droppleman 1971), marital satisfaction (Hudson 1997), and spiritual well-being (Brady et al. 1999), and the patients only filled out the Functional Assessment of Chronic Illness Therapy (FACIT, Version 4), a self-report measure designed for cancer patients to assess various factors associated with well-being (Cella et al. 1993; Webster et al. 1999). Analysis of the demographics indicated that the trained and wait groups were well matched in terms of gender, ethnicity, family history of cancer, income, prior participation in a cancer therapy group, and involvement in a religious practice.

Analysis of the psychosocial data showed no significant differences in well-being, mood, or quality of life between healthy partners in the trained or wait groups. However, trained group patients showed both a *decline* in physical well-being as compared to wait group patients ($p < 0.01$, two-tailed), and an *improvement* in spiritual well-being ($p < 0.01$, two-tailed).[11] We might interpret this apparently contradictory outcome to imply, purely as a metaphor, that distant intentions might act as church bells that are rung incessantly to assist in healing the ill. The benevolent intentions associated with such chimes may be perceived and appreciated by the mind, thereby raising one's spirits, but they may also prevent the body from getting the rest it needs, making the body feel worse.

Table 20.1: Participant demographics for the three groups

Group	Sessions	Couples	S age	R age	S gender	R gender
Control	16	14	7–71 (average 41)	24–58 (39)	11M/7F	5M/13F
Trained	12	12	37–84 (55)	38–78 (54)	7M/5F	4M/8F
Wait	10	10	42–77 (57)	41–79 (53)	9M/1F	1M/9F

Two of the 18 control sessions did not produce usable data

Data conditioning

To reduce the potential biasing effects of movement artifacts, all data were visually inspected and SCL epochs with artifacts were eliminated from further consideration.[12] This analysis slightly reduced the potential total of 1170 to 1140 epochs (97%) as follows: 387/410 trained epochs (94%),[13] 360/360 wait epochs (100%), and 393/400 control epochs (98%).

Electrodermal activity

S's SCL across all epochs, sessions, and groups increased substantially after stimulus onset, confirming the expected activation in S's sympathetic nervous system as a result of the increased mental effort associated with providing DHI (Figure 20.3). About two seconds after stimulus onset S's SCL began to increase, peaking three seconds later at more than $z = 12$ standard errors above the baseline. In addition, as predicted by the DHI hypothesis, R's SCL also significantly increased. A half-second after stimulus onset R's SCL began to rise, peaking by stimulus offset at $z = 3.9$ standard errors over the baseline (p = 0.00009; all p-values cited are two-tailed).

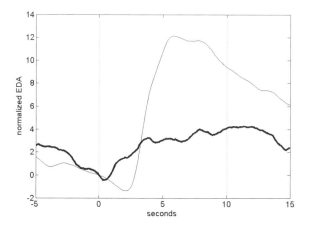

Figure 20.3: Sender (thin line) and receiver (bold line) normalized mean skin conductance levels across all 38 sessions (N = 1140 epochs), from 5 seconds before stimulus onset (at 0 seconds) to 5 seconds after stimulus offset (at 10 seconds) to show the effect in context

Motivated vs. control groups

Figure 20.4 is the same analysis applied to just the motivated group (trained group N = 387 epochs; wait group N = 360 epochs; 747 epochs combined, 22 participants). R's SCL significantly increased to $z = 3.45$ (p = 0.0006) at stimulus offset, peaking at 7.8 seconds at $z = 4.481$ (p = 7.4×10^{-6}).

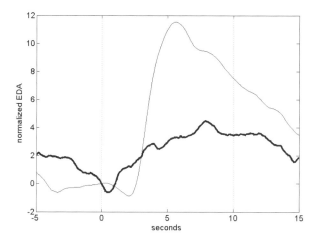

Figure 20.4: Sender (thin line) and receiver (bold line) normalized mean skin conductance levels for all motivated sessions, N = 747 epochs

By comparison, Figure 20.5 shows that R's SCL for the control group (16 sessions, 393 epochs) increased to $z = 2.4$ (p = 0.02) at stimulus offset. The difference between the motivated and control group outcomes at stimulus offset was not significant ($z = 0.73$, p = 0.46). When comparing *effect sizes* per stimulus epoch (where $e = z / \sqrt{N}$, N being the number of epochs) as shown in Figure 20.6, R's SCL at stimulus offset was observed to be about the same magnitude in all of the groups.

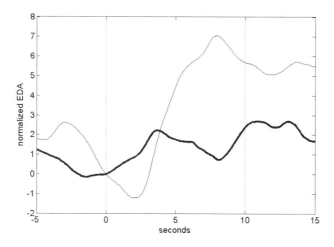

Figure 20.5: Sender (thin line) and receiver (bold line) normalized mean skin conductance levels for control sessions, N = 393 epochs

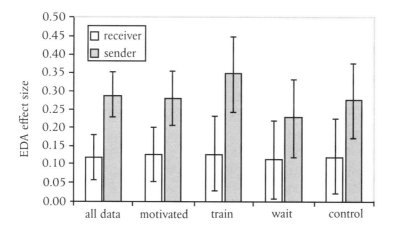

Figure 20.6: Comparison of sender and receiver effect sizes (per epoch) measured at stimulus offset (with ±2 standard error confidence intervals) for all sessions, motivated sessions (trained and wait groups combined), and for trained, wait, and control groups separately

Comparison of the R SCL time course among three groups reveals a more interesting trend, as shown in Figure 20.7. Receivers in all three groups responded quickly at stimulus onset, but (a) the control group's response subsided after four seconds, (b) the wait group's response was initially stronger and subsided after five seconds, and (c) the trained group's response continued to progressively rise for eight seconds, reaching the maximum deviation among all three groups.[14] These differences were not predicted in advance so they must be interpreted with caution. However, if future replications continue to show similar patterns, then training plus motivation would appear to enhance R's response over motivation alone, and motivation would appear to enhance the response over interest alone.

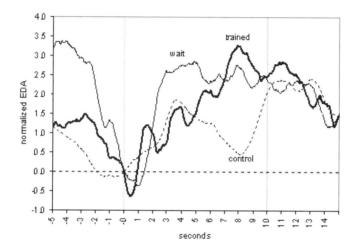

Figure 20.7: Normalized comparison of receiver skin conductance levels in the three groups

Discussion

Analysis of all skin conductance data indicates that S's DHI had a measurable effect on R's autonomic nervous system. Inspection of the time-course of SCL over the average epoch suggests that the trained group had a slower but more sustained effect, followed by a more moderate wait group response, and an even smaller control group response. The overall SCL effect size per session for the motivated groups was $e = 3.45 / \sqrt{22} = 0.74$, some 6.7 times larger than the earlier meta-analytic estimate of $ema = 0.11$, and surprisingly even the control group effect size was some 5.4 times larger than ema ($e = 2.4 / \sqrt{16} = 0.60$). It might be noted that the absolute magnitudes of the observed effects were still rather small, for example for R's SCL the peak changes over baseline amounted to fractions of a microSiemens.[15]

Alternative Explanations

Many artifacts can produce outcomes that mimic DHI effects. In order of decreasing likelihood, they include measurement artifacts, sensory leakage between S and R, R's anticipation of the timing of stimulus epochs, software artifacts, violation of statistical assumptions, selective data reporting, and collusion between S and R.

Potential measurement artifacts include electrical crosstalk that can arise between amplifiers in the same monitoring device, or artifacts induced into the equipment due to electromagnetic (EM) pulses associated with switching the video monitor signal at stimulus onset and offset. The possibility of crosstalk was precluded by using two independent Biopac monitors located 20 meters apart, each with its own data recording computer. Potential effects of EM pulses were significantly diminished by the use of a double steel-walled EM-shielded room and 20-meter separation between S and R. The shielded chamber was designed to effectively block all EM radiation above 10 KHz, but it did not block extremely low frequency (ELF) EM or magnetic fields. Living systems are known to be sensitive to weak EM and magnetic fields, so bio-electromagnetic factors cannot be absolutely ruled out as potential artifacts (Lin 2005). However, prior successful studies (in distant perception tasks) conducted with S on land and R in a submarine under many meters of sea water raise doubts that ELF signals are sufficient to explain this type of "non-local" outcome (Schwartz 2007). Further doubts are raised because of evidence suggesting that DHI effects can be observed even when S and R are displaced in time (Braud 2000; Leibovici 2001; Radin, Machado and Zangari 2000). Sensory leakage artifacts can include conscious or unconscious visual, auditory, or vibratory cues that might pass between S and R. Such artifacts were precluded from the present experiment through the use of separate rooms for S and R, the latter being a heavily shielded chamber, and through prior sound leakage tests. In addition, the experimenters were located between the S and R locations, with no other points of access between the two sites, so any attempt by the couple to communicate through ordinary means would have been detected. Moreover, the physiological condition of both participants was continually monitored during the experiment, allowing detection of the smallest bodily movements in either person. No gross motor movements consistent with attempts at surreptitious signaling were detected in any of the sessions.

For other potential artifacts, could R have anticipated when the stimulus epochs were about to occur, and then respond accordingly? This possibility was prevented through the use of random inter-epoch timing and double-blind conditions. No one knew in advance of a session when each DHI epoch would begin. The random timing and blinded design is also relevant to assessing the impact of a potential bias due to the first author's awareness of which couples were in the control group, and to the fact that most of the data from the control couples were collected by the last three authors. Could different interpersonal styles among these four investigators have influenced how couples responded in this experiment? The question arises because investigators holding different a priori opinions about the likelihood of DHI effects have reported results, even in jointly run experiments, that fell into alignment with their individual beliefs (Wiseman and Schlitz 1997). However, a replication study designed to examine the role of interpersonal interactions in more detail failed to support the earlier results, thus the influences that different investigators may have on DHI outcomes remain uncertain (Schlitz *et al.* 2006). In any case, all investigators in the present study were open to the concept of DHI, so while some interpersonal bias cannot be ruled out, it seems unlikely that the first author's knowledge of which couples participated in the control group would have had much impact on the outcome. Indeed, all three groups showed significant results in the preplanned outcomes.

Potential violations of the assumptions underlying parametric statistics were avoided by using a nonparametric, computational bootstrap procedure to normalize the ensemble averages. To prevent selective reporting biases, data from all usable epochs across all sessions were analyzed and reported for the measure of principal interest (SCL). Collusion between S and R would have been exceedingly difficult to carry out, not only because the EM shielding prevented obvious signaling methods such as sounds and cell phones, but because almost all of the couples participated in only one session, so they did not know what to expect in advance about the laboratory setup or the experimental protocol.

Interpretations

If not due to conventional explanations, then how do we interpret these results? Sloan and Ramakrishnan have asserted that "Nothing in our contemporary scientific views of the universe or consciousness can account for how the 'healing intentions' or prayers of distant intercessors could possibly influence the [physiology] of patients even nearby let alone at a great distance" (Sloan and Ramakrishnan 2005, p.1769).

Is it really true that nothing in science suggests the presence of connections between apparently isolated objects? Quantum entanglement, a far from common-sense effect predicted by quantum theory and later demonstrated as fact in the laboratory, shows that under certain conditions elementary particles that were once connected appear to remain connected after they separate, regardless of distance in space or time. If this property is truly as fundamental as it appears to be, then in principle everything in the universe might be entangled (Radin 2006). Everyday objects and humans certainly do not appear to show such entanglements, and there are non-trivial arguments for why small-scale entanglement would be difficult to sustain in large, living systems. But still, one cannot help wondering, what if this concept *did* apply to humans? In a casual, indifferent, unmotivated couple, entanglements between their minds and bodies may be difficult to detect not only in a fundamental physics sense, but even in an ordinary psychodynamic sense. By comparison, in a long-term, highly motivated, bonded couple, and with S specifically trained to provide compassionate intention, the underlying correlations might be far more evident. Such a relational model is appealing because it does not require anything (force, energy, or signals) to pass between S and R. Instead, it postulates a physical correlation that is always present between people (and everything else) due to the "non-local threads" from which the fabric of reality is woven.

Another possible interpretation is that the outcomes of this and similar experiments were due to precognition on the part of the investigators, who manage to begin each session at just the right time so as to match natural fluctuations in R's physiology with the randomly determined moments of stimulus onset and offset. While such an explanation may seem implausible, independent evidence in favor of retrocausal effects in humans continues to accumulate (May, Paulinyi and Vassy 2005; McCraty, Atkinson and Bradley 2004a, 2004b; Radin 1997, 2004b; Spottiswoode and May 2003); so it is not inconceivable. Indeed, because there are as yet no adequate theoretical models that would predict macroscopic correlations akin to DHI, we are obliged to remain open to a wide range of possible explanations.

A key limitation in the present study was the lack of closely matched demographics among the three groups. Given this limitation, it would be imprudent to draw strong conclusions about performance differences among the groups. However, based on the overall support of the formal hypothesis, it is possible to draw one conclusion: Directing one's attention towards a distant person apparently causes measurable changes in that person's nervous system. This suggests that DHI provides more than a psychological coping mechanism, and that prayer for others is the second most popular CAM modality for a very simple reason: It has an effect on the human body, presumably an effect that is usually perceived as beneficial in some way. Whether it specifically promotes *healing* remains to be seen.

Notes

1. The terms sender and receiver are used for expository reasons. They do not imply a signaling model as the underlying mechanism.
2. Biopac GEL101, Biopac, Goleta, CA.
3. Biopac type TSD203, 8mm Ag/AgCl electrodes.
4. 2μS per volt, or 0–20μS for the full 10-volt range of the EDA amplifier.
5. Biopac M150.
6. Lindgren/ETS, Cedar Park, Texas, Series 81 Solid Cell.
7. SI Tech Models 2809/2010 and Model 2550, Batavia, IL.
8. Model 840028, Sper Scientific, Scottsdale, AZ.

9. The random source in both cases was based on Visual Basic 6.0's pseudorandom algorithm, seeded by the PC's CPU clock at the beginning of each session.

10. Ontrak Control Systems Model ADR-100, Sudbury, Ontario, Canada.

11. Both results survive Bonferroni corrections for multiple tests.

12. Artifacts were identified by the first author, who was not blind to each epoch's underlying condition.

13. The first two trained trials consisted of 25 epochs, the last 10 consisted of 36 epochs, for 410 possible epochs.

14. In this comparison, the number of epochs in each curve is approximately the same, so the normalized curves are not biased by differences in sample size. Trained = 387 epochs, Wait = 360 epochs, Control = 393 epochs.

15. Of course, small magnitude effects do not imply "no effects." Statistically speaking the results are unambiguous.

Chapter 21

THE PINEAL GLAND AND ITS INFLUENCE ON BODY– MIND–SOUL INTEGRATION

Decio Iandoli, Jr., MD, PhD

At the beginning of the twentieth century, a five-year-old Austrian boy began to suddenly grow very quickly and within months looked as if he was 13 years old. Hair grew on his body, his voice became lower, and he showed all the significant signs indicative of puberty. His sexual precociousness was accompanied by mental sophistication beyond his true age. Reportedly, he asked his parents what would be the fate or condition of the soul after death. On another occasion, he observed thoughtfully: "It is strange how I feel better letting the other children play with my toys rather than when I play with them myself." Some other things the child said reflected the maturity of thinking in a way considered normal for a mature adult.

The child died before he was six years old, four weeks after being hospitalized, and the autopsy showed a tumor in the pineal gland. Cases like this one, reported in the medical literature, inspired others to study the pineal gland.

Despite the early studies, little was known about the physiological effects of the pineal gland until recently. According to some researchers from the 1950s and 1960s the pineal was only a phylo-genetic remnant or tissue with no function. During this same era, other researchers saw the pineal gland as having a unique role in transporting particular stimuli to the nervous system, especially after the isolation of melatonin by Lerner in 1958 (Brainard 1978), after which more attention was devoted to the study of melatonin and its effects as well as to the study of the pineal gland as a sensorial organ, and not just an endocrinal one. We came to understand that melatonin is only found in the pineal gland.

Today this small structure is one of the most studied by modern science and the knowledge of its structure and functions grows every day at an incredible speed. In our last review (2007) of the databases of MEDLINE, LILACS, Cochrane Library, and SciElo, we counted 13,256 indexed articles, 4358 written since 2000. We now recognize the pineal gland as the headquarters of cronobiology (the temporal structure of the living being) with important relations to other neuro-endocrine structures.

We find spiritually oriented writers who have discussed the importance of the pineal gland since the mid-nineteenth century. Its importance was also noted clearly by ancient cultures, as well as philosophers who lived centuries ago. Reports dating back more than 2000 years from ancient Eastern cultures such as India named the gland the "third eye," the seat of the "sixth-sense," the "center of power," or "eye of Shiva." Nostradamus (1503–1556) described it as "the highest fine antenna of our nervous system," and "a master vessel." René Descartes (1596–1650), philosopher, mathematician, and "creator" of the Cartesian method of research, said the pineal gland is the "seat of the rational soul" or "the gland of knowledge" that allows the ego to influence the physical self.

Melatonin, Brain Sand, and Mediumship

The main secretion of the pineal gland is melatonin, produced in greater quantity in the evening. The production of this hormone is more abundant in women than in men and its production is enhanced by physical exercise, hypergonadotrophic hypogonadism (a condition in which the gonads, testicles, or ovaries do not respond despite having a large quantity of hormones stimulating them), and long abstinence from food (Bruis, Crasson and Legros 2000). The maximum production of melatonin occurs between 2 a.m. and 6 a.m. and its production decreases with age. There is evidence from research (Brendel, Niehaus and Lerchl 2000; Karasek *et al.* 1998; Rosen, Barber and Lyle 1998) that under the effect of magnetic fields the production of melatonin is reduced and this can create physiological repercussions, including changes in the function of the immune system.

The pinealocyte, a specialized cell of the pineal that creates melatonin, has a cell membrane that contains the receptors of all known neurotransmitters. The pinealocyte has a very irregular nucleus and presents inclusions that may contain granules of peptides with unknown function. Moreover, these granules emit concretions of calcium carbonate, "brain sand," which tend to increase at puberty without, however, changing the activity of the gland's secretions. Thus the appearance of brain sand does not appear to be a degenerative process (Commentz *et al.* 1986).

Brain sand consists of cellular organelles with a specific function in the resonance of the magnetic fields of the body. They convert something within the magnetic fields into neurochemical stimuli (Gould 1984; Harvalik 1978; Semm, Schneider and Vollrath 1980). The nature and distribution of these crystals have been studied by Dr. Sergio Felipe de Oliveira. He believes that brain sand responds to changes in electromagnetic fields of any nature that act upon the human body. (Despite my efforts Dr. Sergio has not provided me with references for his work.) Dr. Sergio does suggest that brain sand crystals, being diamagnetic, would act by resonance, converting electromagnetic stimuli into electrochemical stimuli. A recent study performed in Austria (Schmid *et al.* 2007) confirmed the diamagnetic property of the pineal gland, stating that it is also able to capture radio waves like those emitted by a common cell phone with frequency that ranges between 400 and 1850 MHz and power ranges between 125 and 250 MW.

As a result of his clinical observation, Dr. Sergio also raises the possibility that the highest density of crystal in the pineal body is an indicator of the highest mediumistic capacity, of incorporation of spirits, while the lowest incidence of these crystals might be related to the ability of out-of-body experience (OBE). These notions need to be researched further.

The action of melatonin, in general, suppresses some brain function, allowing an increase of distribution to receptors in the brain. A hormone can only influence tissue through cells that have a receptive protein. The presence of melatonin does not determine its effects, but rather the presence of receptors. Therefore, it is important to study the distribution of receptors to understand melatonin's influence on the central nervous system (CNS), including its effects on mediumship.

The receptors enable the process of mediumship to be established, reasons Dr. Sergio. He relates that the sedative effect of the hormone inhibits certain brain areas, and encourages the expression of specific types of mediumship—such as unconscious mediumship and some types of psychography (automatic writing), among others. In line with this thinking, characteristics in synaptic connections in the thalamic, cortical, and subcortical pineal areas, associated with the distribution of melatonin receptors, would form the neuro-anatomical and functional basis of the mechanisms related to mediumship. This organic function, he believes, is genetically determined. Some more consistent studies are necessary in order to evaluate the function of crystals in mediums' process and their relation to the distribution of mediumship in the population as a whole.

Brain sand does not indicate a greater or lesser capacity for mediumship. It denotes a specific neural organization that may be related to greater or lesser mediumship capacity. We cannot, as yet, make a definite claim in this regard, since we don't yet have sufficient evidence to fully explain the brain's activity during a mediumistic trance.

Prevalence of Brain Sand

Computed tomography (CT) and other diagnostic devices reveal that 33–76 percent of all adults have identifiable concretions (brain sand). Kanta *et al.* (1996) studied 2016 tomographies in sequence in AIDS patients, and found an average incidence of 61.7 percent with a predominance of 6.7 percent in men, while Zimmerman and Bilaniuk (1982) found an incidence of 40 percent in 725 normal adults, and they reported incidences of 8 to 11 percent in children from 8 to 14 years. Children under six years old seldom show such concretions and their presence suggests neoplasias such as pinealomas.

Studies of the melatonin receptors (Jockers and Petit 1998) identified two basic types, Mel1 and Mel2, the first divided into Mel1a, Mel1b, and Mel1c, found in the brain, retina, and many other peripheral tissues. In birds, it was shown that the presence of motor neurons in Mel1b, as well as Mel1c receptors involved in the singing control of the singing birds, linked melatonin with motor function (Jansen *et al.* 2005).

A study at the University of Milan (Mazzucchelli *et al.* 1996) identified the location of these receptors in the human brain, finding them in large quantity in the following structures (listed in descending order of concentration of receptors):

1. cerebellum

2. occipital cortex

3. parietal cortex

4. temporal cortex

5. thalamus

6. frontal cortex

7. hippocampus.

Functions of the Pineal Gland

In humans the pineal is biochemically active for life; however, the functions of the pineal still generate controversy in the medical literature.

We can say that, almost always, the endocrine action of the pineal is suppressing. One notion is that, in humans, melatonin has an inhibitory action on the gonads (as was verified when the pineal tumors were responsible for cases of early puberty). However, research in India in 2006 (Sengupta and Kumar Maitra 2006) showed that the pineal, not melatonin, is responsible for the seasonal pace in the testicular activity in a parakeet found in Africa, India, and China, Psittacula krameri, which opens a new window for research and discussions about the pineal's physiologic mechanism.

Today we know that melatonin is significantly connected with:

• biological cycles

• aging

• phenomenon of jet lag, especially for pilots of aircraft

• sleep disorders

• seasonal affective disorders

• fertility.

Maturation, Aging, and the Pineal Gland

When a fetus is 50 days old, the pineal is already developed, allowing the fetus to capture magnetic and/or superluminal stimuli that provide the development of the brain nuclei, stimulating the neuroblasts that migrate and connect among themselves. Some studies show that the action of the pineal gland is vital to morphology and the development of the CNS (Janjoppi *et al.* 2006; Tunç *et al.* 2006, 2007; Turgut *et al.* 2007). Thus, the pineal is already important in life in utero, and perhaps acting as a lens that receives stimuli that synchronize the individual with the cosmos and the fourth dimension (time). This partially explains the intervention of the perispirit as the blueprint of the physical body.

Calcification of the pineal gland is observed with aging. This would not be due to inactivity and degeneration of the structure, but because of an increase in its "vibrational" activity and resonance, providing trans-ductional crystal with subtle energies, particularly important for our mental receptivity. The term "vibrational" has been used to describe biological energies by Richard Gerber, MD, in his book *Vibrational Medicine* (2001).

The fact that radiological studies show the rarity of these calcifications in children up to six years of age leads us to ponder what was channeled to Chico Xavier in the Spiritist literature by André Luiz, recorded in the 1945 book *Missionaries of Light* (Xavier 2009). Luiz teaches that incarnation is completed only at seven years of age, and up to that age, the individual is highly susceptible to suggestions and traumas from the environment where he or she lives, as if in a hypnotic trance. When the age of seven is reached the connection between the body and the spirit is complete. Then, the definitive development of the conductive pathways of subtle energy begins. This requires a trans-ductional structure and a higher capacity to conduct energy.

Luiz's point of view matches the theories of Freud and several other psychoanalysts that followed him, who observed the importance of this stage (0–7 years) in shaping the character of the individual and the effects of trauma suffered in this period, which could potentially generate neuroses and even psychoses.

At 14 years of age the pineal finally opens to the file of information from its perispirit, bringing memories of past lives. These start to arise as tendencies and impulses adding to the conditioning acquired in childhood which create a new personality for the current life. In addition the development of character is influenced by genes and cosmological aspects. Cosmological influences are seen in biological cycles, as well as during pregnancy, which lasts 40 lunar weeks. They can also be seen in circadian cycles of cortisol that increase in early nighttime. The combination of all of these factors is the start of an adult personality.

If the person finds a positive structure in which to develop and resources to overcome negative tendencies, there can, of course, be increased movement toward developing positive tendencies.

Time and the Fourth Dimension

One can see that most of the activities assigned to the pineal are related to time periods and the cycles of life. Hence its relationship to light/dark, day/night, and cronobiology. This includes the mechanisms and the properties of the recurrent physiological and behavioral changes, and the so-called biological rhythms. Some of these periodicities are clearly identified, such as: respiratory cycles, heart beats, the different cycles of activity–rest in animals or the wake–sleep cycle of human beings, and the menstrual cycles of the animals and superior primates, including humans. Others require the development of specific instruments and methods to better detect and characterize them.

Time, the fourth dimension, is the key that organizes the activity of the biological system; the form itself depends on its relationship to space–time. Medical researchers in cronobiology recognize the pineal as the biological clock acting strongly on the process of sexual maturation. However, other external factors, including cycles of light, influence the biological cycles. Among them are room temperature, availability of food, social factors, atmospheric pressure, electrostatic and electromagnetic fields, and relative humidity (Douglas 2000). These are the external factors, the afferent information which merges with the efferent factors, called endogenous by physiologists, producing the resulting organic cronobiological control.

The biological cycles are divided into four main groups:

1. Circadian Cycles—24 hours, controlled by the sun—day/night cycles.

2. Ultradian Cycles—hormonal peaks related to periods of the day.

3. Infradian Cycles (monthly cycles)—controlled by the moon—e.g. hair, menstruation, pregnancy, pituitary cycles.

4. Cycles related to environmental changes such as tidal changes, moon cycles, and the seasons.

Spirit, Cosmos, and the Pineal

The spirit is manifested in the physical body by controlling the fourth dimension (time), thus organizing the biological system. The pineal gland is the main tool of this control.

Studies in birds and other animals have shown that the pineal acts as a navigation center (Demaine and Semm 1985; Walcott, Gould and Lednor 1988). Migrating birds lose their orientation when they have their pineal damaged or submitted to inverted electromagnetic fields, which demonstrates the capacity of the gland to realize the magnetic north of the planet, confirming its capacity of orienting animals to the magnetic fields.

The magnetic axis of the earth has an influence on all organ systems. Similarly the pineal has magnetic sensors (in its electromagnetic and electrostatic fields), which connect us with the stars and harmonize us with the time of the solar system, placing us biophysically in relationship to it. The pineal does not produce the rhythms, but it organizes them, and therefore integrates the life of the Spirit and the planets and celestial bodies that influence the earth, synchronizing the individual with the cosmos. With these responsibilities of command, the pineal is linked to the Soul, which is the intelligent principle, and therefore the perispirit, which is its intermediary.

The pineal functions as a lens that concentrates the orders of the perispirit and thalamus as a prism distributor. Between these two structures there is a wide range of synapses and neural pathways as already described. It is not difficult to imagine the pineal as the "eye" which communicates the exterior world to the interior, or else, we may say, the one that connects men to the cosmos because it guides us in relationship to the cycles of the stars in the solar system.

The Intelligent Principle

Genes account for a biochemical production that determines characteristics and functions of the physical body, but these structures must be controlled by intelligence, an organizing force that dominates space–time.

We can divide the body into several functional and structural fields: anatomical fields, genetic fields, molecular fields (neurotransmitters, immunoglobulins, etc.), and bio-electromagnetic fields. The pineal acts on all fields, providing the structure in time, the key element needed for the Spirit to take command of its biological structure.

When we analyze the atom on a subatomic level we can see the distances between its material particles. We see that subatomic matter is composed of much more space than particles. In these spaces, scientists have already observed the presence of particles which appear from "nowhere" and disappear into "nowhere," suggesting we are on the edge of a different dimension or frequency.

Those little particles observed subatomically in the vacuum between the particles of the atom were named the "Dirac Sea." They generate quantic-floating energy throughout the so-called vacuum of space. These particles spontaneously appear and can annihilate each other in a flash of energy. The structural nuclei of the DNA molecule may be contained in the Dirac Sea and structure the communication between the physical and spiritual dimensions. Let's call this bridge the "intelligent principle." It is the organizing force of matter and, consequently, the biological system. It also exercises its action through the commands of the perispirit, the body from which it manifests.

The arrival of the pineal gland in the evolutionary scale, occurring in fish, may be the first sign of the individualization in the intelligent principle. This primary connection to spirit, although primitive, has endured for more than 7 million years. It marks a stage of awareness in human evolution that brings the spirit into relationship with the capacity for reason. This higher potential for knowledge increases our responsibility. Learning to manage that responsibility correctly will determine our potential for further evolution.

The Soul, the Chakras, and the Pineal

Certain diseases are clearly related to alterations in the phase of pace, such as depression which causes a slowing down, or anxiety which causes a speeding up of thinking and other functions. These emotional disorders ultimately cause neurophysiologic changes.

The sleep–wake cycle determines the degree of connection between the spirit and body, and the pineal can control the periods of sleep and wakefulness by the secretion of melatonin. According to Spiritualist literature, the pineal is likely interconnected with a "special energy system" that is involved with the chakras (transducers of subtle energy to the physical body). The scientific literature has named these "centers of force," or chakras, and is attempting to measure and study them (Hacker *et al.* 2005). This special system of energy is linked to the rise of the energies of personality to a higher level, meaning with more spiritual awareness. It can release all the creative and evolutionary potential of the individual. Acupuncture is the only accepted medical specialty that is clearly involved with this "special energy system."

Observations of André Luiz, MD

It is interesting to correlate the information of the traditional scientific sources with what André Luiz provided from his observations about the pineal gland as a disincarnate. His observations came through the automatic writing of the medium Francisco Cândido Xavier, beginning in 1945 in the book *Missionaries of Light*— long before the data collected from modern scientific literature, explored in this chapter, was published. He wrote:

> The tiny gland had become a radiating nucleus and its rays formed a
> lotus flower of sublime petals around it. (Xavier 2009, p.23)

Luiz remarked on the great flow of energy that connects to this pathway and says the pineal is very important in communications with the spiritual plane:

> During puberty, it awakens the creative forces in the human organism,
> and thereafter it continues to function as the most advanced

laboratory of a human being's psychic elements. During the period of childhood development—the readjustment phase for this important center of the preexisting perispiritual body—the pineal gland seems to restrain the manifestations of sex; however, these observations need to be rectified. At the age of fourteen, approximately, the pineal gland goes from a stationary state regarding its essential attributes and begins to function again in the reincarnated person. What once represented control now becomes a creative source and an escape valve. The pineal gland readjusts itself to the body's organic order and reopens its wonderful world of sensations and impressions in the realm of emotions. (Xavier 2009, p.25)

Notice the corroboration between what our disembodied author says and data accepted by the scientific community today regarding the endocrine function of the pineal:

As an organ of the ethereal body's highest expression, it presides over the neural phenomena of the emotions. It is the key source of magnetic potential and secretes "psychic hormones" or "power units." By secreting subtle psychic energies, the pineal gland maintains control over the entire endocrine system. Connected to the mind through electromagnetic principles in the vital field—which ordinary science has not yet been able to identify—it commands subconscious powers under the direct determination of the will. The neural webs form its "telegraph wires" for giving immediate orders to all cellular areas and under its direction psychic energies are supplied to all the autonomous storage areas of the organs. (Xavier 2009, pp.25–26)

André Luiz was the first to remark on the relationship between the pineal and the autonomic nervous system and the endocrine system. His observations turn our attention to the relationship of psychic activity in mediumistic processes with the evident adrenergic reaction observed in mediums in trance.

With regard to sexuality and mental health, Luiz writes:

Sex as an expression of love is in conformity with spiritual harmony and in accordance with the law of God, yet when it manifests itself restricted to the sexual area alone (for sensual pleasure only), the creative force and comprehensive energy is reduced and restricted, generating energetic disturbances that may be manifested by physical disease and psychological maladjustments. (Xavier 2009)

Regarding the action of the pineal in mediumship, Luiz writes: "In the exercise of any psychic modality, the pineal gland plays the most important role" (Xavier 2009).

Although André Luiz provided us precise and accurate information about the pineal gland which, at the time of publication (1945), was overlooked by science, corroboration of his point of view has subsequently been increasingly found by scientists. This can alert us to paths that may be valuable to follow for further scientific investigation in the future, for example scientifically researching other things told to Chico Xavier by disincarnate doctors.

> The pineal can be compared to a powerful plant that should be utilized in a controlled way to enlighten, refine and generally benefit the personality. It should not be allowed to drain its supply of psychic energy in coarse emotions that are not uplifting. Virtuous activity is the occupation of the soul and brings about mental health. Accepting the elevated path of personal sacrifice is as important to individuals as pruning trees correctly to help them grow strong and healthy. We need to use our assets with respect, taking a dignified approach to life, and thus lift ourselves up. As we do this, it is important to distinguish between harmony and balance. (Xavier 2009)

Bringing together current scientific observations with those of André Luiz we conclude that the pineal gland is a crystalline-like structure that receives information from the soul, or the intelligent principle, and from the subtle bodies, or perispirit. It may be a biological imperative that we open our minds to allow this information to flow into consciousness and inform our decisions and our growth. We will feel better for it. This may be more true for those gifted with powerful abilities as mediums. When they do not listen to the information from the intelligent principle, they may be expending energy holding back an extremely creative force for good, and resisting it may be detrimental (more on that in Chapter 5, about a cause of mental illness being repressed mediumship). But even those of us who are less gifted can adopt the idea that the pineal is like an antenna, capturing wisdom from the Universe and spiritual realms, allowing us to become adjusted to our environment and more balanced. It may be especially important in improving our health and well-being and nurturing our spiritual development.

Part IV

THE INTERNATIONAL IMPACT OF SPIRITISM

Editor's Note

As we next contemplate how Spiritist ideas and practices may be both relevant and helpful to people outside Brazil, it is interesting to reflect on how receptive non-Brazilian people might be. How open are we to notions of the afterlife, reincarnation, mediumship, and discarnates communicating with people? Do we believe that the mind has healing power that can effectively contribute to health protocols?

In 1991 a poll was conducted in 17 Christian countries (not including Brazil) by the International Social Survey Programme (Robinson 2007a), asking about a definite belief in the afterlife. North Americans ranked highest with 55 percent confidence that an afterlife exists. The UK ranked 11th with 23.8 percent believing in an afterlife. The poll suggested that those believing in an afterlife tended to focus more on reunion with loved ones rather than union with God.

B.A. Robinson (2007b) of Ontario Consultants on Religious Tolerance consolidated some recent findings and updated this 1991 study making the following reports:

- In 1999 a poll was done in North America by the Survey Research Center of the University of California at Berkeley. That poll discovered that 86 percent of Protestants, 83 percent of Roman Catholics, 74 percent of Jews, and 58 percent of those with no religious affiliation believe in an afterlife.

That's an increase from 55 percent of all North Americans just eight years earlier! Has belief in an afterlife continued to rise in the twenty-first century at such a rapid rate? Also from Robinson (2007b):

- A Harris Poll from January 21–27, 2003 found that 51 percent of all North Americans, 58 percent of women, and 65 percent of people age 25–29 believe in ghosts.

- This same Harris Poll found that 27 percent believe in reincarnation, with 40 percent of those aged 25–29 believing in reincarnation.

The June 2005 Gallup Survey on how many people in the USA believe in at least one aspect of the paranormal is another indicator. David Moore (2005) reported in an article, "Three in Four Americans Believe in Paranormal":

- 41 percent believe in extra-sensory perception
- 32 percent believe that spirits of dead people can come back to communicate with those in body
- 21 percent believe that people can communicate mentally with someone who has died
- 9 percent believe in allowing a "spirit-being" to temporarily assume control of the body, as in channeling
- 55 percent believe in the healing powers of the mind
- 31 percent believe in telepathy, that is, communication between minds without using traditional senses.

In December 2010 a Gallup poll discovered that 7 in 10 North Americans say that religion is losing its influence on American life. Fifty-four percent say religion is "very important" in their lives (down from 75% in 1952). The current 61 percent of Americans who report being a church or synagogue member is as low as has been measured by Gallup since the 1930s (Newport 2010).

Those who do not identify fully with conventional religion and have strong beliefs in the paranormal may be wondering where they can go to be part of a supportive community group who share these beliefs (or at least want to explore them) and practice the healing powers of the mind. A 22-year-old woman recently posed this question to me: "Where do you go in the USA if you want to improve your life and you don't identify with any Church? Many of my generation want self-improvement, but don't know where to look. The answer can't be psychotherapy: It's just too expensive!"

Could an "outside Brazil" form of Spiritist Center provide an answer?

Chapter 22 describes what one might find in a Spiritist Center in the UK, from the perspective of a woman who has been a Spiritist for decades. Chapter 23 recounts travels in Brazil and how two North Americans consider bringing home to North America the resources they found at Spiritist Centers in Brazil.

Chapter 22

WHAT SPIRITIST CENTERS OFFER OUTSIDE BRAZIL

Janet Duncan

Introduction

The United Kingdom is a country with a tradition of haunted houses and ghosts, of creepy crawly things that go bump in the night. Strangely few seem to want to know what this is, or what it is about. Most just go on feeling goose pimples and their hair stands on end, so they quickly run in the opposite direction.

Before today there have been few people interested in discovering what is going on in spiritual terms in the UK. Spiritualists tend only to want to know more and more about psychic phenomena, especially the "messages from loved ones who have passed on" and materializations, with the idea of proving that there is life after death, but they shy away from any profound questions. Even the most basic ones, such as: What am I? Where have I come from? What am I doing here? Where will I go later on? People of all walks of life seem to be afraid to even think these questions, let alone ask them.

Strangely enough Spiritualists have constantly refused to consider what so-called "life after death" is composed of. If these people consider traveling abroad they usually look up travel brochures, etc. and make some inquiries about the country they plan to visit. But it seems these same people are quite happy to go blindly into the next world without any desire to prepare themselves for what they will find, even believing they will be sitting on a fluffy white cloud playing a harp or something similar. Quite extraordinary!

Spiritism in the UK

Despite these attitudes the Spiritist movement was started in the UK in 1983. Today there are a number of Spiritist Groups in and outside London holding regular meetings open to the general public, as well as the British Union of Spiritist Societies (BUSS), now a registered charity. The Spiritist teachings are penetrating, being accepted and understood by an ever-increasing number of people, very importantly including those from within the medical profession.

But finally the word is beginning to spread outside Brazil that we are immortal spirits by nature, temporarily enclosed within a material body, the purpose for which the Spiritist teachings have a clear, rational, and logical explanation, proved many thousands of times over by people across the world. Now these facts are also starting to be accepted by science and a number of highly qualified and respected researchers, medical doctors, alternative therapy workers, and a large number of nursing staff in varied working situations, in several countries, and to some degree also here in the UK.

One of the most baffling happenings within the medical profession has always been the frequent occurrence of mental problems, when the patient not only hears voices but is often taken over by these same voices (as in schizophrenia), and is sometimes thrown into a convulsive state, perhaps followed by unconsciousness (as in epilepsy). These so-called "illnesses" are now being recognized by some more spiritually aware doctors and researchers as possibly having an "outside" cause. So finally a deeper understanding is beginning that here we may be dealing with "outside influences" and not merely bodily illness or disease, although when these influences are suffered over a prolonged period of time they can provoke bodily dysfunction, even severe.

Chapters 15 and 16 of this book were written by two British psychiatrists working in this field here in the UK. Another psychiatrist, Peter Fenwick, MD, from the Royal College of Psychiatry in London, is researching and studying various aspects of approaching death and the frequent accompanying "effects" (Fenwick 2008). In his opinion there is a need for training to be given to workers in this field, so they are more prepared to help the dying person to make the transition into the next world. As he continues his research into death-related sensory experiences (DRSE) it becomes clear that these are spiritually transforming experiences, often with the appearance of a messenger beyond the visible observable universe, coming to guide a dying person through the process. These DRSEs have been reported to occur most commonly among those dying from terminal illness. Communication frequently takes place between the dying person and the apparition that brings comfort and serenity. Reportedly the DRSEs are intense spiritual experiences. So we see the spiritual world about us, on different dimensions, but nevertheless totally aware of the occurrences on our material level of life. In these circumstances there is always a conveying of loving compassion, seeking to offer guidance and assurance of the immortality of the soul. Peter Fenwick feels that special preparation and training for all medical staff working in these areas, especially within the hospice area, is greatly needed (2008).

Since the middle of the 1800s spiritually based information has been received from the spiritual world in many places, but especially in Brazil, by well-recognized and proven mediums. Today the Brazilian Spiritist library totals several thousand books, many of which have been translated into various languages. In the last 30 years these teachings have begun to spread far beyond the boundaries of Brazil and South America, up through the Americas, and over to Europe. Now they are infiltrating slowly into Russia, Asia, Africa, China, New Zealand, Australia, Japan, and beyond, to reach all four corners of our planet. Stemming from the study and practice of all this information are some remarkable results.

We see that Spiritist teachings begin to take root due to the constant sufferings and anguish of people in all countries, in all walks of life, be they rich or poor. The Spiritist Centers begin to spring up and develop as people of all ages and needs find they receive loving comfort, as well as spiritual healing, for both their bodies and minds within these centers. All of which is always offered free of charge! Therefore, these healing opportunities are available to everyone, without distinction of wealth, education, race, or religion. The teachings comfort and aid without encroaching on anyone's beliefs.

Spiritism understands that help needs to be available in varying forms, so there will always be something to suit every circumstance and need. All Spiritist Centers, following the lines marked out by Allan Kardec, work on many levels, from philosophical, scientific, and medical understanding to moral concepts of spiritual progress. The use of prayer as a powerful instrument for good is taught during the various processes of guidance in these groups and non-contact spiritual healing is offered in all circumstances. There is also an atmosphere of welcome and friendship, together with a real sense of fellowship.

Let me make one thing very clear at this point. To be a Spiritist worker is not a profession, no! These are merely ordinary people working in normal jobs to earn their wages and pay their rent. They only work in their Spiritist Center in their spare time. Therefore they have no need to charge or demand payment. These are very charitable people doing their best to help and befriend anyone in need or distressed. Their attitude has come about because they have really studied the Spiritist teachings and come to fully understand the meaning of one of its most important concepts: "Without charity there is no salvation!" It is also known that the healing energies really come from the spiritual level and that the so-called spiritual healer is actually little more than a useful channel through which the energies are transmitted under controlled conditions directly to the patient.

Understandably the Spiritist worker must learn to be a kind and loving friend, as well as needing skills in giving guidance using a great deal of discernment and intuition. Each person who approaches is a unique individual requiring individualized help and guidance.

As knowledge and acceptance of the spiritual aspect of our lives widens, it will gradually become apparent to the professional medical worker that they also need the same spiritual study as those working in Spiritist Centers, so as to be more discerning during diagnosis and about life in general. The ideal situation, already beginning to occur in many places, is for all levels of workers in the field of spiritual understanding to study together and exchange experiences and views. This greatly facilitates spiritual awareness, especially when referring to the complexities of obsession and all disturbances of the mind.

Each properly organized Spiritist group offers regular study periods, and spiritual healing as their working basis, together with lectures and various specialized courses. Centers of longer standing also offer the opportunity to make an appointment for individual spiritual guidance, referred to as "fraternal guidance." During these sessions, conducted by a responsible medium, the person may ask for advice on spiritually related matters and guidance for daily living.

Education of Mediums

Many people, including scientists and medical workers, are very skeptical regarding our psychic potentials. However, science has long known about the pineal gland and today admits that it does continue to function even after the period of so-called "crystallization," when it was thought to become inactive. This is merely the reaching of maturity of this very important organ, which in fact is known to be our natural antenna, allowing us access to the vibratory waves that are all around us on many levels. However, this gland is not necessarily active as an antenna in every person. It is frequently found to be in a latent state, and may never become psychically active in a particular life. Nevertheless, it can sometimes be provoked into action by meditation and specific exercises. The Spiritist teachings advise us that care should be taken as, if artificially or forcefully provoked into activity, it could become a source of serious problems, unable to find a happy solution.

When the pineal gland awakens naturally, even in only a slight degree, this is the time when we can sometimes hear the spiritual voices or see those in the spiritual world. We should not be surprised at this, as technology today is constantly inventing electrical apparatus capable of capturing many noises and sounds we cannot normally hear or see. This is our own "built-in apparatus," allowing us at times to tune in and even view people and animals on a spiritual level. So let us understand once and for all that not all people who hear voices and see things outside the normal range of vision are mad. Many may be mediums who can learn how to use their sensitivities to improve their quality of life as well as help others.

A well-run and firmly based Spiritist Center will offer highly specialized courses for mediumship education. These Mediumship Education Courses are of varying duration, from two to five years, followed by rigorously disciplined Mediumship Practice Sessions held in private on a regular weekly basis. These practical sessions deal with "rescue work," utilizing trance mediumship to receive needy spirits, many of whom are lost and frequently not even aware of their departure from the material world. These suffering spirits are given guidance and healing and helped to come to terms with their varying situations, so as to be able to find peace and be reunited with their family members in the spiritual world.

Sometimes within a Spiritist Center there is a Mediumship Practice Session of very long standing, meaning for perhaps some ten years. If this session has always been held on a regular day, with the very same well-prepared people, it can happen that this private group may be given the opportunity to deal with cases of "disobsession." This will happen only with the authorization and under the guidance of the spiritual mentors of that particular center. At the moment (June 2011), within Kardec-oriented Spiritist Centers, there are no disobsession sessions being held in the UK.

Guidance is Offered

The guidance that can be received in all well-organized and established Spiritist Centers or groups will be given by prepared mediums on matters related to spiritual well-being. We are never told to do this or do that, but rather we receive general guidance towards the areas in our life that we need to reconsider. Attitudes and behavior are often mentioned because it is here we have most work still to do. Life is a constant action and reaction; what we do or say will cause an obvious reaction for the person we are talking to. If our words are calm and friendly, they will reply in like terms. But the moment we lose our calm and shout, they will reply in like manner. We all know this but take no notice, so we continue to repeat the same pattern of approach to everyone and come to wonder why the world is so angry. Remember, one of the laws of life is "like attracts like." So, in easily understood ways, during guidance we will be gently shown how we can make our life better and happier, and how we can resolve many of our problems.

The more mature UK Spiritist Groups offer fraternal guidance (by appointment) for those wishing to receive help with problems of an emotional nature or possibly relating to psychic faculties that have blossomed and are not understood, causing anxieties and disturbances. This form of guidance can also be useful with health problems, which does not substitute for normal medical attention, however. But it can often clarify if there is spiritual interference as well as physical imbalance. Spiritualism does not operate in this way and apparently has no understanding of it. At least the few who possibly do understand seem to make a point of not disclosing this helpful information to their followers.

Another aspect of Spiritist teachings, within groups in the UK and elsewhere, is centered around the existence of a very powerful energy that most people are seldom aware of, or refuse to take the trouble to learn about. Many even declare that it is of no use at all, because they tried it and it never worked. To what am I referring? What else but prayer. These days attention is gradually awakening as we are constantly being told to "think positively" so as to avoid negative consequences. People are becoming aware that thought is a force that can be either positive or negative. Within Spiritist Groups the art of prayer is explained and demonstrated, and joined to our thought process to create positive changes that can result in great improvements in our lives, especially when linked to the powerful energies existing on a higher level of vibration. Thus prayer takes on a new role and becomes a daily tool for protection and spiritual well-being within our homes and workplaces.

Outside Brazil, in the UK and across Europe, it is becoming known that a Spiritist Center is somewhere to go for help when life seems too hard to bear, a place where everyone will be well received by caring and loving people, happy to offer help of various kinds, that can bring back peace of mind and tranquility. The study of life's reality is a constant in all groups. It creates an atmosphere of calm, filled with hope for a better future. The dedicated workers in these centers are constantly studying life in all of its aspects, not merely for their own benefit but so that they may help all the many troubled people who come to seek their aid.

This depth of understanding of what life is all about can turn people away from negative ideas, such as suicide, euthanasia, and abortion. It shows us through reasoning and logic that we must rethink our ideas if we wish to find peace and happiness. Physical life is not meant to be one big holiday, no! In fact it is given to us so we may right the many wrongs we have committed in the past and also learn new lessons for the future. We need to learn about the natural laws that are eternal and how to live within them, so we can finally find that blessed haven we call heaven.

Studying the Meaning of Life

Therefore the main work within Spiritist Centers around the world is centered on the teaching of the meaning of life itself, as put forth in Allan Kardec's works. The student then continues their studies with the five wonderful books received by Chico Xavier from the Spirit Emmanuel, starting with the title *Two Thousand Years Ago*, recently translated into English (2007). It is then essential to continue with more of the works received by Chico Xavier, especially the series of 11 books received from the Spirit of André Luiz. This spirit had been a medical doctor in his last incarnation and he describes how he found life in the world of spirit, starting with his arrival and continuing with his subsequent discoveries. As a qualified doctor he is surprised when he asks to continue with his profession to be informed that on that level of life his services are not at all appropriate. This is a series that, once begun, inevitably carries you through to the very end. Happily it is now being translated into English and half of the series is already available in Spiritist Centers.

Superstitions, spells, ceremonies, elaborate robes or rituals, etc. have no place within Spiritist teachings. Neither are there any designated superior authorities, only people in leadership through their obvious spiritual progress. Let it be seen also that Spiritism is not a religion, but rather "a way of life," doing the very best to follow the teachings of Christ on a daily basis.

On a More Personal Note

I was born in August 1928, in a house near the Royal Botanical Gardens of Kew, London, UK, and received a post-Victorian education from my very strict English mother. I had my first psychic experience at the age of four and a half, which left a very vivid memory; even today, it is as if it had happened only yesterday. Over the years I have continued periodically to receive help and guidance from my spiritual friends. In my early twenties I immigrated to Brazil together with my husband and spent the next 30 years based in the great metropolis of São Paulo. As a teacher of English and methodology for language teaching I had the opportunity to travel extensively from the north to the south of Brazil, lecturing in most of the universities and many language schools, so coming to know and understand Brazilian people.

At the end of the 1960s I bought a copy of *The Spirits' Book* by Allan Kardec, which immediately rang a loud bell for me. Then in July 1971 I was led to visit Brazil's most famous medium, Francisco Candido Xavier (Chico), who later became a friend. At that first meeting Chico guided me to where I should begin the study of the Spiritist teachings and start the education of my psychic faculties, in São Paulo near where I lived. After an intense study period of ten years I was called back to London in 1981 and in February 1983 I began the Allan Kardec Study Group-UK, Center for Spiritist Teachings, in a suburb of London.

Now at the age of 82 I am finally able to meditate and look back over my life. I clearly remember the headstrong young girl who fervently declared that she could not change her character because she had been born that way, so it was quite impossible! I was not happy with some of my characteristics, but felt entirely unable to do anything about them. It was not until 1971, when I discovered the Spiritist teachings, and received guidance from Chico Xavier, that I came to realize it was possible to make whatever changes one desires. However, it takes a lot of willpower and some considerable time; it does not happen overnight.

As I look back I recognize the importance of 1971 and that special initial meeting with Chico. They say that wisdom only comes with age. I quite agree, although I profess only to have a very small amount of wisdom. Nevertheless, now having the understanding of what life is really all about, I feel like a new person. Knowing from whence I came and to where I will be going in the not too distant future has made all the difference. When my time comes I will be happy to return to my spiritual homeland and be reunited with members of my spiritual family. Until such time, however, I have every intention of continuing to work as long as possible, to serve Spiritism, and continue my studies; also to continue to work to become a better person. This is because I am now fully aware that it is only in this that spiritual progress is to be found—consequently enabling the finding of ever-greater happiness. And who does not want to be happier?

The following lines came to me through inspiration:

> If we are all faith and no reasoning we become fanatics!
> But if we are all intellect and no faith we become as robots!
> The password then is equilibrium at all times!

Chapter 23

CONTRIBUTIONS OF BRAZILIAN SPIRITIST TREATMENTS TO THE GLOBAL IMPROVEMENT OF MENTAL HEALTH CARE

Stanley Krippner, PhD, and Emma Bragdon, PhD

Introduction

This chapter provides an account of our observations of Spiritist healing centers we have independently visited. The main focus is on the one center we both visited, that of John of God, a healer who has attracted international attention. Several implications of these institutions for improving global health care are cited at the end of the chapter.

Stanley Krippner's Journey
The House of St. Ignatius of Loyola

Krippner arrived in Brasilia, the capital city of Brazil, on July 29, 2005, when friends drove him 70 miles to the Casa do Dom Inácio de Loyola (The House of St. Ignatius of Loyola), in the hamlet of Abadiânia. There were more than 1000 people at the Casa, as this date marked the birthday of Dom Inácio (St. Ignatius of Loyola) who would, at times, be "incorporated" by João Teixera de Farias, better known as "João de Deus" (John of God). Although he only had two years of formal education, the medium, João, when an entity is incorporated, has successfully performed complicated surgeries apparently without causing pain or infection, without using conventional anesthetics or antibiotics.

João Teixera claims to work with some 35 "spirit guides" or "entities of light," the principal guide being Dom Inácio. St. Ignatius of Loyola is an appropriate choice of an entity for alleged "incorporation" as he selected the first Jesuit priests, recognizing their discipline, dedication, flexibility of perception, and their powers of mental imagery.

A colleague of Krippner's had taken Krippner's photograph to the Casa in 2001, shortly after Krippner had been diagnosed with prostate cancer. At that time João de Deus said there was no need for Krippner to make a personal visit to Abadiânia because he would make a satisfactory recovery, and sold Krippner's colleague six weeks' supply of herbal capsules (pulverized passionflower said to carry "subtle vibrations" of healing specifically tailored for Krippner) with the instructions that they should be taken three times each day with water, praying before ingesting them.

The Casa has brought prosperity to Abadiânia, where a number of hotels and restaurants have been constructed to accommodate the steady stream of visitors who are attracted by stories of João de Deus' abilities. Some are drawn by a desire to learn more about healing, others to become healed from physical and mental illnesses. Most visitors are impressed with the Casa's soup kitchen and dental clinic that provide free food, clothing, toys, and dental care to the poorer residents of Abadiânia.

During his 2005 visit, Krippner joined the line of people awaiting João de Deus' consultation, briefly thanked João for his assistance in 2001, and was given another prescription for a herbal remedy. He went to the onsite "pharmacy," bought (at a nominal fee) the prescribed bottles of capsules, and received instructions not to drink alcohol or eat hot peppers and pork products during the six weeks it would take to deplete the supply. As he had in 2001, Krippner followed the instructions.

Krippner found the assembly hall of the Casa to be fairly large; a small cement stage at one end of the room allowed people to watch João de Deus if he happened to come out to do "physical operations" in front of the audience. It was noticed that João de Deus usually remained in his meditation and "Current room," ministering to each visitor one by one, and, periodically, entered the Casa's "blessing room" to complete various "spiritual surgeries." The "spiritual operations" given some visitors involve manipulation of what the French author Allan Kardec called the "perispirit," or one's "spiritual body." Kardec's books, written in the mid-1800s, created a sensation in Brazil, leading to the founding of "Spiritism," a movement based on Kardec's insights.

In the assembly room, speakers provide inspirational testimonials about "cures" they have received at the Casa or discuss the Spiritist philosophy that underlies the Casa's activities. Krippner viewed another small storage room filled with crutches, wheelchairs, and prosthetic aids said to have been left by visitors following their recoveries.

The Casa also has a "recovery room" where people can rest following physical surgery, and before returning to their hotel for a longer rest period of 24 hours or more. The main building is surrounded by a lush garden, and near the parking area a pathway leads away from the sanctuary to a waterfall that, with the permission of João de Deus, can be used for "purification." In addition, there are several rooms adjacent to the garden where guests can receive "crystal bed" treatments whereby one lies on a cot and receives colored light rays that are pulsed through specially cut crystals suspended from a frame above the body. These 20-minute treatments are accompanied by soft music and are meant to relax, clear, and balance one's "subtle energy" bodies.

In the main complex of the Casa there are three meditation rooms where hundreds of people meditate and pray along with trained mediums. These rooms are the heart of the Casa and they are felt to be important for one's personal transformation. People sit in these rooms, eyes closed, without interruption for 2–4 hours in the morning, and then again in the afternoon. Some participants feel guided to send "positive energies" to João de Deus in order to help him in his healing endeavors. This exercise of charity encourages *reforma intima*, or personal transformation, which, in itself, is thought to cleanse the "subtle bodies." After sitting in "the current," people have reported such experiences as interactions with spiritual guides, of being unburdened of their emotional and physical problems, and/or feelings of being bathed in the "Light of the Divine."

As a teenager, João Teixera de Farias (João de Deus) had a vision of a luminous woman who directed him to a nearby Spiritist Center. Following his vision, he located the center, a place he had never visited before, and began to heal people, even though later he did not recall these healing activities. However, the people at the center told him that he had apparently gone into a "trance" and incorporated King Solomon, and that many people had benefitted from his ministrations.

Because João insisted that God did the healing, he was dubbed "John of God," a name that has stayed with him over the decades. He himself prefers to be called "the medium, João." The various "entities" that he incorporates range from deceased Brazilian and German physicians, who insist they want to continue to heal people, to St. Ignatius of Loyola, who was born in Spain.

During his healing procedures João de Deus does not wear surgical gloves, nor wash with hot water and soap between surgeries. Water "blessed by the entities of light" is used in place of antiseptics after a physical surgery is done. Interestingly, in 2000, three physicians undertook an onsite investigation of 30 "operations," finding no signs of infection even after three days of follow-up (Almeida, Almeida and Gollner 2000).

Bragdon, in her book about the Casa (2002), repeats a position first published by Robert Pellegrino-Estrich (1997, p. 100) that João de Deus "has been studied by teams of legitimate scientists from Russia, Germany, Japan, France, and the United States. [Pathology tests reveal that] the tumors, substances, and tissues the Entity removes from the sick are indeed human tissues from the individuals operated upon." A 1997 thesis by Savaris, published in Portuguese, details a number of purportedly successful interventions, yet from our perspective an article in an English-language journal that is peer-reviewed is long overdue.

In regard to her own account, Bragdon wrote, "Nothing in this book is meant to replace the advice of a physician… No healer, physician, or disembodied entity that makes him or herself available for [this] healing is perfect" (2002, p.10). This cautionary statement should be kept in mind and seriously considered by visitors intending to go to Abadiânia.

The Frei Luiz Shrine

The Frei Luiz Shrine is a healing center outside of Rio de Janeiro that attracts many Brazilians as well as visitors from other countries. The work at this center has been influenced by the writings of Allan Kardec; it is named after a Franciscan monk, Teodoro Henrique Reinke (later known as Frei Luiz), who lived and worked in the Brazilian state of Minas Gerais, until 1937. Like João de Deus, Frei Luiz was venerated for his kindness, for his devotion to charitable projects, and for his healing powers.

Immediately after leaving John of God's sanctuary, Krippner flew to Rio on August 2, 2005, and was taken to a private home. He had suffered an insect bite a few days before leaving for Brazil, which left him with a fever and a large abscess on his neck. Antibiotics had brought the fever under control, and his traveling companion, Dr. Yanez, had brought medication to reduce the swelling. In addition, another friend, Maria Lucia Sauer, had arranged for him to be seen by Fernando Gilberto Arruda, the chief medium of the Frei Luiz Shrine.

Krippner reclined on a long padded table while Arruda incorporated the spirit of Frederic von Stein, an alleged Nazi physician who died in the final months of World War II. "Dr. Frederic" reportedly regrets the wartime role that he had played, and now works from "the other side" to bring healing and restoration to people who are sick or suffering. Krippner was told that "Dr. Frederic," working through Fernando Gilberto Arruda, directed a team of half a dozen "associates" also affiliated with the Frei Luiz Center. "Dr. Frederic" allegedly "drew from the channel" to bring about the desired outcome, utilizing a non-contact healing intervention.

Krippner expected the team to work on his abscess, which was still highly visible. Instead, they focused on his groin area. One of the members of the team, Luiz Augusto de Queiroz, directs the House of Padre Pio, which Krippner and Yanez were to visit the following night. During the healing session, Luiz Augusto de Queiroz claimed that Padre Pio had told him that Krippner's abscess would disappear in a few days but that he still had prostate cancer in his "perispirit." As a result, the healing session focused on the prostate gland. Krippner had not told anyone in this group about his 2001 treatment for prostate cancer (but it was no secret to his friends and colleagues in the United States).

The procedure was performed under soft lights while recorded music was playing. Luiz Augusto de Queiroz chanted, in Portuguese, "We are giving our brother our love so that he will be free of prostate cancer." Krippner closed his eyes and listened to the chants and the music. About half an hour later, the session came to an end. "Dr. Frederic" left Arruda, and the room's normal lighting was restored. Luiz Augusto de Queiroz told Krippner that his "perispirit" was now free of cancer and that it would not return. When Krippner opened his eyes, he noticed that his white shirt was stained with a red and yellow fluid.

The House of Padre Pio

Padre Pio, a Capuchin priest from San Giovanni Rotondo, Italy, was said to have manifested a variety of unusual phenomena. Among them were stigmata, bilocation, prophecy, conversion, anomalous scents of perfume, and remarkable healings (Mary 1999). Although he died in 1968, his Brazilian supporters claim that people are still being healed through his intercessions. They also feel a connection with the American seer Edgar Cayce, and derive inspiration and direction from his "readings" and from books about his life and work. Padre Pio was canonized in 2002 as a result of so-called "miraculous healings" that supposedly resulted from his postmortem intercession.

Maria Lucia Sauer works at the House of Padre Pio where she practices "lightbody infusion." She describes this treatment as a type of "mind–body–spirit healing" that was introduced to her by the Brazilian medium Luiz Gasparetto in 1979 at the Esalen Institute in California. She now teaches this technique in seven countries, including the United States.

A Casa do Padre Pio (The House of Padre Pio) is supported by a group of about 200 patrons. Krippner and Yanez were told that a hospital is being planned by the Members of the Association, and that 20 percent of the beds will be reserved exclusively for people who are unable to pay for their medical treatment. Members of the Association believe that spiritual work needs to be accompanied by social work.

The director of the Padre Pio Center, Luiz Augusto de Queiroz, claims to incorporate several spirits including that of a Chinese master, Chung In-Lang. In 1996, after he heard a voice identifying itself as that of Padre Pio, de Queiroz began to "talk" with Padre Pio through intuition, clairvoyance, and—on occasion—verbally. In 1997 de Queiroz started meeting weekly with friends who were interested in spiritual matters and these conversations led to the establishment of the healing center.

On August 3, 2005, Krippner and Yanez visited de Queiroz at a bank that he owns in Rio de Janeiro. He continues to work in the bank because he says it helps him remain a "balanced person." On Mondays, his spiritual group holds study sessions that involve discussions as well as "energizing therapy" treatments. The group studies the Kabala and other spiritual systems, such as the work of Swami Yogananda.

Krippner recalled: "We went to the House of Padre Pio that evening at 7:00 pm. Maria Lucia suggested that we pray as we sat in the waiting room to experience 'light infusion' so that we would have 'a more intense experience.'" Soft, relaxing music was played while 13 women and 10 men waited, all praying. Yanez recalled:

> I was sitting against the wall, and a beautiful painted landscape named "Hope" was in back of me. I could see the face of "Hope," which thrilled me. I was so overcome with emotion that I closed my mouth and began to cry softly… During the two-hour waiting time, I closed my eyes and experienced a light show. There was a sudden flash of lights, the same lights that have appeared in my prayers on several occasions. When I went into the healing room, I counted a total of 16 healers. Once I reclined on the table, they began some sort of examination followed by the restoration of my energy. They started touching some of my acupuncture points, with subtle gentleness and love. Specifically, they touched my 3-thumb point, my thymus point, my liver and spleen point, and a point in my ankle. They proceeded to touch areas all over my body. At times, when they touched me, their arms started to vibrate. It felt really wonderful… They paused before touching my nose, passing their fingers up and down the very place where I once had surgery due to a chronic allergy. The "light show" continued until I was told that I could go back to the waiting room.

Krippner also saw several "lights" once he was on the bed in the healers' area. He recalled: "I assumed that the tiny lights were painted on the ceiling with some sort of phosphorescent substance. However, I closed my eyes and the lights were as vibrant as ever." Krippner and Yanez had the opportunity to speak to some of the mediums after the sessions had ended. Each spoke of the inspiration they derived from Padre Pio, either through what they knew about him or from a sense of "presence" when they entered the Casa.

Stanley Krippner's Reflections: Post-Trip

Yanez took Krippner's stained white shirt with him to Mexico to have it analyzed at a Mexican medical laboratory. It was found to contain no trace of blood. However, the healer had claimed that the stains were, in part, "physical emanations of spirit" from ectoplasm, allegedly a semi-material substance disembodied spirits use for appearing and healing when interacting with the physical world.

In March 2006 Krippner received his prostate examination report from Kaiser Permanente Hospital, where he had been tested twice a year since his radiation treatment in 2001. His PSA level was 0.5, about the same as it had been for four years. The report concluded with the statement, "We will now check you only once a year since you are remaining stable." The effectiveness of the Spiritists' treatment cannot be measured by PSA levels, of course, because "Dr. Frederic" and João de Deus had worked with the "perispirit," not the physical body. In September 2010 Krippner's PSA still remained at the same low level.

Emma Bragdon's Reflections

Over the last ten years, since 2001, I have seen an increase in international travelers coming to Brazil to be healed, or to improve their own abilities as healers by studying with various Brazilian healers. As happens when one visits medical doctors, one might be to your liking, yet another you don't find appealing in the least. Similarly, if you visit three health care providers over a period of a few days—on tour in a culture that is exotic, and where you don't speak the language—you will perceive one aspect of one healer, and another aspect of another. One visitor may feel emotionally touched by one healer, while another may find the deep reservoir of their subconscious mind being stimulated. Unless a friend or a guide encourages them to do so, rarely do tourists stop to meditate for long periods of time, afraid they will miss some of the action. Why close your eyes and go inward when there is so much to see, and so many people to meet?

This is also why João de Deus recommends letting the healing work done in his sanctuary integrate for 40 days before one visits another healer or has other energy balancing done. There are many subtle energy adjustments in the work of his Casa that could be interrupted or neutralized by other forms of energy work. Clearly choosing to pay attention to one message at a time allows the body to have a consistent clear message, and solidify the inner transformation that has been stimulated by the visit.

My own experience over ten years of travel to more than 30 Spiritist Centers and Hospitals has taken me from fascination and awe to being more objective, and then becoming more a part of the "family." Through readings, study, focused meditation, and a deeper engagement with the mediums of Brazil, I have increased my ability to observe as well as deepened my respect for these healing methods.

Guiding over 40 groups, writing books, and narrating films has also demanded that I define and articulate my observations. I acknowledge the medium João de Deus for pointing me in the direction of Spiritism, and the vital importance of working on my own personal transformation. The spirits, angels, and saints we may interact with can only lend a helping hand; we are the ones who must do the work that will change our lives.

Conclusion

There are several principles and protocols that both Krippner and I have observed in Spiritist Centers that are worth bringing back to our home countries with the hope that they can augment our ailing health care systems.

Brazilian healing practitioners represent a new paradigm that encompasses spiritual reality and the effects of evolution over lifetimes as a direct source of illness and wellness. They recognize that karmic issues from the past can be the source of both emotional and physical issues in this lifetime. They practice ways of healing that attend to energies that may be both invisible and more powerful than the material reality. The best of these healers also make use of intuitive abilities in a disciplined as well as charitable manner.

- *Diagnosis.* Our standard medical protocols could be complemented by the diagnostic procedures of well-trained mediums and healers who utilize medical intuition to diagnose the illness and the source of the illness. Illuminating this type of diagnosis to the patient, when appropriate, would allow him or her to address the karmic issues directly, and thus be proactive in "righting the balance." The processing could be assisted by trained counselors who give fraternal support for "lifestyle changes" that facilitate personal transformation. Ideally, medical intuitives who have the gift of seeing the impact of disincarnates would also check patients with psychiatric disturbances once a week and add their diagnostic perceptions into medical case reports to empower a truly integrative structure of care.

- *Treatment.* An important source of both health and illness lies in the "subtle bodies," aka informational bodies that carry the records of the past. In order to heal the very source of the problems they are having, patients need to work on personal transformation to remove the source of problems existing in these "subtle bodies." We could add well-trained body workers who know how to work with "subtle energies" to complement and in some cases substitute for standard treatments that may not fully address the true origin of disease states. These "energy workers" could also be available to energize the health professionals who become weary or face burnout at work.

- Allan Kardec carefully mapped the interaction of the spiritual realms with the human realm. His books are still highly relevant for anyone wanting to understand this cosmology, and the practical information needed to understand the role of being a medium working with spirits. On entering this realm, it is vitally important to choose to align oneself with highly evolved spirits, instead of those who are still driven by addictions, fear, and anger.

- Psychics and mediums need to be well trained and have a social support system. Those with intuitive and mediumistic abilities have a responsibility to use these gifts to benefit other people's spiritual evolution—not to satisfy frivolous, mercenary, or self-centered goals. The best spiritual centers and hospitals in Brazil are careful to train mediums and healers thoroughly, and watch that they do not overwork. Mediums need social support, continued supervision, healthy lifestyle habits, and regimes that involve voluntary control of internal states, such as meditation and prayer. Becoming a working medium does not happen during a weekend workshop, but is a disciplined way of life developed over years.

- Spiritual work needs to be accompanied by social work. Spiritism has been called "a way of practical Christianity." Being charitable towards others is not only the suggested way of life that brings happiness, but is the most direct path toward spiritual evolution and well-being.

- Spiritual work—being a medium or healer, or a friend to someone in need—is given freely, without charge. There is no financial requirement, and nothing is expected in return for the service. This attitude allows the "giver" to disengage from his or her basic drives, and to be motivated by compassion and a sense of union with others—a more evolved motivation. "Receivers" can be greatly uplifted by such compassionate interaction.

- A typical Brazilian Spiritist Center is filled with volunteers who want to have the opportunity to serve those who are suffering—without obstructing the health providers in charge of medical intervention. These volunteers have been trained to sit quietly, to listen, and to offer compassion and empathy to the patients—as well as to play, when it is time to laugh and have fun. This could be adapted into Western hospitals that care for the physically and mentally ill, orphanages, and other institutions for people with disabilities.

- A typical way of saying goodbye to someone in Brazil who practices Spiritism is *Vai com Deus*, Go with God, or *Fica com Deus*, Be with God. This is an abbreviated way of forgiving, letting go of animosity, and merging with that beautiful, sacred energy, or Light, that transcends the small human ego. Let's find a way to integrate this perspective in the way we interact personally and in institutions dedicated to health care.

- It is time to enhance a cross-cultural exchange:

    (1)   To help Brazilians conduct research they are involved in focusing on the effectiveness of Spiritist protocols, as well as to evaluate and refine programs for training mediums and healers.

    (2)   To offer students of health care outside of Brazil opportunities to come to Spiritist Healing Centers and Psychiatric Hospitals for further study and training.

Approaching these practices with an open mind will likely produce insights that improve the quality of life for health providers and the people they serve in clinics and hospitals.

Part V

EDUCATION AND RESEARCH

Chapter 24

TRAINING MEDIUMS WHO TREAT PSYCHIATRIC PATIENTS

Gerald Magnan

Working as a Medium and Healer: First Encounter

My first experience with mentally ill people happened when I joined a group of mediums that worked inside the Spiritist Hospital of Porto Alegre in 1995. The purpose of that group was to help the patients by comforting and calming them through laying-on of hands ("*passé*" in Portuguese). Below are the steps we took together.

The mediums would first gather alone together in a quiet room and concentrate for a few minutes. The person leading the work would say a few opening prayers so as to further harmonize the group, and then we would all walk in silence to a previously designated hospital ward. There we would find the patients seated on chairs arranged in long rows, and our action would begin. One of us would tell a short story, something of spiritual and moral value, so as to create harmony in the room. Then the mediums, one by one, would perform laying-on of hands on each of the individuals present. The task was simple: We would place our hands just above the patient's head, radiating energies of peace and love. When that was over, we would all hold hands, mediums and patients together, and say the Lord's Prayer, and then say goodbye and leave the ward. Back in the quiet room, we would concentrate again, say a thank-you prayer, and end our activities.

I remember that, the first few times I did this, my heart would beat fast and strong, but with time and understanding that excitement transformed into a sense of well-being. This allowed me to better understand that those brothers and sisters who were there as patients were going through difficult trials in their lives. Although simple, in those brief moments of our work we had to give our very best; our purest love was invoked so that those vibrations would embrace the person there at that moment and bring him or her some relief from the torments he or she was undergoing.

Some time later, I was named coordinator of that group and also head of the Department of Spiritual Assistance (DAE) of the hospital.

Challenges to Mediums

With regard to the group of people who administered the laying-on of hands, I faced the problem of the high turnover of mediums. We had a small core of faithful ones, but most others couldn't manage to stay in this activity for long. Mediums of the latter group rarely stayed with us for more than a year, despite the care I took. I always spoke with them after the work was over, gave them verbal encouragement, and had group conversations about any delicate situations that might have come up during the laying-on of hands. I tried to understand why mediums would leave. Even though there were a myriad of excuses that justified each of those workers leaving, I knew there had to be something else, something I wasn't seeing.

The day came that that "something" came to meet me. We all have a side that is darker than we wish it was, a side that we attempt to forget and bury, so that it will not annoy our thoughts. In a psychiatric hospital, however, working directly with the patients, sooner or later we have to face situations that wake up that undesirable side in us. At that moment, those of us who have not yet consolidated the emotional side of ourselves suffer a devastating inner conflict. The day I met my darker side through a patient, I felt an awful impact on my chest, everything inside me trembled, and all my alarm signs went off at the same time. I felt the urge to run out the door. I breathed deeply, reminded myself of my commitment to helping the ones in need, and stood firm.

Discipline

Discipline is indispensable for a medium; without it serious work cannot be done. It is acquired through reading, study, exercises, good will, mediumship work dedicated to helping others, and exchange of experiences with other mediums. Human beings are by nature quite fragile, and mediums, because of their sensitivity, need a lot of help in overcoming the troubles of a messy and disordered mediumship and harvesting the fruits of a disciplined mediumship. I do not speak here of military discipline—the discipline I mean here is the one that gives us peace, that prevents abuses of all sorts, that polices our thoughts and drives away all mental rubbish; I mean the discipline of humility that tilts our heads down and does not retaliate over offenses, the discipline that leads our footsteps towards others so as to alleviate their troubles.

A medium who works directly with mentally ill people must learn to keep quiet and concentrate, speak only when necessary, and if possible say nothing at all. In our group, only one person would address the patients. This was done so as to keep concentration as focused as possible among the mediums. But it was also done because we were aware that, if an unqualified medium were to talk to a patient, the latter might misinterpret what was said, or take it the wrong way, or even adjust the words said to his or her distorted way of viewing life. Hence, whenever a medium felt something strange or uncomfortable during the laying-on of hands, he or she would discreetly speak to the coordinator, who would then take whatever measures seemed necessary.

One day, while I was walking along a hospital corridor, a nurse called me and requested laying-on of hands for the patients of his ward twice a week, instead of only once. He claimed that following our weekly visits the patients would remain calmer than usual for as long as three or four days. On another occasion, while speaking with the chief nurse, it became clear that we needed to help one of the wards for alcoholics and chemically addicted patients. That ward was notorious for its violent patients, who were frequently psychotic. I accepted the challenge and invited the most reliable of the mediums who practiced laying-on of hands with me, explaining to them the situation. We scheduled a date and time, and there we were, knocking at that ward's door. Our hearts were all beating fast; we had no idea how we were going to be received. We went to the dining hall of the ward and arranged the chairs in rows. The nurses and the social assistant, who had already announced our arrival, then called the patients. We explained to them some of the many benefits of the laying-on of hands, and immediately began our work, which was accompanied by absolute silence. We ended with a prayer, asking everyone to hold hands in a circle for the "Lord's Prayer." Walking out of the ward, the anxiety of the first time gave way to a smile of satisfaction in each medium's face. The following week, when we walked into the dining hall we were surprised to see the chairs already arranged, and most of the patients already seated and waiting for us. I worked as coordinator of this group of very reliable and trustworthy mediums for a few years, and then passed that task on to the person who replaced me, because other tasks awaited me.

Healing at a Distance

One of them was that of setting up a group for spiritual assistance at a distance. By email, the hospital office receives a large number of requests for help every month. Those requests were usually forwarded to Spiritist Centers independent of the hospital. When I read these emails I was moved by the individual cases and also by the trust that people dedicated to us. After a period of reflection, we decided to answer some of those requests, which came from all over Latin America and even Europe, so as to try to comfort those people in their suffering. I addressed the Hospital's Department of Spiritual Assistance explaining the idea, and tried to find out whether there were any mediums interested in the project. We scheduled a date for the beginning of our activities after 12 mediums volunteered.

Prior to actually attending people's requests, I had to find out more about the mediums with whom I was working. Even though their faces were all familiar to me, I did not know how they were going to behave together as a group. I also did not know how much they knew about obsession and disobsession.

Before moving on, perhaps I should say something about disobsession meetings, so as to make clear what I mean. Suely Caldas Schubert's book *Obsessão/Desobsessão* (Obsession/Disobsession) (2008) defines these meetings as follows:

> It is to this appropriate environment, sheathed with the adequate vibrations and requiring special care from Higher Spirituality, that the spirits who are ill are brought in from space to receive the treatment of love. No other medication exists, more adequate or better suited. Moral wounds, pain entrenched into the core of one's being, the torture of hatred that burns those who fuel it, the hearts that have rejected God and are caged within themselves, suicidal spirits who feel they live and die in great pain, unhappy spirits chained to their addictions, in other words, all who display the procession of human agonies, they will only find relief and treatment, answers and guidance through the universal medication of LOVE!
>
> So it follows that a disobsession meeting will only be successful and fruitful once the whole team of mediums learns how to cultivate this "medicine" in their hearts, so that they can then donate it to those who need it. The spiritual team that guides the mediums, to be sure, awaits this kind of cooperation and expects it in our actions… Mediumship work represents for the disembodied spirits both the possibility of getting in contact with those who are still on Earth and of receiving from them the magnetic vibrations for which they long… (p.158)

In the book *The Messengers* (2008), channeled from André Luiz, MD, to C. Xavier, Luiz says that, "with this kind of contact, [the disembodied spirits] experience the awakening of new strengths" (p.249). The pure love, as we have seen, is indispensable in the treatment of suffering spirits.

I had to continually ask myself, "Was it present in each of the members of our group? What was the quality of our magnetic vibrations? Could it be of any help to our suffering brothers and sisters?"

A rather lengthy work of observation and training was then started. We began by first establishing internal rules for the group:

- Fixing the time at which mediumship work would begin was important. At that time, the doors would be locked and no one else could come in or leave, so as not to disturb concentration.

- Because Brazilians have the nice and healthy habit of hugging and kissing each other each time they meet, and of greeting each other in a loud tone of voice, I asked that these demonstrations of affection be made outside the room.

- I also asked that the mediums all come into the room at least ten minutes ahead of time, and that they remain in silent prayer or reading something akin to our activities until work began. At the scheduled date and time of our first actual work, we found ourselves seated around a table, rather concerned but also calm.

- Some competence in what we were about to do was also needed. Allan Kardec wrote in *The Mediums' Book* (1986) that "a meeting is a collective being, whose qualities and properties result from those of its members and make up a sort of bundle. The more harmonious the group is, the greater its strength will be" (p.392). Based on that, we understood the significance of concentrating before and during our work.

- We also understood the importance of knowing the medium next to you and of trusting him or her and the others of the group, and of the friendship among the members of the group, so that when failures happen, everyone knows that no one will be singled out for criticisms nor will anyone be judged. This kind of harmony is indispensable; without it the mediums will not feel at ease or have the self-confidence needed to devote themselves completely to the job at hand.

Prior to the first session devoted to the messages we received by email, I had asked that each of the mediums bring the name of a family member or of someone else they knew and who was in need of disobsession work, a person on whom we could test the efficacy of our work, as we could note how he or she was both before and after the session. This was to be a sort of practice session. We opened with a prayer, and once the group was "harmonized," we began to work. I observed the reactions and abilities of each medium, as each has a unique way of practicing mediumship. It is important for the smooth flowing of the session that these peculiarities are recognized.

At the end of that session, I already knew what task most of the mediums would be performing from then on. But after our final prayer, before leaving, we each made an assessment of our work, and this would, with time, become a common practice among us. Because the people treated were known to at least one member of the group, I asked if what was felt regarding the person corresponded to that individual's personality and his or her needs. The replies were very encouraging, and most of the mediums had indeed gotten hold of the most striking aspects of the personality and difficulties of the individuals being treated from a distance. They had also accurately perceived the physical problems of the patients, for example those who had internal organs irritated, inflammations, etc.

After a few months of this practice, we had acquired a lot of experience. I continued to watch over the efficacy of the group, by placing names of individuals whom I knew well on the list without telling the others of the group, so as to see if the group's mediumship was not weakening or wearing out.

Animism

There was also the problem of "animism." Within Spiritism (Kardec 1986), this is the term used for the influence that the medium's soul imposes on the communications by the spirits. In most mediumship sessions this is not too relevant, but in the disobsession of mentally ill people it needs to be watched for and very controlled. Having identified that this problem was increasing in our sessions, I had to do something to mitigate its effects.

I searched the Spiritist literature, which is vast and serious in Brazil, for indications on how to proceed, and gathered all information available on this matter. I wrote up a summary and took it to the group. We read it together and— to my surprise—the mediums whom I wished to enlighten anonymously through that reading identified themselves spontaneously, and each pointed out in the text descriptions which fit the sensations they had had and also what needed to be done to mitigate the problem. Ignorance really is the worst of our enemies.

In the next few sessions the percentage of animistic influences in the channeled messages decreased significantly. I adopted that manner of proceeding for most of the problems faced by the mediums of our group. Of course, if that was insufficient, I would then speak privately to each of the mediums who, I perceived, was having a problem.

Self-Care of Mediums

Because ours is a disobsession group, it is frequently challenged by that portion of the spiritual world that has not yet faced up to love. Therefore it is fundamental to the medium to take good care of his or her personal life.

Spiritism teaches us to "watch and pray" (Kardec 1987, 1996). Pray so as to become attuned to the spiritual world, guided by the unconditional love of Jesus. Watch so as to avoid all kinds of excesses. How can you help someone who is mentally ill if you are out of balance?

Physical health is as important as mental health. Taking good care of our bodies without being selfish is a duty. Likewise, avoiding getting too tired, without being sedentary. Healthy food and beverages, frequent contact with nature, especially trees, which have the power to clean and recharge our energies, bathing in the sea, walking on the sand, gentle sunlight on the skin…these are all resources that Mother Nature has provided for us.

The leader of a mediumship group has to know as much as possible of the life of his or her colleagues, not by meddling into their private businesses, but by observing their reactions, their language, their gaze, and their behavior. Very rare are those who manage to hide serious problems for long.

The Role of the Group Leader

The role of the leader is to care for the homogeneity and harmony of the group of mediums. If he or she runs across any difficulties in a medium, the leader must talk to him or her privately and offer help. This brother or sister may be going through a hard time in his or her life, and might need to be supported. It is the leader's job to take care of the environment where the group works, and his or her authority in this regard has to be based on his or her own example. The leader must also know the Spiritist philosophy, and how to give love to our neighbors. He or she must have faith and be gentle and firm, among other qualifications. This is acquired after a significant amount of work and readings, and plenty of study of Spiritism and other philosophies.

Developing Automatic Writing

When, in the group, voice channeling had become sufficiently trustworthy, we began exercises aiming at the development of channeling through writing. There are three kinds of channeling in writing: mechanical, where the medium lends his or her arm and hand to the Spirit without knowing what will be written (the hand writes without him or her controlling it); intuitive, in which the medium has full control over the hand, hearing in his or her mind a voice that dictates what will be written; and quasi-mechanical, a mixture of the former two in which the medium feels a drive in his or her hand but at the same time knows what is being written.

For a few months, we practiced exercises for the development of channeling through writing. At the day of the practice session, after the disobsession work, each medium had a blank sheet of paper and a pen on the table in front of him or her. We asked the spiritual mentor of each medium to come closer and act according to the capacities of the medium. At the end, I would collect the writings, store them in my briefcase, and read them at night calmly, analyzing each one.

Channeling in writing is a very delicate business; it can arouse the medium's pride and vanity if the message is signed by someone famous or carries pompous advice. We did lots of tests. Some mediums wouldn't write anything; others felt a discomfort on his or her hand and would immediately start writing. Some would write what their hearts felt, while others received advice from an alleged spiritual brother or sister. But how can we know if it really is a spiritual brother or sister that is writing, and not something we made up in our own minds? The answer is simple: what is written down must be analyzed by people other than the one who channeled the message.

During constructive criticisms in group discussion, an honest medium will acknowledge whether what he or she wrote corresponds to his or her own thoughts or something he or she read recently. Still, that does not mean that the message is completely animistic. A disembodied spirit may use part of the medium's knowledge to express him- or herself. What really counts is the content of the text. Many times I analyzed "messages" that were full of beautiful words and written in impeccable grammar, but when the blah-blah-blah was over, it had nothing helpful for the group, nor any constructive advice: rubbish. We also have to be cautious against authoritarian messages containing weird commandments. An evolved spirit does not give out orders: he or she advises, and does not obligate; he or she suggests, and does not get bogged down in sterile paraphrasing; the messages are objective and clear.

The spirits themselves, through the work of Allan Kardec, alert us: "It is best to refuse ten truths than to accept a lie." An evolved spirit does not take offense in seeing his or her text barred by a judgment that it may be false and will try to pass on the message some other way, so as to be more clear and accessible to those it wants to reach. But if a group is careless enough to take in any writing received through channeling, without submitting it to criticism or study, then it will be vulnerable to mystification, fraud, and ridiculous and even humiliating situations, and it will be susceptible to the application of norms that are senseless or lack good sense. Without an analysis of the texts channeled, the group may become an instrument of frivolous spirits, who will control that group shamelessly, and may use it to sow disagreements and create imbalance within a Spiritist Center. As we have seen, the job is simple, but it is not easy.

Examples of Concrete Results

To wrap up this chapter, I would like to convey some examples of concrete results of several of the topics mentioned above: magnetic laying-on of hands, voice channeling, and channeling in writing.

In the magnetic laying-on of hands given to patients who are mentally ill or suffer from chemical addictions, we felt that the environment where the activity took place would become spiritually more ethereal. Some patients also felt that. The permanent agitation, common in those places, would quickly cease or decrease. While they were receiving the laying-on of hands, many patients would silently pray, moving only their lips. The nurses, who often received the laying-on of hands alongside the patients, were also benefitted by these energies, which remained with them for a long time after we had left, rendering the environment more serene and calm.

In our disobsession group, while still in its testing phase, the name of a child who had abruptly changed her behavior was brought to us. She was about ten years old, and had become demanding, aggressive, and excessively sensual. During the disobsession, she was seen by mediums as spiritually crying and desperate. Suddenly I had the intuition that this was a case of sexual abuse. I kept my silence until another medium said it out loud, and from then on the picture gradually became clear. An old man was seen coming closer to the girl near her home. I immediately contacted the adult responsible for the girl, and explained what we thought could be the cause for the girl's change in attitude. That person then subtly questioned the girl, gradually narrowing in on the problem, until the girl acknowledged that a construction worker from a building next door had lured her to an isolated place and caressed her. Steps were then taken to avoid anything worse from happening, and the girl received professional psychological counseling.

Regarding channeling in writing: throughout my years of experience I have never had before my eyes a message from a group member worthy of being reported here. Some contained judicious advice on how to proceed with our disobsession work, which was analyzed and discussed by our group, and was confirmed by the Spiritist literature, but there were also many wastebaskets full of paper.

You cannot be too careful when the matter is spirituality. We are human beings and are still very much influenced by the vapors of pride, vanity, and selfishness. The goal of inner transformation advanced by Spiritism means the overcoming of those vices, which is to be achieved by the acquisition of virtues. This, in turn, requires both a struggle against our own ignorance and the performing of charity in favor of brothers and sisters who need our help and are either here with us, incarnated, or in the spiritual realm.

Chapter 25

TEACHING HEALTH PROFESSIONALS HOW TO SUPPORT PERSONAL TRANSFORMATION IN PATIENTS

Gelson Roberto, Psychologist

The importance of a broader view of health, which accounts for spiritual aspects of health as well as physical, emotional, and social (as proposed by the World Health Organization in 2003), is becoming more and more evident. Nowadays, the number of studies about the effects of spiritual practices on healing processes is on the increase (Moreira-Almeida 2010). In Brazil, we call the combination of conventional medical treatment and complementary therapies that include attending to spiritual life "integrative medicine."

The increasing importance assigned to the religious aspects in human life and to the vastness of our psychological universe brings man closer to the unknown and unexplored realities of himself. In light of this, we value the study of current-day themes regarding issues dubbed spiritual.

Spirituality assists in improving health due to several factors. According to some studies (Saad and de Medeiros 2008), it brings about a better psychological state (e.g. bringing hope, forgiveness, altruism, and love) and, therefore, improved strategies to deal with problems and a reduction of stress. This generates balance in the organic functions controlled by the nervous system, such as the production of hormones and strengthening of immunity. Moreover, other ways that spirituality may affect health include increasing respect for the body, as taught by many religions, which generates better nutrition and general life habits, and the optimization of psychoneuroimmunological, psychoneuroendocrinological, and psychophysiological pathways.

In addition to the above factors, it's important to consider the moral aspects of life and the spiritual dynamic involved in them. This is a step further, and important in a global view of health that involves spirituality. Every health professional should be aware of the significance of these aspects. The transformation process demands that the professional work with the patient's internal world, a work that is directly related to moral aspects of thinking and behavior. Therefore, a better analysis of the relation of the internal processes with morality and the spiritual dynamic must first be made.

Morality

Moore wrote:

> A moralistic attitude, which is yet another by-product of materialism and egotism, sees everything in terms of black and white, good and bad. It fills courtrooms and builds prisons instead of clinics and hospitals. It is blind to the complexities of a life… It can't distinguish between bad behavior and sickness of a soul.
>
> A moral attitude…considers the conditions under which people make bad decisions and dally with criminality and resort to violence. It sorts out the context of bad behavior and tries to heal conflicted emotions, twisted histories, and misguided views. Rather than punish individuals, it works toward a healed society. (Moore 2010, pp.66–67)

When speaking of morals, more than just external actions, we refer to an internal attitude: an attitude that involves spiritual values and feelings. Therefore, we have in morality not only behaviors, but living forces that act directly on our life and interact with the whole universe. These manifest as subtle vibrations and spiritual forces that operate on several levels of existence.

Moral forces are involved in a dynamic interaction within us in three ways.

First, morals can give a form that balances the spiritual dynamic, providing the appropriate conditions for inner transformation to occur. Morals lend quality and establish the means to handle the other spiritual forces and the spirits' influence.

Kardec (1985, p.249) asks the spirits, in question 459, "Do spirits influence our thoughts and actions?" They answered that "They influence much more than we imagine, to a point where sometimes they may govern our lives." That means we are constantly interacting, influencing, and under the influence of spirits and mental forces.

André Luiz notes:

> The lamp in whose bulb is produced light, casts off photons which are living elements of nature which then vibrate in [physical space], through the movements that are particular to them; and, in the intimacy of our soul, we process the ideas that radiate out to others, with or without spiritual principles, condensed in the multiple force of thought. It is through these principles that we influence

> the [mental space]. Thus the worlds act upon one another through their radiations and souls mutually influence each other through the mental agents they produce. (Xavier 1991, p.48)

We have in morals not only a shield, but a harmonic field—the factor with the greatest benevolent power to transform the spirits and the field of subtle forces that surrounds us. This confirms Jesus' affirmation that the best way of teaching is through example, not only by way of external gestures, but through an authentic expression of what one feels. The radiation of these true feelings can motivate beneficent action in others.

The second point to consider is that psychosomatic processes and all aspects of becoming ill are profoundly influenced by one's previous karma. When referring to karma, we are not expressing anything more than the expression of the negative aspects that are registered in our memory and still live in our subtle bodies. It is the lack of understanding of the importance of morality and its relationship to life that generates a disharmony with the internal cosmos and with the whole. (Morality is nothing more than the natural laws governing Life.) This disharmony imposes a search for reconciliation that will then be manifested in karmic processes.

Working with karma requires understanding and change within one's moral attitude:

> This way we possess the valuable observations of the earth, alluding to the chemistry of dense matter, relating it with atomic units. The field of the mind offers broad studies of their combinations… Thoughts of cruelty, anger, sadness, love, understanding, hope and joy have natural differences, with their own characteristics and weights, condensing the soul, or purifying it, and further defining its magnetic qualities… To possess certain mental wave force coefficients in silent concentration, the external verb, or the written word… We are naturally victims, or benefits of our own creations, according to our current mental projections. They enslave us to bend to the consequences of our experiences, or free us to the forefront of progress, conforming our deliberations and activities in harmony, or disharmony, with the universe. (Xavier and Vieira 1999, pp.48–49)

The third aspect is that mortality gives meaning to existence; it enables us to understand that we have a personal myth and that life has an end. We are thus in a moral commitment with ourselves, and with life. Jung summed up this idea when he wrote:

> The conscience of man was created with a finality so that one must recognize that one's existence comes from a higher power. Each

of us thus has a debt dedicated to this source. When, after careful consideration, we choose to execute orders emanating from this source which has an intelligent and responsible form, we are provided an optimum life and the possibility of developing the psyche in its totality. (Jung 1982, p.156)

This conscience is not of an intellectual nature, an activity of cerebral mechanisms, but rather is the force that propels them. At first we possess an egoic consciousness, and make contact with our reality on a cognitive and reflexive level. Later, we receive knowledge through others, and we acquire a relational consciousness where feeling is established in a relationship with all aspects of the cosmos, and finally, we become generators and bearers of a more integrated consciousness.

Mind and Morality

André Luiz affirms through Xavier (1991, p.118), appropriately, that our soul resides where the heart puts it. He relates the following four themes to sum up the processes between mind and morality found in the book *Mecanismos da Mediunidade* (Mechanisms of Mediumship).

1. Wherever we go in life we proceed under the influence of our creations. Gravity in the mental field is as decisive as it is in the realm of physical experience. The Divine Law is dedicated to the good of all. To collaborate in the execution of its wise purposes is to illuminate the mind and brighten life. To obstruct Divine Law in order to cultivate whims that cause harm is to obscure reason and cause the shadow to solidify around us.

2. In the domains of the spirit there is no neutrality. We evolve with the eternal light, according to God's designs, or remain stationary in the dark, according to the free determination of our ego self. Every day, the forms come together and fade away. We must pursue our inner transformation with increasing vision, so that we may carry on with the true notion of the eternity in which we move in time.

3. To imagine is to create. Every creation—even though it is only an image held in the self—has life and movement, fleeting though it may be. The consciousness that manifests the creation has responsibility for it, and it's indispensable to analyze that which we give, so that we may judge what we shall receive. Can one who is caught up in anguish and crime, misery and perturbation, find reflections in the mirror of his or her own soul on any images other than those of disharmony and suffering?

4. The wings of angels and the shackles of the condemned are forged in ideas that are created in the mind. Thought exteriorizes and projects itself,

forming images and suggestions that it casts over the objectives it seeks to accomplish. When benign, it conforms to the Laws that govern us, creating harmony and happiness, but when unbalanced and depressing, establishes affliction and ruin. Mental chemistry is at the root of all transformation, because we really evolve in deep telepathic communion with all those incarnate or disincarnate that attune to us.

Nowadays, we are more conscious that there are multiple levels of reality that are simultaneously connected in a global and dynamic process. When considering the work of psychology, we cannot limit ourselves to seeking behavioral transformations but, rather, we must conceive of a psychic reality where the mind and its complex relation to the body must be considered as a whole. Here we find the potentials for inner reform, that is to say, the commitment to morality implies nothing more than a total transformation, where not only one's personal reality matters, but also reality itself. Jung informed us that moral attitude is a real factor that must be assessed by a psychologist, without which he or she might incur tremendous mistakes. Thus, each one of us needs a spiritual life that speaks to our own heart, giving life meaning, a meaning that is not to be found in the outer circumstances of academia and the material world:

> The physician's recognition of the spiritual factors in their true light is vitally important, and the patient's unconscious helps him in his need by producing dreams whose contents are undeniably religious. Not to recognize the spiritual source of such contents means faulty treatment and failure. (Jung 1994, p.686)

The general spiritual representations are indispensable elements of the constitution of psychic life, and are to be found in all people who have some level of a developed consciousness.

The task of psychology in the future will be to study the spiritual determinants of psychic process (Jung 1994, p.687). Spiritual is everything that implies, in any degree, the hypothesis of a dimension that's not separate from the material reality that points to manifestations of a psychic order. This may seem obvious and even redundant, but freeing the psyche from becoming an epiphenomenon of the brain is a recent effort, and one of vital importance so that advances may be made in the field.

Supporting Psi Man through Group Activity

We may call the new stage we are entering that of "Psi Man." This stage is characterized by an increasing awareness of the spiritual reality and of the values that seek to develop our inner potentials. In this psychological stage we no longer emphasize the world and outer conquests, but rather the challenge of conquering ourselves.

We have, then, an important commitment, not only to our patients but also to the teams of spirit guides that work with them. It was bearing this in mind that we created groups in the Spiritist Hospital of Porto Alegre to study Psychology and Spiritism as well as Medicine and Spiritism. Through these meetings, the participants increase their understanding of the spiritual reality and also undergo a process of increasing self-awareness, which they can, in turn, apply to their patients.

This approach has no direct relation to a religion in and of itself, but rather seeks to shed light on objective elements of spiritual reality. We encourage each person to articulate what he or she learns according to the context of his or her own life. An example is the use of prayer and meditation, which may be performed in different ways. What matters is acknowledging that these practices are enlightening, whereby we assimilate superior currents of mental force that help us towards redemption (or ascension) and towards health and inner harmony.

We are working with the concept of two centers in personality. One, formed by the ego, identifies itself as the center of consciousness, but is limited. The other, the Self, truly bears witness to the wholeness of the life process. In *The Spirits' Book* (Kardec 1985) we find this reflected in question 612, when Kardec asks, "Where is the law of God inscribed?" The spirits replied, "In consciousness." We have, thus, two concepts of consciousness: one being egoic, partial, and unilateral, the other, transpersonal, deep, and integral.

In this profound process of acknowledging our spiritual essence and its moral commitment for the fullness of all aspects of being, we must free ourselves of two bonds: one is materialism, with its tendency to focus on what is literal, and the other is egocentrism with its tendency for self-centered subjectivity.

Self-discovery is, at this moment, a basic requirement. There is no way to advance without acknowledging who we are. Thus, it's important that we are always conscious of the elements of which our being consists—the mind. The mind is the very manifestation of the spirit and is formed by thought, feeling, and will. These are the forces of the spirit that we must cultivate for our spiritual development.

The first step in this work of knowing ourselves is to start where we stand. This means looking at reality as it is, accepting ourselves without guilt and without complying with a sense that we are inferior. We must also avoid evading through justifications from our past or empty expectations for the future. It's important to acknowledge that the past still bears fruit in the present, and that the future points to new ideas, but this must be done in a balanced way, without forgetting the work that is done in the present instant, within current reality.

To acknowledge oneself as a whole being, with all of one's characteristics, difficulties, and potentials, is the first step; opening oneself up for change, for overcoming oneself, and making personal growth possible is the second. Being conscious of both, we may utilize several resources in order to achieve a wholeness of being.

It's our mental attitude through its reflection that determines the state of our lives and our bodies. We are the result of this mental state where thought, guided by will and the intensity of our feelings, has the power to build or destroy in all moments of our lives.

The Three Elements of Inner Transformation

The psychological work of transformation may be formed by three elements:

1. *Predisposition*: the individual ideally presents an awareness that healing or transformation is possible and desirable, starts accepting and acknowledging his or her own reality, and begins improving him- or herself without ceasing.

2. *Sense of Self*: the person is aware that his or her healing is part of something bigger than him- or herself, that he or she is experimenting with the effects of Divine power and the spiritual dimension of his or her reality. Total attunement with the Self comes with maintaining mental harmony with the Source of spiritual power.

3. *Transformation*: the individual acknowledges that he or she must change basic cognitive, affective, and behavioral patterns, that the transformation does not take place from the outside, but one must change from the inside. One must treat not just the pathology but make changes in one's way of life to promote positive change. One is not only treating symptoms, but becoming whole as an existential process. The healing experience is an experience of wholeness, and operates on multiple levels.

Through this liberating work one recognizes oneself in one's spiritual dimension, a son or daughter of the Father, bearing immense creative potential. From the book *O Ser Consciente* (The Conscious Being):

> The conscious being must always work, starting from the initial point of its own psychological reality, and accepting itself as it is, and improving without ceasing. This clarity can only be achieved by he who analyzes himself, willing to find himself without disguises. For that, one does not judge nor justify, does not accuse or blame, but only discovers oneself. (Franco 1995, p.10)

The Three Operational Levels for Transformation

In this psychological work of transformation there are three operational levels:

1. *Procedure:* involves the instruments, practices, and attitudes used to elicit healing, which are techniques and creative processes of interaction and mental directing, meditation and visualization techniques, prayer, self-love, and the development of self-esteem programs, relaxation, mental control techniques, and breathing and body exercises; as well as the psychology of love that addresses affective maladjustments.

2. *Process:* the nature of the patient's experience in relation to the holy and the healing action involves: episodes of insight; changes in thoughts, emotions, attitudes, meanings, and behaviors; conditioning the subconscious by removing the accumulated strata and substituting these with optimistic ideas and higher aspirations; correction of habits, abandoning the victim mentality, and a tranquil analysis of occurrences replacing habits of avoiding them; and the constant self-evaluation of conduct and the content of thoughts.

3. *Disposition:* effort and a positive or negative attitude facing the factors that involve healing and change of behavior.

To summarize: We have offered general guidelines about the necessity of constant work within supportive groups in order to give both a basis for understanding the spiritual realities but also to support necessary changes in attitude and inner transformation with the goal of integral health.

Chapter 26

RESEARCHING THE INVISIBLE
Entangled Minds, Psychiatry, and Psychology

William Braud, PhD

Editor's Note

> The comparative benefits and risks of biomedical and nonconventional treatments in mental health care have not been clearly established, and at present there are no evidence-based or expert consensus guidelines for the use of non-conventional treatments alone or in combination with conventional biomedical treatments. However, these very problems underscore the necessity for rigorous clinical trial evaluation and data review for the diverse therapies that are regarded as being alternative or complementary. (Lake and Spiegel 2007, p.xxii)

Chapter Overview

Previous chapters have addressed, in detail, the major principles and practices associated with the work of Spiritist Hospitals and their inter-relationships with psychiatry, psychology, and science in general. Here I'll present additional empirical evidence relevant to important Spiritist concepts and claims, the nature of the research approaches that have yielded these findings and ways that similar research might be improved and expanded in future, what we have learned about the accompaniments and aftereffects of Spiritist-related experiences, and the implications and possible applications of these findings for psychiatry, psychology, and the healing professions.

Parapsychological and Related Parallels to Spiritist Principles and Practices

In addition to the more conventional procedures employed in Spiritist Hospitals, the most important distinctively Spiritist practices and principles involve spirituality in general, medical intuition, mental treatments, work with mediums, past life considerations, and addressing a subtle, spiritual body. Parallels of each of these six practices have been subjected to careful scientific study outside the Spiritist tradition. Most of the relevant work has been done within the fields of psychical research and parapsychology, but this has been supplemented by increasing contributions from more established scientific fields such as consciousness studies and neuropsychology.

Spirituality Considerations

Spirituality is notoriously difficult to define but, generally, describes values, attitudes, ways of knowing and being, and practices that transcend and improve upon our familiar egoic ways and concerns (Braud 2009). *Spiritual* also can be used to describe qualities, realms, or realities other than or beyond those recognized in materialist and deterministic worldviews. *Spiritual* and *religious* are related but not identical: The former emphasizes individual experiences whereas the latter emphasizes formalized institutions, structures, and beliefs. In the context treated in this book, *spirit* and *spiritual* tend to refer to a subtle, nonmaterial aspect of oneself, of the deceased, and of the world. Spirituality in general has become an increasingly popular topic in areas of scholarship, disciplined inquiry, and science, and among medical and psychological practitioners. Content related to spirituality is being taught in an increasing number of medical schools and is being studied in an increasing number of research projects in neuropsychology and the new field of *neurotheology*. As such interest and studies continue and deepen, they might begin to address aspects that are less general and more specifically related to the particular form of *spirit* as this is treated in Spiritist Hospitals.

Research on Direct Knowing

In the practice of *medical intuition*, one becomes directly aware of the internal condition of another person's body or of the mental state of another person. In some cases, this "intuition" might involve the sensing of subtle clues in the patient's appearance or behavior and a coordination of subtle but conventional knowing with a vast store of information and patterns that the healer may have acquired through a lengthy history of observations. Much of this might occur in an "unconscious" manner. However, this more familiar form of intuition can be augmented by a much more direct form of knowing, which need not depend upon sensory information or logical inference. Here, aspects of the health condition of a patient are directly, and usually effortlessly and automatically, apprehended and the healer becomes aware of these through his or her sensations, feelings, imagery, and thoughts. Most of us are familiar with direct knowing as it appears in our resonance with the thoughts and feelings of loved ones, in the effortless coordination of musical and athletic performances, and in intuitions about good or bad business deals or about safe or dangerous individuals or environments (Murphy and White 1995; Dean *et al.* 1974).

However, direct knowing has been studied most extensively and most carefully in the field of experimental parapsychology. Here, it has been explored in the forms of telepathy (direct mind-to-mind interactions), clairvoyance (direct mind–external object and mind–external event interactions), and precognition (accurate foretelling of future events that cannot be conventionally expected) which, like medical intuition, seem to be three particular instances of a more general direct knowing process. These three forms of direct knowing, collectively known as *psi* (short for psychic functioning), have been documented in countless careful laboratory investigations. In all of these, research participants are asked to accurately describe targets or events that are beyond the reach of the conventional senses. The targets are randomly selected (so that they cannot be rationally predicted) and made conventionally inaccessible by shielding them or placing them at a distance in space or time. Results are evaluated statistically, to rule out chance coincidence. A great variety of experimental designs have been used to explore telepathy, clairvoyance, and precognition. These have included guessing the nature of hidden cards or drawings, testing under sensory restriction (*Ganzfeld* procedure) and other altered conditions of consciousness (such as relaxation and hypnosis), describing remote geographical sites visited by another person (*remote viewing*), and predicting future events that are randomly determined. All of these designs have yielded statistically significant and reliable evidence for accurate direct knowing. The studies are not always successful, and the obtained effects often are small. However, researchers have effectively countered methodological objections of critics and have presented convincing cases for the reality of these forms of direct knowing. Details of these experiments cannot be described here but can be found in many published overviews (Braud 2002, 2008; Radin 1997).

These types of studies are mentioned because they indicate that persons are indeed able to accurately describe, under well-controlled conditions, things and events invisible to the conventional senses, and this makes more plausible the claims of medical intuitives that it is possible to directly know what is happening inside the bodies and minds of patients—that is, to successfully perform psychic diagnoses or intuitive assessments of medical or psychological/psychiatric conditions. Outside the context of Spiritist investigations, direct experimental studies of psychic diagnosis or intuitive assessment have been conducted, although such studies have been quite few in number compared to the much larger number of studies of telepathy, clairvoyance, and precognition, and have not been as successful as studies of these latter three processes. However, sufficient evidence does exist to make it reasonable to entertain claims of the reality of psychic, intuitive, spiritual, or mental diagnosis (Benor 1992, n.d.).

Research on Direct Mental Influence

As opposed to the relative paucity of studies of psychic or intuitive medical diagnosis, there exist many more studies relevant to psychic, mental, or spiritual healing. The number of such studies can be expanded even more greatly if remote or distant healing can be viewed as a particular form of a more general process of *direct mental or intentional influence*. Direct mental influence has been studied very extensively, within the field of experimental parapsychology, in the form of *psychokinesis* (mind–matter interaction). Hundreds of studies have been conducted in which it has been shown that research participants are able to successfully influence—mentally, at a distance, and through the use of focused attention, intention, and "wishing"—a great variety of physical, biological, and psychological processes, events, and outcomes. The mentally influenced "targets" have included bouncing dice, the outputs of radioactivity-based electronic random event generators (electronic coin flippers), biological target systems (bacteria, fungi, cellular preparations, plants, behaviors of small animals), and the physiological activities of other persons (e.g. autonomic nervous system activity and brain activity) (Radin 1997). The successful research outcomes for inanimate target systems indicate "proof of principle" of the direct mental influence process, and the studies using various biological target systems can be considered healing analog studies. Space allows mention of only a few of these *healing analog* studies. One of these involved impressive results in a study of mental and laying-on of hands healing of skin wounds in mice (Grad 1965). Another involved distant healers' successful influence of brain activity of distant persons whose brain activity was being measured via functional magnetic resonance imaging (Achterberg *et al.* 2005). A great number of studies have demonstrated successful mental influences of the autonomic nervous system activity (assessed by skin conductance measurements) of distantly located target persons (Braud 2003). Of greater relevance to the possible role of direct mental influence in working with psychological or psychiatric conditions, rather than bodily conditions, are studies in which helpers were able to aid the concentration and attention-focusing abilities of other persons, mentally and at a distance, by concentrating themselves and intending for the distant person's concentration to improve during certain periods (Braud *et al.* 1995). These studies indicate that psychological processes can be psychically influenced and, in turn, suggest that psychological/psychiatric disorders might be targeted and alleviated in this manner.

There also have been a relatively large number of actual mental, spiritual, or psychic healing studies involving medical monitoring of patients, and enough of these studies have been successful to suggest the reality of a true distant healing process. To these, we can add studies of intercessory prayer, if prayer is viewed as involving at least the possibility of direct mental (intentional) influence by the person praying. These direct healing and prayer studies have focused on serious medical conditions such as cardiovascular conditions, AIDS, and others. The details of such studies can be found in a number of thorough overviews and meta-analyses (Dossey 2008; Krippner and Achterberg 2000).

In addition to these laboratory studies and clinical trials, direct mental influence in the form of mental, psychic, or spiritual healing is being used as an adjunctive treatment in various hospitals and medical facilities. This is well described, for Brazil, in other chapters of this book. The use of spiritual healers is now quite common in the United Kingdom. Doctors are allowed to recommend this form of complementary and alternative treatment to their patients, and spiritual healers may treat patients in National Health Service hospitals, should patients request such services.

One of the most fascinating findings regarding direct mental influence is that it seems possible for such intentional influences to work not only in "real time" but also to act retroactively ("backward in time") to influence what initially happened in the past. This suggests the possibility of using such processes in truly preventive medicine (Braud 2000). These time-defying properties, however, also greatly complicate our approaches to studying these processes scientifically.

An important bottom-line conclusion to be drawn from the findings of the many direct knowing and direct mental influence studies is that there exists a profound *non-local interconnectedness* (or *entanglement*, as a similar process in quantum physics has been named) among all things—of each of us with one another and with all of nature (Radin 2006).

Work with Mediums

Mediums are persons who seem able to contact, interact with, and obtain information from "spirits of the deceased" (*discarnates*). Serious research has been carried out with mediums since at least the middle of the 1800s. Individuals seek out mediums with the hope that the latter might provide communications from deceased loved ones, affirming their continuing existence in some form. Modern mediumship research includes projects that explore the possible role of mediumistic communications in helping individuals move more effectively through their grief/bereavement process. Researchers study mediums chiefly to learn whether they might contribute evidence relevant to the possibility of the survival of consciousness or personality after physical death. Countless investigations have yielded evidence that mediums can indeed provide sitters with accurate information about the deceased that they could not have known in conventional ways. What remains unclear, however, is whether this information originates in discarnates themselves or whether it might be accessed from some vast extra-physical reservoir of information or obtained through the medium's unconscious use of telepathy, clairvoyance, precognition, or retrocognition, from existing living or physical sources (Beischel 2007–2008; Beischel and Rock 2009; Beischel and Schwartz 2007; Fontana 2005; Gauld 1984; Schouten 1994).

Past Life Considerations

Aligned with the Spiritist emphasis on past lives are research studies of instances variously called *reincarnation, cases suggestive of reincarnation, cases of the reincarnation type,* or simply *past life recall* or *past life experiences.* The leading researcher in this area was the psychiatrist Ian Stevenson who published extensively on this topic. Stevenson and others have investigated and reported on a large number of cases in which children, usually between the ages of 2–3 and 7–8 years, spontaneously reported memories, exhibited appropriate behaviors and skills, or even had birthmarks or birth defects that appeared to match those of another person who died before the child was born and with whom the child seemed to identify (Mills and Lynn 2000). Past life experiences also have been reported by adults, usually elicited in the context of hypnosis sessions. These hypnosis-facilitated past life experiences generally are considered not as reliable as the spontaneous cases reported by children, because of the increased likelihood that bias, suggestion, and expectancy effects may occur in hypnosis conditions.

Other Survival Evidence

One interpretation of past life experiences is that something akin to an individual personality might survive the death of one person and later "incarnate" into another person. Psychical researchers have identified other phenomena suggestive of survival of death. These include after death communications or encounters (in which persons spontaneously experience what seem to be messages or other types of communication from the deceased), feelings of presence (of the deceased), apparitions (perception of something that has the visual appearance of the deceased, commonly called *ghosts*), hauntings (unusual sights, sounds, or feelings associated with a certain location and taken to be manifestations of the deceased), poltergeist occurrences (physical disturbances sometimes attributed to some surviving "spirit"), electronic voice phenomena and instrumental trans-communication (in which the voice or appearance of the deceased is reported to have been heard or seen by means of electronic equipment such as radios, tape recorders, telephones, televisions, or computers), deathbed visions (of the deceased), and near-death and out-of-body experiences (in which one has perceptions and other experiences that suggest to the experiencer that there is an aspect of one's personality or identity other than the physical body—a subtle spiritual body?—and that this aspect may survive physical death).

A Subtle, Spiritual Realm?

Spiritist teachings, beliefs, and practices emphasize the existence of a separate spiritual realm with which the living can interact. If the types of experiences mentioned in the three preceding subsections really are manifestations of the surviving deceased (discarnates), then the latter must exist in another realm that is ordinarily invisible and unknown to us, except for these relatively rare incursions into our world. However, an alternative explanation for these appearances and actions attributed to the deceased is that these may be due, instead, to the psychic functioning of the living persons involved in these instances. Knowledge attributed to discarnates may have been gained through the telepathic, clairvoyant, and precognitive processes of the living persons involved in these cases, and physical phenomena attributed to discarnates may have occurred through psychokinetic influences of the living—all of this having occurred without the living persons' conscious awareness that they may have been the sources of these happenings. Our current research tools do not yet allow us to determine which of these two types of explanations—activities of discarnates versus psychic functioning of the living—is the correct one, or whether each may account for certain cases but not others. The plausibility of each of these alternative interpretations could be explored on a case-by-case basis. An interesting twist is that, even if survival evidence is really psychic functioning of the living in disguise, that functioning itself might indicate or require a separate "spiritual" realm in which to operate.

The Need for Expanded Research Approaches

In their efforts to track the tantalizing yet usually invisible phenomena described in this chapter, investigators have thus far limited themselves to a rather narrow range of research approaches. Most of what we have learned has come from studies using experimental, quasi-experimental, causal-comparative (i.e. other types of group statistical studies), correlational, individual case study, and case collection designs, supplemented sometimes by clinical observations. To more fully and adequately address the reality and nature of these phenomena, it will be necessary for us to extend and expand our methods and approaches. Rhea White (1992) has provided a thorough, detailed review of the limitations of the methods just mentioned and has suggested a variety of additional approaches that could be used. These include cross-cultural, longitudinal, psychological, phenomenological, archetypal, folklorist, active imagination, and social constructionist approaches. In addition to these, a number of less familiar qualitative research approaches could be employed, including experiential, heuristic, narrative, life story, feminist, ethnography, auto-ethnography, grounded theory, textual analysis, discourse analysis, hermeneutical, field study, and action research approaches. These can be further supplemented by approaches developed more recently within the field of transpersonal psychology: intuitive inquiry, organic inquiry, and integral inquiry (Braud and Anderson 1998).

Exceptional Human Experiences and Their Nature, Accompaniments, and Outcomes

Besides suggesting methodological expansions, Rhea White has also made an important substantive contribution by developing a useful general framework for the types of occurrences treated in this chapter and in this book as a whole. She called these *exceptional human experiences* (EHEs), which might be characterized as anomalous experiences that, if worked with sufficiently, can foster beneficial and transformative changes in the experiencer. She identified nine classes of such experiences: mystical and unitive, psychical, encounter, unusual death-related, peak, exceptional human performance/feats, healing, desolation/nadir, and dissociative experiences. White's EHE approach is of great value because it inter-relates a great variety of experiences that had previously been treated in isolation and because it emphasizes the accompaniments and aftereffects of these types of experiences (White 1997).

Research on EHEs has identified many transformative and health—and well-being—accompaniments and outcomes of a variety of EHEs, including the types of psychical experiences emphasized in Spiritist practices. There is space only to briefly summarize these findings here.

Risks

There are risks associated with these types of experiences. These include feelings of puzzlement, confusion, and fear, especially when these are experienced for the very first time or when the experiencers have had very limited or erroneous knowledge about these experiences. Additional distress can occur if reports of these experiences elicit negative reactions from others (disbelief, suggestions that these are unhealthy or dangerous experiences), and keeping such experiences secret can result in low-grade stress of lengthy duration.

Benefits

The mentioned risks can be outweighed by the great number of benefits that arise as accompaniments and outcomes of EHEs. Here, space limits allow only a brief summary of reported health and well-being benefits. These include decreases in "negative" feelings and emotions such as depression, anxiety, isolation, loneliness, stress, future concerns, and fear of death; increases in "positive" feelings and emotions such as amazement, surprise, curiosity, joy, elation, happiness, confidence, wonder, connectedness, feeling confirmed and validated, gratitude, and love; changed attitudes and beliefs regarding human potential, spirituality, the meaning of life, purpose, the self, and death; changes in one's worldview; greater broadening, expansiveness, and openness; greater mindfulness, awareness, and understanding; increased ecologically supportive actions and positive environmental attitudes; and enhanced physical, psychological, and spiritual health and well-being. In addition to these influences for individuals, various types of EHEs have influenced society and culture at large by informing the great spiritual and wisdom traditions; inspiring practically useful insights, discoveries, and inventions; and informing great works of literature, art, and music (Braud and Associates 2007; Palmer and Braud 2002, 2010).

Psychiatric and Psychological Relevance

The risks and benefits just mentioned already point to the psychiatric and psychological relevance of these experiences. Ordinarily, such experiences are neglected by physical and mental health care professionals because they are believed to be unreal, real but not relevant to their areas of concern, dangerous, or not a politically correct focus of their attention. Whereas it was once a common view that having such experiences might be symptomatic of mental illness, practitioners are increasingly recognizing that this is not so. It is possible, of course, to have a psychological or psychiatric disorder and also experience psychic and other EHEs, but these are not identical and may not be associated. It also is recognized that EHEs can be signs of spiritual growth, development, and transformation (spiritual emergence), but that these experiences also can be psychologically overwhelming if they occur without adequate preparation or support (spiritual emergencies). What is needed is for persons in the healing professions to become better informed about the nature of these experiences and their possible accompaniments and outcomes, so that they might be better able to adequately work with persons who report such experiences. As we have seen in other chapters, health practitioners in Spiritist Hospitals are unusual in that they facilitate the training and use of these experiences for promoting health.

Beyond these practical application considerations, EHEs have important implications for psychiatry and psychology at large because they highlight the limitations of established conceptualizations and theories in these areas and point to the need of revising and expanding these to accommodate and honor the facts and findings that have been uncovered regarding these experiences.

Need for Additional Research and Support

The scientific study of these unusual experiences is still in its infancy and our understandings of their true nature and operation are quite limited. There is a great need for further research, better education, and greater practical applications regarding these experiences. Advances in these areas face three major challenges. The first involves the very nature of the phenomena: They are unusual, operate invisibly and in curious ways, and require novel and creative research approaches if we are to address them adequately. Another challenge is overcoming the widespread biases and misunderstandings that are present in researchers, practitioners, and the general public about these experiences. Still another challenge is the very limited funding for research and application and the relatively small number of researchers who are active in this area. It is problematic to do research because research monies that are available are usually geared toward patenting products for sale rather than toward furthering our understanding of these sorts of experiences and of human potential and consciousness itself. It is encouraging that, despite these challenges, some headway is being made toward these research and application goals in the Spiritist Hospitals of Brazil. It is hoped that these efforts will continue, expand, and spread to other hospitals and to other parts of the world. If this happens, there might be an eventual marriage of science and spirit of the type envisioned a century and a half ago by Allan Kardec.

The Contributors

Carlos Appel, **MD** (General Practice) has been exploring diagnosis through Kirlian photography. He has been deeply associated with several Spiritist Centers in Brazil. He lives near Porto Alegre, Brazil.

Tania Appel, MA (Nutrition) is a medium and leader at the Sanctuary, The Casa de Dom Inácio (The House of Saint Ignatius), where John of God works in Brazil. She lives in Abadiânia, Brazil.

Emma Bragdon, PhD (Psychology) is the Director of the Foundation for Energy Therapies. Since 2001 she has been traveling through Brazil researching Spiritism and Spiritist Psychiatric Hospitals. She is the author of *Kardec's Spiritism: A Home for Healing and Spiritual Evolution* and the executive producer of the documentary film *Spiritism: Bridging Spirituality and Health*. She lives in Vermont, USA, and Brazil. www.SpiritualAlliances.com

Camilla Casaletti Braghetta, MA is an occupational therapist at HOJE, a Spiritist Psychiatric Hospital in São Paulo. She also is the Coordinator of their Spiritual Assistance Program. She lives in São Paulo, Brazil. www.hoje.org.br

William Braud, PhD (Psychology) is Professor Emeritus, Institute of Transpersonal Psychology, Palo Alto, California. William has been a researcher and writer in areas of consciousness studies, research methods, and spirituality for four decades. He is the author of *Distant Mental Influence* and co-author of *Transpersonal Research Methods for the Social Sciences* and *Transforming Self and Others Through Research*. He resides in Texas, USA. www.inclusivepsychology.com

Janet Duncan studied in Brazil for 30 years and has been active in setting up many groups to study Spiritism in the UK. She is a founding member of the International Spiritist Council. From 2000 to 2002 she was President of the British Union of Spiritist Societies, BUSS. She is dedicated to translating Spiritist books into English. www.buss.org.uk

Shahram Eskandarnejad, MD is currently working for the Sonoma County Academic Foundation for Excellence in Medicine in California, USA.

Decio Iandoli, Jr., MD, PhD is a Professor of Medicine at UNIDERP, Mato Grosso do Sul (Brazil), and is the President of the Medical Spiritist Association of Mato Grosso do Sul (AME-MS). He lives in Brazil. www.luzespirita.com/biografias-decio.htm

Joan Koss-Chioino, PhD (Medical Anthropology) is Professor Emerita in the School of Human Evolution and Social Change at Arizona State University, where she developed the program in Medical Anthropology. She is also Visiting Professor of Psychiatry and Neurology at Tulane Medical Center in New Orleans and Research Professor in the Department of Psychology, George Washington University. She lives in Maryland, USA.

Gail Hayssen is an international shaman liaison, clairvoyant, medical intuitive, and researcher from Sebastopol, CA. www.smallmediumatlarge.net

Stanley Krippner, PhD (Psychology) is a professor at Saybrook University, and past-president of two divisions of the American Psychology Association. He is the co-author and co-editor of many books including *Varieties of Anomalous Experience: Examining the Scientific Evidence* (2000). He lives in California, USA. http://stanleykrippner.weebly.com

James Lake, MD (Psychiatry) is the author of the *Textbook of Integrative Mental Health Care* and co-editor with David Spiegel, MD of *Complementary and Alternative Treatments in Mental Health Care* (2007). He is Chair of International Network of Integrative Mental Health, Inc. and Clinical Assistant Professor at the Arizona Center of Integrative Medicine, University of Arizona College of Medicine. Dr. Lake is in private practice in Monterey, California, USA. www.progressivepsychiatry.com

Frederico Camelo Leão, MD, PhD (Psychiatry) is the CEO of Hospital João Evangelista and Coordinator of the program for Health, Spirituality and Religion at the University of São Paulo's Medical School. He was formerly Director of the Spiritist Center of Our Spiritual Home, André Luiz, a 650-bed residence for those with mental disabilities. He lives in São Paulo, Brazil. www.hoje.org.br

Ellen Levine, PhD is a clinical social worker, psychoanalyst, and expressive arts therapist in Ontario, Canada.

Giancarlo Lucchetti, MD (Geriatrics) is the Research Executive Coordinator of the Spirituality and Mental Health Integration Program at Hospital João Evangelista, and the Coordinator of the Research Department at São Paulo's Spiritist Medical Association. He lives in São Paulo. www.hoje.org.br

Gerald Magnan was recently the supervisor for 150 mediums who worked exclusively in the Department of Spiritual Assistance at the Spiritist Psychiatric Hospital of Porto Alegre. As a result of his intense dedication to spiritual work, Gerald Magnan does not work under a license conveyed by an academic or professional licensing board, even though he earned diplomas in the past. He lives in Porto Alegre, Brazil.

Dorothy Mandel, PhD is adjunct faculty at Santa Barbara Graduate Institute and a clinical psychologist in Santa Rosa, CA, specializing in heart based attachment and trauma repatterning therapies. www.dorothymandel.com

Alexander Moreira-Almeida, MD, PhD (Psychiatry) is a Professor of Psychiatry at the Medical School of Juiz de Fora and the University of São Paulo. He is the director of the Center for Research in Spirituality and Health at the Federal University of Juiz de Fora School of Medicine. He lives in Juiz de Fora, Brazil. www.ufjf.br/nupes-eng

Melvin Morse, MD (Pediatrics) was an Associate Professor of Pediatrics at the University of Washington for 20 years, retiring in 2007 to concentrate on research and writing. He published the only study of near-death experiences in children in the medical literature, and one of the first case-controlled prospective studies of near-death experiences. He lives in Delaware, USA. www.spiritualscientific.com

Marlene Nobre, MD (Gynecology) specializes in cancer prevention. She is the President of the International Medical Spiritist Association (AME-Int); President of the Brazilian Medical Spiritist Association (AME-Br), São Paulo; and President of the Spiritist Centers G.E. Cairbar Schutel and Creche Lar do Alvorecer. She is the author of several books and Editor in Chief of *Folha Espírita*. She lives in São Paulo, Brazil. www.amebrasil.org.br

Julio Peres, PsyD, PhD is a Clinical Psychologist with a PhD in Neuroscience and Behavior. He is a Researcher at the Program for Health, Spirituality and Religiosity (ProSER) at the Psychiatry Institute, University of São Paulo School of Medicine, where he also teaches. He lives in São Paulo, Brazil. www.julioperes.com.br

Andrew Powell, MD (Psychiatry) is a psychiatrist and psychotherapist who has held consultant and academic appointments in London and Oxford. He is Founding Chair of the Spirituality and Psychiatry Special Interest Group of the Royal College of Psychiatrists, UK, with now over 2500 psychiatric members (www.rcpsych.ac.uk/spirit). He is co-editor of the book *Spirituality and Psychiatry* (2009). He lives in Oxfordshire, England.

Dean Radin, PhD (Psychology) is Senior Scientist at the Institute of Noetic Sciences and Adjunct Faculty at Sonoma State University, California. For over two decades he has been engaged in consciousness research. He is the author of several books including *The Conscious Universe* and *Entangled Minds*. He lives in California, USA. www.DeanRadin.com

Gelson Roberto, Psychologist, is an advisor to the Spiritist Psychiatric Hospital of Porto Alegre, and has a private clinical practice. He teaches classes in continuing professional education on Spirituality and Health at the Hospital. He is the Director of a Spiritist Center, and resides in Porto Alegre, Brazil. www.hepa.org.br

Gilson Roberto, MD (General Practice/Homeopathy) is the Medical Director of the Spiritist Psychiatric Hospital of Porto Alegre, Brazil, and the Vice President of the Medical Spiritist Association for Rio Grande do Sul. He is the director of a Spiritist Center, has a clinical practice as an MD, and lectures internationally on spirituality and health. He lives in Porto Alegre, Brazil. www.hepa.org.br

Jaider Rodrigues e Paulo, MD (Psychiatry) works as a psychiatrist at the Spiritist Hospital André Luiz of Belo Horizonte, Brazil. He lives in Belo Horizonte, Brazil. www.heal.org.br

Beverly Rubik, PhD (Biophysics) founded and directs the Institute for Frontier Science. She is a consultant, teacher, researcher, and author on the frontiers of science and medicine. She serves on the editorial board of several journals, including the *Alternative Health Practitioner*, *Alternative Therapies in Health and Medicine*, and the *Journal of Complementary Therapies in Medicine* (UK). Beverly resides in California, USA. www.frontiersciences.org

Linda Russek, PhD was Assistant Clinical Professor of Medicine in the Department of Medicine at the University of Arizona. She was co-founder and co-director of the Human Energy Systems Laboratory. She directs the Heart Science Foundation and has a clinical psychology holistic practice in Arizona, USA. www.heartsciencefoundation.com

Alan Sanderson, MD (Psychiatry) is a hypnotherapist, spirit-release therapist, and President of the Spirit Release Foundation. He lives in London, England. www.spiritrelease.com

Marilyn Schlitz, PhD is President and CEO of the Institute of Noetic Sciences, Petaluma, CA.

Mario Sergio Silveira, PhD is an administrator at Bom Retiro, a Spiritist Psychiatric Hospital in Curitiba, Brazil, and in private practice as a psychologist. He lives in Curitiba, Brazil. www. hospitalbomretiro.com.br

Jerome Stone, RN, MA is the author of *Minding the Bedside: Nursing from the Heart of the Awakened Mind.* www.mindingthebedside.com

Candido Pinto Vallada, MD (Psychiatry) is the Vice President of the Council of Directors and General Coordinator of the Spirituality and Mental Health Integration Program at Hospital João Evangelista. He is a Jungian Analyst and founding member of the Jungian Association of Brazil and the Jung Institute of São Paulo. He lives in São Paulo. www.hoje.org.br

Homero Vallada, MD (Psychiatry) is the President of the Council of Directors at the Hospital João Evangelista, and an Associate Professor at the University of São Paulo's Medical School. He lives in São Paulo. www.hoje.org.br

Roberto Lucio Viera de Souza, MD (Psychiatry) is the Director of the Spiritist Hospital André Luiz of Belo Horizonte, Brazil. He is a psychiatrist and therapist at the Renascimento Psychic Assistance Institute and a Vice President of the Spiritist Medical Association (AME) of Brazil. He lives in Belo Horizonte, Brazil. www.heal.org.br

Alan Wallace, PhD (Religious Studies) has specialized in training of attention in Tibetan Buddhism and its relation to modern psychological and philosophical theories of attention and consciousness. He is President and founder of the Santa Barbara Institute for Consciousness Studies. He resides in California, USA. www.alanwallace.org

Further Reading and Viewing

The Companion Book

Emma Bragdon (ed.) (2012) *Resources for Extraordinary Healing: Schizophrenia, Bipolar and Other Serious Mental Illnesses* is available as an ebook or in print. It briefly reflects on current needs for integrative mental health care in the USA vis à vis Spiritist resources in Brazil with particular attention paid to the spiritual aspects of care. More importantly, the book gives up to date contact information for resources for both non-residential support (clinics and individual practitioners who collaborate) and residential care facilities for those needing integrative care with serious mental health issues including withdrawing from psychiatric medications, when necessary. Further information can be found at www.ResourcesForExtraordinaryHealing.com.

Books on Integrative Mental Health, Obsession, and Disobsession

Cook, C., Powell, A. and Sims, A. (eds) (2009) *Spirituality and Psychiatry*. London: RCPsychPublications.

Franco, D.P. (2004) *Obsession*. São Paulo: Livraria Espirita Alvorada Editora.

Franco, D.P. (2005) *Understanding Spiritual and Mental Health*. São Paulo: Livraria Espirita Alvorada Editora.

Lake, J. (2006) *Textbook of Integrative Mental Health Care*. New York: Thieme Books.

Lake, J. (2009) *Integrative Mental Health Care: A Therapist's Handbook*. New York: W.W. Norton.

Lake, J. and Spiegel, D. (eds) (2007) *Complementary and Alternative Treatments in Mental Health Care*. Washington, DC: American Psychiatric Publishing.

Monti, D.A. and Beitman, B.D. (2009) *Integrative Psychiatry*. New York: Oxford University Press.

Xavier, F.C. and Vieira, W. (2005) *Disobsession*. Brasilia: ISC.

Original Texts on Spiritism

Kardec, A. (1999) *Introduction to the Spiritist Philosophy*. Philadelphia: Allan Kardec Educational Society. (Original work published 1859.)

Kardec, A. (2004) *The Gospel According to Spiritism*. Brasilia: ISC. (Original work published 1864.)

Kardec, A. (2007) *The Mediums' Book*. Brasilia: ISC. (Original work published 1861.)

Kardec, A. (2008) *The Spirits' Book*. Brasilia: ISC. (Original work published 1860.)

Kardec, A. (2008) *Heaven and Hell*. Brasilia: ISC. (Original work published 1865.)

Kardec, A. (2011) *Genesis*. Brasilia: ISC. (Original work published 1868.)

Electronic Library of Articles on Spirituality and Health

Coordinated by Alexander Moreira-Almeida, MD, and available both in English and Portuguese: www.hoje. org.br/site/elsh.php.

Films (recommended for discussion groups and classroom use)

Chico Xavier (2010): full-length documentary of the life of the Brazilian, Francisco Xavier, who channeled more than 400 books in his lifetime, and was thought of as a living saint and ambassador of Spiritism. There is no other film that shows the development of a mature medium who began afraid of his gift and, through the guidance of his mentors, became both well balanced and highly successful.

Healing: Miracles, Mysteries and John of God (2011): a full-length film that captures some of the remarkable stories of John's healing and explores inexplicable but well-documented instances of miraculous intervention.

I Do Not Heal; God Is the One Who Heals (2006): a 30-minute documentary introducing the work of John of God and his healing sanctuary in Brazil.

Mothers of Chico Xavier (2011): a full-length film documenting the interaction between Chico Xavier and three mothers who faced the death of their children. Viewers are aware of the great healing power of mediums who can help with depression associated with grief, abortion, and miscarriage. In Portuguese with English subtitles.

Nosso Lar (2010): full-length film dramatizing the book written by Francisco Xavier about one of the astral colonies spirits go to after death of the body. A profoundly moving film that follows a popular book channeled by a spirit who was a physician in his last life, who describes what he experienced in his transition of death.

Spiritism: Bridging Spirituality and Health (2008): a 30-minute documentary which introduces the viewer to the work of Spiritist Centers in Brazil and the USA. A professionally done film with groundbreaking intimate footage of disobsession work.

Organizations Supporting the Integration of Spirituality and Psychiatry

Center for Research in Spirituality and Health
Federal University of Juiz de Fora, Brazil
www.ufjf.br/nupes-eng

Center for Spirituality and Healing
University of Minnesota, Minneapolis, MN, USA
www.csh.umn.edu

Center for Spirituality, Theology and Health
Durham, North Carolina, USA
www.spiritualityandhealth.duke.edu

Division of Perceptual Studies
Department of Psychiatry and Neurobehavioral Sciences
University of Virginia, Charlottesville, VA, USA
www.medicine.virginia.edu/clinical/departments/psychiatry/sections/cspp/dops

George Washington Institute for Spirituality and Health
Washington, DC, USA
www.gwumc.edu/gwish

The Spirituality and Health Online Education and Resource Center (SOERCE) at George Washington's Institute for Spirituality and Health aims to be the premiere online location for educational and clinical resources in the fields of spirituality, religion, and health: www.gwumc.edu/gwish/soerce/index.cfm

International Medical Spiritist Association
São Paulo, Brazil
www.ameinternational.org/site

International Society for the Study of Subtle Energies and Energy Medicine (ISSSEEM)
Lafayette, CO, USA
www.issseem.org

PRISME—Spirituality and Mental Health Integration Program
São Paulo, Brazil
prisme@hoje.org.br
www.hoje.org.br

Progressive Psychiatry
Monterey, CA, USA
http://progressivepsychiatry.com/index.php?main_page=page&id=7

Scientific and Medical Network
Gloucestershire, UK
www.scimednet.org

Spirit Release Foundation
London, UK
www.spiritrelease.com

The Spirituality and Psychiatry Special Interest Group
Royal College of Psychiatrists, UK
www.rcpsych.ac.uk/spirit

US Spiritist Medical Association (SMA-US)
www.sma-us.org

Research Institutes

Institute of Noetic Sciences
Petaluma, CA, USA
www.noetic.org

Núcleo de Pequisa do Espiritismo e Psiquitria (NUPESP)—Center for Research of Spiritism and Psychiatry
Hospital Espirita Eurípdes Barsanulfo
www.casadeeuripedes.com

Samueli Institute
Alexandria, VA, USA
www.siib.org

Windbridge Institute for Applied Research in Human Potential
Tucson, AZ, USA
www.windbridge.org

Glossary

aura: a light or radiance, sometimes perceived as an "energy" that emanates from the physical body, visible to those with psychic powers of clairvoyance. The aura is a general term that may contain the light, color, and energy of several subtle bodies associated with one physical body.

bilocation: the ability of a person to be in two locations at the same time. The person bilocating has the ability to view both locations and retains memory of both locations. The person viewing the bilocating person may or may not see them "in the flesh."

brain sand: concretions of calcium carbonate, which are not markers of degeneration, that are emitted by granules of peptides within the pineal gland. Brain sand consists of cellular organelles with a specific function in the resonance of the magnetic fields of the body. They convert something within the magnetic fields into neurochemical stimuli. It could be that the highest density of brain sand in the pineal body is an indicator of the highest mediumistic capacity (see Chapter 21).

catalepsy: a seizure or abnormal condition characterized by postural rigidity and mental stupor.

channeling: to convey verbal or written messages from a disembodied source.

clairvoyance: the paranormal power of seeing objects or actions beyond the normal range of vision.

control: a psi research term which means an honest person who observes the medium and the researcher in order to ascertain that no sleight of hand or other fraudulent behavior occurs which would skew research (see Chapter 19).

ectoplasm: a viscous substance that emanates from the body of a medium usually through an open mouth. It can be used as a healing substance in spiritual healing and can also be used by disincarnate spirits to attain a form to facilitate interaction in the physical world.

etheric double: also called the "etheric body," this is our vital body, mediating the functions of the physical and spiritual bodies. Esoteric philosophies have perceived it as the first or lowest layer in the "human energy field" or aura. It is said to be in immediate contact with the physical body, to sustain it and connect it with "higher" bodies. At death, after the etheric body has maintained the physical body's form, it separates from the physical body, and the physical reverts to natural disintegration.

faith-healing: the use of religious faith or prayer to bring about healing.

fluidify: to magnetize or send a flow of pure spiritual energy into water so that it becomes "blessed" (fluidified) and can help heal and uplift those who drink it.

group field: the energy that is built up in the environment when a group meets for a certain purpose. A group that meditates and prays together has a field full of positive intent to bring out the best in themselves and others.

hypnotize: to influence or control by suggestion when the subject is in an altered state of consciousness caused by a process known as induction. Contemporary research suggests that hypnotized subjects are fully awake and are focusing attention, with a corresponding decrease in their peripheral awareness. These subjects show an increased response to suggestions.

incorporate: to allow a disincarnate to use one's body, speech, and mind for purposes of communication and interaction with the material world.

informational field: another name for the "aura" or "subtle bodies" that surround the physical body; the field that holds information about the body's health and all past memories.

karma: the universal law of cause and effect; when applied to describe a life situation it is said that negative acts in the past may result in challenges in the present in order to learn lessons that were previously not learned with the ultimate goal: To become more wise and loving.

magnetism: the properties of attraction or molecular properties possessed by magnets; the properties of attraction possessed by people who have developed spiritual attributes that can assist in healing others.

magnetize: to transmit pure spiritual energy for the purpose of healing.

materialism: 1. preoccupation with or emphasis on valuing material objects, comforts, and considerations as opposed to invisible, spiritual, emotional, or intellectual values; 2. the philosophical theory that regards matter as constituting the universe and all phenomena including those of mind.

medium: a person through whom the spirits can contact those in body; an interpreter for the spirits.

mediumship: the practice of being a medium whereby other sources of intelligence, e.g. spirits not in body, can articulate themselves through the mind (telepathically) or voice of the medium to non-mediums. Mental mediumship (also called "clairvoyant" mediumship) occurs in a conscious and focused waking state. In contrast, during trance mediumship, the medium may be unconscious of surroundings, his or her normal personality is not present, and the intruding or invited intelligence replaces it. In the latter situation the medium retains little or no recollection of what has been said or done in the absence of his or her regular personality. In either case the spirit may use the medium to do healing work or transmit thoughts through writing (automatic writing or psychography).

mentor: a wise and trusted counselor, benefactor, or teacher that may be in body or disincarnate. Spiritual mentors are spiritual guides with great authority because they have evolved great wisdom and compassion. They may be associated with individuals, places, groups, and/or organizations such as hospitals. Each disobsession group has a human director and a spiritual mentor.

miasma: a Portuguese term meaning a congestion of energy located in the subtle body that originates in negative thinking or negative intention. Spiritists consider miasms are often the seed that leads to illness in the mind or the physical body.

passé: a Portuguese term for the laying-on of hands, where there is a donation of spiritual energies from a healer to a recipient/patient. Spiritism recognizes three types of passé: 1) *Magnetic*, in which the energy source is the medium; 2) *Spiritual*, in which the energy source is the Spirit; and 3) *Mixed*, in which the energy comes from both the medium and the Spirit.

perispirit: a subtle, ethereal, nearly mass-less covering, a kind of energy body that serves as a blueprint for the human form (see p.15). This etheric body permeates the physical body in every detail, creating an exact duplicate of every organ and limb. Its main function is to transmit energy to the physical body.

psi: psychic phenomena including clairvoyance, telepathy, precognition, and psychokinesis.

psychic surgery: a non-physical intervention typically done by a medium/healer whereby the auric field is open and miasms cleared from the perispirit. This can effect healing of the physical body and mind immediately or over time.

psychosphere: the energetic ambience that carries certain emotional qualities that surround a person, group, or place.

somnambulist: one who has the ability to walk during sleep and may come to harm as a direct result.

soul: a spiritual aspect of human beings which carries the level of its moral development and the capacity for reason it has attained. The seat of human feelings that are preserved from one life to the next. The soul is believed to survive physical death and continue from lifetime to lifetime, having the opportunity to develop both in and out of physical life.

stigmata: marks or wounds resembling the wounds of the crucified body of Christ said to emerge spontaneously on the bodies of certain people in elevated states of consciousness.

subtle body: living beings have a series of psycho-spiritual envelopes that surround them, give them energy, and connect them with specific subtle realms. Each of these subtle bodies corresponds to a subtle plane of existence, e.g. the astral body is connected to the astral realm. The perispirit is a general term that encompasses many of these psycho-spiritual envelopes which are given more distinct names in other metaphysical and religious traditions.

syntony: a harmony between two or more that is so profound that people report feeling "at one" with each other.

trance medium: mediums who enter into an altered state of consciousness in order to allow a spirit to speak through them. The medium still exerts complete control over him- or herself so as to choose to accept the influence of the spirit or not. Example: Trance mediums receive the spirits of obsessors during disobsession work or the advice of the spiritual mentor guiding the group.

xenoglossy: speaking in a language unknown to the medium.

xenography: writing in a language unknown to the medium.

References

Foreword

Achterberg, J., Cooke, K., Richards, T., Standish, L.J., Kozak, L. and Lake, J. (2005) "Evidence for correlations between distant intentionality and brain function in recipients: a fMRI analysis." *Journal of Alternative and Complementary Medicine 11*, 6, 965–971.

Anderson, J., Anderson, L., and Felsenthal, G. (1993) "Pastoral needs for support within an inpatient rehabilitation unit." *Archives of Physical Medicine and Rehabilitation 74*, 574–578.

Astin, J.A., Harkness, E., and Ernst, E. (2000) "The efficacy of 'distant healing': a systematic review of randomized trials." *Annals of Internal Medicine 132*, 903–910.

D'Aquili, E.G. and Newberg, A.B. (2000) "The neuropsychology of aesthetic, spiritual, and mystical states." *Zygon: Journal of Religion and Science 35*, 1, 39–51.

Hamburg, D., Elliott, G., and Parron, D. (eds) (1982) *Health and Behavior: Frontiers of Research in the Biobehavioral Sciences.* Washington, DC: National Academy Press.

Hebert, R.S., Jenckes, M.W., Ford, D.E., O'Connor, D.R., *et al.* (2001) "Patient perspectives on spirituality and the patient–physician relationship." *Journal of General Internal Medicine 16*, 10, 685–692.

Jonas, W.B. and Crawford, C.C. (eds) (2003) *Healing Intention and Energy Medicine: Science, Research Methods and Clinical Implications.* New York: Churchill Livingstone.

King, D. and Bushwick, B. (1994) "Beliefs and attitudes of hospital inpatients about faith-healing and prayer." *Journal of Family Practice 39*, 349–352.

Koenig, H., Ford, S., George, L., Blazer, D., *et al.* (1993) "Religion and anxiety disorder: an examination and comparison of associations in young, middle-aged and elderly adults." *Journal of Anxiety Disorders 7*, 321–342.

Levin, J. (1996) "How religion influences morbidity and health: reflections on natural history, salutogenesis and host resistance." *Social Science and Medicine 43*, 849–864.

Levin, J. (2003) "Spiritual determinants of health and healing: an epidemiologic perspective on salutogenic mechanisms." *Alternative Therapies in Health and Medicine 9*, 6, 48–57.

MacLean, C.D., Susi, B., Phifer, N., Schultz, L., *et al.* (2003) "Patient preference for physician discussion and practice of spirituality: results from a multicenter patient survey." *Journal of General Internal Medicine 18*, 1, 38–43.

Mitchell, L. and Romans, S. (2003) "Spiritual beliefs in bipolar affective disorder: their relevance for illness management." *Journal of Affective Disorders 75*, 3, 247–257.

Neeleman, J. and King, M.B. (1993) "Psychiatrists' religious attitudes in relation to their clinical practice: a survey of 231 psychiatrists." *Acta Psychiatrica Scandinavica 88*, 6, 420–424.

Olive, K. (1995) "Physician religious beliefs and the physician–patient relationship: a study of devout physicians." *Southern Medical Journal 6*, 274–279.

Sageman, S. (2004) "Breaking through the despair: spiritually oriented group therapy as a means of healing women with severe mental illness." *Journal of the American Academy of Psychoanalysis and Dynamic Psychiatry 32*, 1, 125–141.

Samano, E.S., Goldenstein, P.T., Ribeiro Lde, M., Lewin, F., *et al.* (2004) "Praying correlates with higher quality of life: results from a survey on complementary/alternative medicine use among a group of Brazilian cancer patients." *São Paulo Medical Journal 122*, 2, 60–63.

Schlitz, M. and Braud, W. (1997) "Distant intentionality and healing: assessing the evidence." *Alternative Therapies in Health and Medicine 3*, 6, 62–73.

Sloan, R.P., Bagiella, E., and Powell, T. (1999) "Religion, spirituality and medicine." *Lancet 353*, 9153, 664–667.

Standish, L.J., Johnson, L.C., Kozak, L., and Richards, T. (2003) "Evidence of correlated functional magnetic resonance imaging signals between distant human brains." *Alternative Therapies in Health and Medicine 9*, 1, 128.

Sullivan, W.P. (1993) "'It helps me to be a whole person': the role of spirituality among the mentally challenged." *Psychosocial Rehabilitation Journal 16*, 3, 125–134.

Yankelovich Partners Inc. (1996, June 12–13) for *Time/CNN*.

Introduction

Benson, H. (1996) *Timeless Healing*. New York: Simon and Schuster.

Berger, W., Mendlowicz, M.V., Marques-Portella, C., Kinrys, G., *et al.* (2009) "Pharmacologic alternatives to antidepressants in posttraumatic stress disorder: a systematic review." *Progress in Neuropsychopharmacology and Biological Psychiatry 33*, 2, 169–180.

Birks, J. and Harvey, R.J. (2006) "Donepezil for dementia due to Alzheimer's disease." *Cochrane Database of Systematic Reviews 1*, CD001190.

Bragdon, E. (2002) *Spiritual Alliances: Discovering the Roots of Health at the Casa de Dom Inácio*. Woodstock, VT: Lightening Up Press.

Bragdon, E. (2004) *Kardec's Spiritism: A Home for Healing and Spiritual Evolution*. Woodstock, VT: Lightening Up Press.

Bragdon, E. (2005) "Spiritist healing centers in Brazil." *Seminars in Integrative Medicine 3*, 2, 67–74.

Bragdon, E. (2006) *I Do Not Heal, God Is the One Who Heals*. [Documentary film.] Woodstock, VT: Old Dog Documentaries and Spiritual Alliances.

Bragdon, E. (2008) *Spiritism: Bridging Spirituality and Health*. [Documentary film.] Woodstock, VT: Old Dog Documentaries and Spiritual Alliances.

Bragdon, E. (2010) "South American Spiritism: Spiritist Hospitals and Healing Centers in Brazil." In M. Micozzi (ed.) *Fundamentals of Complementary and Integrative Medicine*, 4th edn. St. Louis, MO: Saunders/Elsevier Press.

Breggin, P. (2008) *Medication Madness*. New York: St. Martin's Press.

Breggin, P. (2010) "The Study of Empathic Therapy: Human Connection versus Psychiatric Control." *Huffington Post*, available at www.huffingtonpost.com/dr-peter-breggin/the-center-for-the-study-_b_706253.html (September 7), accessed December 15, 2010.

Dixon, L.B., Dickerson, F., Bellack, A.S., Bennett, M., *et al.* (2010) "Schizophrenia patient outcomes research team (PORT)." *Schizophrenia Bulletin 36*, 1, 48–70.

Ferreira, I. (1993) *Novos rumos à medicina*. São Paulo: FEESP. (Original work published 1945.)

Fountoulakis, K.N. (2008) "The contemporary face of bipolar illness: complex diagnostic and therapeutic challenges." *CNS Spectrums 13*, 9, 763–774, 777–779.

Fournier, J.C., DeRubeis, R.J., Hollon, S.D., Dimidjian, S., *et al.* (2010) "Antidepressant drug effects and depression severity: a patient-level meta-analysis." *Journal of the American Medical Association 303*, 1, 47–53.

Hervé, I. (2006) *Reencarnação: A Única Explicação [Reincarnation: The Only Explanation]*. Porto Allure, Brazil: Editora Age.

Hervé, I., de Silva, S., Borges, R., Tejada, V., *et al.* (2003) *Apometria: A Conexão Entre a Ciência e O Espiritismo [Apometry: A Connection Between Science and Spiritism]*. Porto Alegre, Brazil: Dacasa Editora/Livraria Palmarinca.

Hyman, S. (1996) "Initiation and adaptation: a paradigm for understanding psychotropic drug action." *American Journal of Psychiatry 15*, 151–161.

Institute of HeartMath (2003) *Emotional Energetics, Intuition and Epigenetics Research*. Boulder Creek, CO: Institute of HeartMath.

Kardec, A. (2004a) *Spiritism in Its Simplest Expression*. Philadelphia: AKES.

Kardec, A. (2004b) *Introduction to the Spiritist Philosophy*. Philadelphia: AKES.

Katzman, M.A. (2009) "Current considerations in the treatment of generalized anxiety disorder." *CNS Drugs 23*, 2, 103–120.

Kirsch, I. (2008) "Challenging received wisdom: antidepressants and the placebo effect." *McGill Journal of Medicine 11*, 2, 219–222.

Lacasse, J. (2005) "Serotonin and depression: a disconnect between the advertisements and the scientific literature." *PLoS Medicine 2*, 1211–1216.

Lam, R.W., Kennedy, S.H., Grigoriadis, S., McIntyre, R.S., *et al.* (2009) "Canadian Network for Mood and Anxiety Treatments (CANMAT): clinical guidelines for the management of major depressive disorder in adults. III. Pharmacotherapy." *Journal of Affective Disorders 117*, Suppl. 1, S26–43.

Moreira-Almeida, A. and Moreira, A. (2008) "Inacio Ferreira: the institutionalization of the integration between medicine and paranormal phenomena." A presentation at the Convention of the Parapsychological Association and the Society for Psychical Research.

Shealy, N. and Church, D. (2008) *Soul Medicine: Awakening Your Inner Blueprint for Abundant Health and Energy.* Santa Rosa, CA: Energy Psychology Press.

Shoenfelt, J.L. and Weston, C.G. (2007) "Managing obsessive compulsive disorder: in children and adolescents." *Psychiatry (Edgmont) 4*, 5, 47–53.

Tajima, K., Fernández, H., López-Ibor, J.L., Carrasco, J.L., *et al.* (2009) "Schizophrenia treatment: critical review on the drugs and mechanisms of action of antipsychotics." *Actas Españolas de Psiquiatría 37*, 6, 330–342.

Tandon, A., Murray, C.J.L., Lauer, J.A., and Evans, D.B. (2000) *Measuring Overall Health System Performance for 191 Countries.* Geneva, Switzerland: World Health Organization.

Thase, M.E. (2008) "Do antidepressants really work? A clinicians' guide to evaluating the evidence." *Current Psychiatry Reports 10*, 6, 487–494.

US Department of Health and Human Services (1999) *Mental Health: A Report of the Surgeon General.* Washington, DC: Department of Health and Human Services.

Whitaker, R. (2010) *Anatomy of an Epidemic.* New York: Crown Publishers.

Chapter 1: A Brief History of Spiritism

Dossey, L. (1997) *Healing Words.* New York: HarperOne.

Dossey, L. (2008) "What we know and don't know." *Explore: The Journal of Science and Healing 4*, 6, 341–352.

Ellis, A. and Blau, S. (2000) *Albert Ellis Reader: A Guide to Well-Being Using REBT.* New York: Citadel.

Ingerman, S. and Harner, M. (2006) *Soul Retrieval: Mending the Fragmented Self.* New York: HarperOne.

Koenig, H. (2007) "Religion, spirituality and psychotic disorders." *Revista de Psiquiatria Clínica [Journal of Clinical Psychiatry] 34*, Suppl. 1, 95–104.

Krippner, S. and Villoldo, A. (1987) *Healing States: A Journey into the World of Spiritual Healing and Shamanism.* New York: Simon and Schuster.

Morse, M. and Perry, P. (2001) *Where God Lives.* New York: HarperOne.

Spiritist Medical Association (2010) Available at www.amebrasil.org.br, accessed on December 10, 2010.

Sri Sathya Sai Institute of Higher Medical Sciences (2008) Available at www.sathyasai.org/saihealth/pnhosp.htm, accessed on 6 July, 2011.

Weisberg, B. (2004) *Talking to the Dead: Kate and Maggie Fox and the Rise of Spiritualism.* San Francisco: HarperCollins.

Chapter 2: A Brief Overview of the Philosophy and Development of Spiritism's Methodologies

Aubrée, M. and Laplantine, F. (1990) *La Table, le Livre et les Esprits [The Table, the Book, and the Spirits].* Paris: Éditions Jean-Claude Làttes.

CEI (Conselho Espírita Internacional—International Spiritist Council) (2011) "Países Membros do CEI." Available at www.intercei.com/es/paises-membros-do-cei.html, accessed on January 27, 2011.

Chibeni, S.S. (1999) "The spiritist paradigm." *Human Nature 1*, 2, 82–87.

Fernandes, W.L.N. (2004) "Allan Kardec e os mil núcleos espíritas de todo o mundo com os quais se correspondia em 1864." *La Revista Espírita.* Available at www.larevistaespirita.com/noticia.php?CodNoticia=287, accessed on June 6, 2011.

Gauld, A. (1968) *The Founders of Psychical Research.* London: Routledge and Kegan Paul.

Hufford, D.J. and Bucklin, M.A. (2006) "The Spirit of Spiritual Healing in the United States." In J.D. Koss-Chioino and P. Hefner (eds) *Spiritual Transformation and Healing.* Lanham, MD: Altamira.

Kardec, A. (1858) "Introduction." *Revue Spirite—Journal d'Études Psychologiques 1*, 1, 1–6.

Kardec, A. (1860) "Manifestations physiques spontanées." *Revue Spirite—Journal d'Études Psychologiques 3*, 1, 77–81.

Kardec, A. (1864) "Le Spiritisme est une science positive." *Revue Spirite—Journal d'Études Psychologiques 7*, 11, 321–328.

Kardec, A. (1868) *La Genese, les Miracles et les Predictions Selon le Spiritisme.* Paris: Union Spirite Française et Francophone.

Kardec, A. (1986) *The Mediums' Book.* Rio de Janeiro: FEB. (Original work published 1861.)

Kardec, A. (1987) *The Gospel According to Spiritism.* London: The Headquarters Publishing Co. (Original work published 1864.)

Kardec, A. (1996) *The Spirits' Book*, 2nd edn. Rio de Janeiro: FEB. (Original work published 1860.)

Kardec, A. (1999) *What is Spiritism?* Philadelphia: Allan Kardec Educational Society. (Original work published 1859.)

Moreira-Almeida, A. (2008) "Allan Kardec and the development of a research program in psychic experiences." *Proceedings of the Parapsychological Association and Society for Psychical Research Convention*, 136–151.

Moreira-Almeida, A. and Lotufo Neto, F. (2005) "Spiritist views of mental disorders in Brazil." *Transcultural Psychiatry 16*, 61 (Pt 1), 5–25.

Myers, F.W.H. (2001) *Human Personality and Its Survival of Bodily Death.* Charlottesville, VA: Hampton Roads Publishing. (Original work published 1903.)

Sampaio, J.R. (2004) "Voluntários: um estudo sobre a motivação de pessoas e a cultura em uma organização do terceiro sector [Volunteers: a study about people's motivation and the culture of a third sector organization]." PhD dissertation, Faculdade de Economia, Administração e Contabilidade. São Paulo: Universidade de São Paulo.

Stoll, S.J. (2003) *Espiritismo à Brasileira [Spiritism in Brazil].* São Paulo (Edusp) and Curitiba: Editora Orion.

Chapter 3: The Spiritist View of Mental Disorders

Almeida, A.A.S. and Moreira-Almeida, A. (2009) "Inácio Ferreira: institutionalizing the integration of medicine and paranormal phenomena." *Journal of the Society for Psychical Research 73*, 4, 223–230.

Almeida, A.M. de and Lotufo Neto, F. (2004) "A mediunidade vista por alguns pioneiros da área mental." *Revista de Psiquiatria Clínica 31*, 3, 132–141.

Ellenberger, H. (1970) *The Discovery of the Unconscious.* New York: Basic Books.

Franco, D. (1993) *O Ser Consciente.* Salvador: Livraria Espírita Alvorada.

Franco, D. (1995) *Autodescobrimento: uma Busca Interior.* Salvador: Livraria Espírita Alvorada.

Franco, D. (1997) *Vida: Desafios e Soluções.* Salvador: Livraria Espírita Alvorada.

Franco, D. (1999) *Dias Gloriosos.* Salvador: Livraria Espírita Alvorada.

Franco, D. (2000a) *O Despertar do Espírito.* Salvador: Livraria Espírita Alvorada.

Franco, D. (2000b) *Desperte e Seja Feliz.* Salvador: Livraria Espírita Alvorada.

Franco, D. (2002) *Elucidações Psicológicas à Luz do Espiritismo.* Salvador: Livraria Espírita Alvorada.

Haraldsson, E. (2003) "Children who speak of past-life experiences: is there a psychological explanation?" *Psychology and Psychotherapy 76*, 1, 55–67.

Hess, D. (1991) *Spirits and Scientists: Ideology, Spiritism and Brazilian Culture.* Philadelphia: Pennsylvania State University Press.

Janet, P. (1889) *L'Automatisme Psychologique.* Paris: Félix Alcan.

Jones, S.R. and Fernyhough, C. (2007) "A new look at the neural diathesis–stress model of schizophrenia: the primacy of social-evaluative and uncontrollable situations." *Schizophrenia Bulletin 33*, 5, 1171–1177.

Kardec, A. (1858) "Introdução." *Revista Espírita 1*, 1, 1–6.

Kardec, A. (1861a) "Ensaio sobre a teoria da alucinação." *Revista Espírita 4*, 7, 208–215.

Kardec, A. (1861b) "Fenômenos psico fisiológicos: das pessoas que falam de si mesmas na terceira pessoa." *Revista Espírita 4*, 8, 239–243.

Kardec, A. (1862a) "Estatística de suicídios." *Revista Espírita 5*, 7, 196–202.

Kardec, A. (1862b) "Epidemia demoníaca na sabóia." *Revista Espírita 5*, 4, 107–111.

Kardec, A. (1863) "Estudo sobre os possessos de morzine." *Revista Espírita 6*, 2, 33–40.

Kardec, A. (1864) "Cura de uma obsessão." *Revista Espírita 7*, 2, 45–46.

Kardec, A. (1865a) "Nova cura de uma jovem obsedada de marmande." *Revista Espírita 8*, 1, 4–19.

Kardec, A. (1865b) "O fumo e a loucura." *Revista Espírita 8*, 5, 142–144.

Kardec, A. (1866) "Monomania incendiária precoce." *Revista Espírita 9*, 6, 171–177.

Kardec, A. (1868) *La Genese, les Miracles et les Predictions Selon le Spiritisme.* Paris: Union Spirite Française et Francophone.

Kardec, A. (1869) "A carne é fraca—estudo fisiológico e moral." *Revista Espírita 12*, 3, 63–67.

Kardec, A. (1986) *The Mediums' Book*, transl. A. Blackwell. Rio de Janeiro: FEB. (Original work published 1861.)

Kardec, A. (1996) *The Spirits' Book*, transl. A. Blackwell. Rio de Janeiro: FEB. Word file version. (Original work published 1860.)

Kardec, A. (1999) *What is Spiritism?* Philadelphia: Allan Kardec Educational Society. (Original work published 1859.)

Koenig, H., Larson, D., and Larson, S.S. (2001) "Religion and coping with serious medical illness." *Annals of Pharmacotherapy 35*, 352–359.

Koss-Chioino, J.D. (2003) "Jung, spirits and madness: lessons for cultural psychiatry." *Transcultural Psychiatry 40*, 164–180.

Moreira-Almeida, A. (2008) "Allan Kardec and the development of a research program in psychic experiences." *Parapsychological Association and The Society for Psychical Research Convention Proceedings of Presented Papers 51*, 327–332.

Moreira-Almeida, A. and Lotufo Neto, F. (2005) "Spiritist views of mental disorders in Brazil." *Transcultural Psychiatry 42*, 4, 570–595.

Stevenson, I. (1977) "The explanatory value of the idea of reincarnation." *Journal of Nervous and Mental Disease 164*, 305–326.

Stevenson, I. (1983) "Do we need a new word to supplement 'hallucination'?" *American Journal of Psychiatry 140*, 1609–1611.

Tucker, J.B. (2008) "Children's reports of past-life memories: a review." *Explore 4*, 4, 244–248.

Chapter 4: The Relationship of Mediumship to Mental Disorder

Almeida, A.M., Neto, L.F., and Cardeña, E. (2008) "Comparison of Brazilian Spiritist mediumship and dissociative identity disorder." *Journal of Nervous and Mental Disease 196*, 5, 420–424.

Andrade, H.G. (1983) *Poltergeist: algumas de suas ocorrencias no Brasil.* São Paulo: Editora Pensamento.

Aspect, A. (2007) "To be or not to be local." *Nature 446*, 866–867.

Benson, H. and Stark, M. (1996) *Timeless Healing: The Power and Biology of Belief.* New York: Simon and Schuster.

Capra, F. (1982) *The Turning Point.* New York: Bantam.

Ferreira, I. (1993) *Novos rumos à medicina.* São Paulo: FEESP. (Original work published 1945.)

Grey, M. (1985) *Return from Death: An Exploration of the Near-Death Experience.* London: Arkana.

Greyson, B. and Flynn, C.P. (1984) *The Near-Death Experience: Problems, Prospects, Perspectives.* Springfield, IL: Charles C. Thomas.

Goswami, A. (1995) *The Self-Aware Universe.* New York: Tarcher.

Goswami, A. (2001) *Physics of the Soul.* Charlottesville, VA: Hampton Roads Publishing.

Goswami, A. (2004) *The Quantum Doctor.* Charlottesville, VA: Hampton Roads Publishing.

Igreja, V., Dias-Lambranca, B., Hershey, D.A., Richters, L.R.A., and Reis, R. (2010) "The epidemiology of spirit possession in the aftermath of mass political violence in Mozambique." *Social Science and Medicine 71*, 3, 592–599.

Kardec, A. (2003) *The Mediums' Book.* Brasilia: FEB.

Koenig, H.G. (2005) *Spirituality in Patient Care: Why, How, When and What.* Philadelphia: Templeton Foundation Press.

Koenig, H.G., McCullough, M.E., and Larson, D.B. (2001) *Handbook of Religion and Health.* New York: Oxford University Press.

Kübler-Ross, E. (1996) *A morte: um amanhecer.* São Paulo: Pensamento.

Larson, D.B., Swyers, J.P., and McCullough, M.E. (1998) *Scientific Research on Spirituality and Health: A Consensus Report.* Rockville, MD: National Institute for Health Research.

Miller, W. (1999) *Integrating Spirituality into Treatment.* Washington, DC: American Psychological Association.

Moody, Jr., R. (1977) *Life after Life.* New York: Bantam Books.

Morse, M. (1990) *Closer to the Light.* New York: Villard.

Nobre, M. (1997) *Obsessão e suas máscaras.* São Paulo: FE.

Nobre, M. (2006) *A alma da matéria [The Soul of Matter].* São Paulo: FE.

Nobre, M. (2007) *O dom da mediunidade.* São Paulo: FE.

Parnia, S.W. and Fenwick, P. (2001) "A qualitative and quantitative study of the incidence, features and aetiology of near death experiences in cardiac arrest survivors." *Resuscitation 48,* 149–156.

Puchalski, C.M. and Romer, A.L. (2000) "Taking a spiritual history allows clinicians to understand patients more fully." *Journal of Palliative Medicine 3,* 129–137.

Ring, K. (1984) *Heading toward Omega.* New York: Quill.

Sabom, M. (1982) *Recollections of Death: A Medical Investigation.* New York: Harper and Row.

van Lommel, P., van Wees, R., Meyers, V., and Elfferich, I. (2001) "Near-death experience in survivors of cardiac arrest: a prospective study in the Netherlands." *Lancet 358,* 9298, 2039–2045.

Venkataramaiah, V., Mallikarjunaiah, M., Chandrasekhar, C.R., Vasudeva Rao, C.K., and Reddy, Narayana C.N. (1981) "Possession syndrome—an epidemiological study in West Karnataka." *Indian Journal of Psychiatry 23,* 3, 213–218.

Xavier, F. (1943) *Obreiros da vida eterna.* Rio de Janeiro: FEB.

Xavier, F. (1947) *No mundo maior.* Rio de Janeiro: FEB.

Xavier, F. (1969) *Estante da vida.* Rio de Janeiro: FEB.

Xavier, F. (1986) *Mediunidade e sintonia.* São Paulo: CEU.

Xavier, F. (2005) *In the Domain of Mediumship.* Brasilia: IEC.

Xavier, F. (2009) *Missionários da luz / Missionaries of Light.* Brasilia: IEC.

Xavier, F. and Vieira, W. (1958) *Evolução em dois mundos.* Rio de Janeiro: FEB.

Chapter 5: Case Studies of Those with Serious Diagnoses

Bragdon, E. (1990) *The Call of Spiritual Emergency: From Personal Crisis to Personal Transformation.* San Francisco: HarperSanFrancisco.

Bragdon, E. (2004) *Kardec's Spiritism: A Home for Healing and Spiritual Evolution.* Woodstock, VT: Lightening Up Press.

Bragdon, E. (2006) *A Sourcebook for Helping People with Spiritual Problems.* Woodstock, VT: Lightening Up Press. (Original work published as *A Sourcebook for Helping People in Spiritual Emergency,* 1988.)

Bragdon, E. (2011) *Resources for Extraordinary Healing.* Woodstock, VT: Lightening Up Press.

Kardec, A. (1986) *The Mediums' Book.* Rio de Janeiro: FEB. (Original work published 1861.)

Kardec, A. (1996) *The Spirits' Book.* Rio de Janeiro: FEB. (Original work published 1860.)

Kardec, A. (2004) *Spiritism in Its Simplest Expression.* Philadelphia: AKES.

Robinson, J.M. (ed.) (1977) *The Nag Hammadi Library.* New York: Brill.

Chapter 6: Three Spiritist Psychiatric Hospitals
Editor's Note

Azevedo, J.L. (1997) *Spirit and Matter: New Horizons for Medicine.* Los Angeles, CA: New Falcon Publications.

Bragdon, E. (2011) *Resources for Extraordinary Healing.* Woodstock, VT: Lightening Up Press.

Chapter 6C: João Evangelista Hospital

Almeida, A.A.S. (2007) "Uma fábrica de loucos: Psiquiatria e Espiritismo no Brasil (1900 a 1950)." Tese de Doutorado apresentado ao Departamento de História do Instituto de Filosofia e Ciências Humanas da Universidade Estadual de Campinas.

Bragdon, E. (2005) "Spiritist healing centers in Brazil." *Seminars in Integrative Medicine* 3, 2, 67–74.

Braghetta, C.C., Leao, F.C., Vallada, H., and Cordeiro, Q. (2010a) "Perfil da religiosidade e espiritualidade em pacientes com transtornos mentais graves internados em hospital psiquiátrico na cidade de São Paulo." In *XXVIII Congresso Brasileiro de Psiquiatria.* Fortaleza: Anais do Congresso.

Braghetta, C.C., Leao, F.C., Vallada, H., and Cordeiro, Q. (2010b) "Aspectos éticos e legais da assistência religiosa em hospital para tratamento de pacientes com transtornos mentais graves." In *XXVIII Congresso Brasileiro de Psiquiatria.* Fortaleza: Anais do Congresso.

Campetti, G. (2010) *Espiritismo de A a Z,* 4th edn. Brasilia: Federação Espírita Brasileira.

Kardec, A. (1987) *The Gospel According to Spiritism.* London: The Headquarters Publishing Co. (Original work published 1864.)

Kardec, A. (2005a) *O Livro dos Espíritos: Princípios da Doutrina Espírita,* 86th edn. Rio de Janeiro: FEB.

Kardec, A. (2005b) *O que é o Espiritismo: Noções Elementares do Mundo Invisível, pelas Manifestações dos Espíritos,* 52nd edn. Rio de Janeiro: FEB.

Leão, F.C. (2004) "Uso de práticas espirituais em instituição para portadores de transtornos mentais." Master's dissertation presented to Departamento de Psiquiatria da FMUSP.

Lucchetti, G., de Almeida, L.G.C., and Granero, A.L. (2010a) "Espiritualidade no paciente em diálise: o nefrologista deve abordar?" *Jornal Brasileiro de Nefrologia 32,* 128–132.

Lucchetti, G., Granero, A.L., Bassi, R.M., Lattaca, R., *et al.* (2010b) "Espiritualidade na prática clínica: o que o clínico deve saber?" *Revista da Sociedade Brasileira de Clínica Médica 8,* 154–158.

Lucchetti, G., Lucchetti, A.L.G., and Koenig, H.G. (2010c) *Impact of Spirituality/Religiosity on Mortality: Comparison with Other Health Interventions.* New York: Explore.

Moreira-Almeida, A. (2007) "Espiritualidade e saúde: passado e futuro de uma relação controversa e desafiadora." *Revista de Psiquiatria Clínica 34,* suppl. 1, 3–4.

Moreira-Almeida, A., de Almeida, A.A.S., and Lotufo Neto, F. (2005) "History of spiritist madness in Brazil." *History of Psychiatry 16,* 1, 5–25.

Moreira-Almeida, A., Lotufo Neto, F., and Koenig, H.G. (2006) "Religiousness and mental health: a review." *Revista Brasileira de Psiquiatria (São Paulo) 28,* 3, 242–250.

Moreira-Almeida, A., Pinsky, I., Zaleski, M., and Laranjeira, R. (2010) "Envolvimento religioso e fatores sociodemográficos: resultados de um levantamento nacional no Brasil." *Revista de Psiquiatria Clínica 37,* 12–15.

Puttini, R.F. (2004) "Medicina e Religião no espaço hospitalar." Doctoral thesis em Saúde Coletiva, Faculdade de Ciências Médicas da Unicamp.

Editor's Note for Chapters 7–12

Moore, T. (2010) *Writing in the Sand: Jesus, Spirituality and the Soul of the Gospels.* Carlsbad, CA: Hay House.

Chapter 7: Magnetic Healing, Prayer, and Energy Passes

Filho, R. and Curi, K. (1995) "Benoit Mure." In S. Hahnemann, *Organon da Arte de Curar.* São Paulo: GEHSP.

Hahnemann, S. (1995) *The Organon of the Healing Art.* Bethesda, MD: Classics of Medicine Library.

Kardec, A. (1996) *A Gênese.* Rio de Janeiro: FEB.

Kardec, A. (2006) *Livro dos Espíritos.* Rio de Janeiro: FEB.

Michaelus (1983) *Magnetismo Espiritual.* Rio de Janeiro: FEB.

Xavier, F. (1982) *No Mundo Maior.* Rio de Janeiro: FEB.

Xavier, F. (1984) *Mecanismos da Mediunidade.* Rio de Janeiro: FEB.

Xavier, F. (1995) *Missionários da Luz.* Rio de Janeiro: FEB.

Xavier, F. (1998a) *Evolução em Dois Mundos*, 16th edn. Rio de Janeiro: FEB.

Xavier, F. (1998b) "Passe magnético." In *Evolução em Dois Mundos*, 16th edn. Rio de Janeiro: FEB.

Chapter 8: Psychotherapy and Reincarnation

Andrade, H.G. (1990) *Reencarnação no Brasil: Oito Casos que Sugerem Renascimento*. Matao: Casa Editora O Clarim.

Athappilly, G.K., Greyson, B., and Stevenson, I. (2006) "Do prevailing societal models influence reports of near-death experiences? A comparison of accounts reported before and after 1975." *Journal of Nervous and Mental Disease 194*, 3, 218–222.

Azari, N.P., Nickel, J., Wunderlich, G., Niedeggen, M., *et al.* (2001) "Neural correlates of religious experience." *European Journal of Neuroscience 13*, 8, 1649–1652.

Beauregard, M. (2007) "Mind does really matter: evidence from neuroimaging studies of emotional self-regulation, psychotherapy, and placebo effect." *Progress in Neurobiology 81*, 4, 218–236.

Beauregard, M. and Paquette, V. (2006) "Neural correlates of a mystical experience in Carmelite nuns." *Neuroscience Letters 405*, 3, 186–190.

Bergner, R.M. (2005) "World reconstruction in psychotherapy." *American Journal of Psychotherapy 59*, 4, 333–349.

Bohart, A.C. (2000) "The client is the most important common factor: clients' self-healing capacities and psychotherapy." *Journal of Psychotherapy Integration 10*, 2, 127–149.

Brune, M., Haasen, C., Krausz, M., Yagdiran, O., Bustos, E., and Eisenman, D. (2002) "Belief systems as coping factors for traumatized refugees: a pilot study." *European Psychiatry 17*, 8, 451–458.

Cadoret, R.J. (2005) "Book review: 'European Cases of the Reincarnation Type,' by Ian Stevenson, M.D." *American Journal of Psychiatry 162*, 4, 823–824.

Creamer, M., McFarlane, A.C., and Burgess, P. (2005) "Psychopathology following trauma: the role of subjective experience." *Journal of Affective Disorders 86*, 175–182.

Data Folha (2007) "97% dizem acreditar totalmente na existência de deus; 75% acreditam no diabo." Available at http://datafolha.folha.uol.com.br/po/ver_po.php?session=446, accessed on March 21, 2011.

Davidson, J.R., Connor, K.M., and Lee, L.C. (2005) "Beliefs in karma and reincarnation among survivors of violent trauma—a community survey." *Social Psychiatry and Psychiatric Epidemiology 40*, 2, 120–125.

Gallup (2003) *The Gallup Poll: Public Opinion 2003*. Wilmington, DE: Scholarly Resources.

Greyson, B. (2000) "Dissociation in people who have near-death experiences: out of their bodies or out of their minds?" *Lancet 5*, 355, 9202, 460–463.

Greyson, B. (2007) "Consistency of near-death experience accounts over two decades: are reports embellished over time?" *Resuscitation 73*, 3, 407–411.

Haraldsson, E. (1991) "Children claiming past-life memories: Four cases in Sri Lanka." *Journal of Scientific Exploration 5*, 2, 233–261.

Haraldsson, E. (2003) "Children who speak of past-life experiences: is there a psychological explanation?" *Psychology and Psychotherapy: Theory, Research and Practice 76*, 1, 55–67.

Haraldsson, E. (2006) "Popular psychology, belief in life after death and reincarnation in the Nordic countries, Western and Eastern Europe." *Nordic Psychology 58*, 2, 171–180.

Haraldsson, E. and Stevenson, I. (1975) "A communicator of the 'drop-in' type in Iceland: the case of Runolfur Runolfsson." *Journal of the American Society for Psychical Research 69*, 33–59.

Haraldsson, E., Fowler, P., and Periyannanpillai, V. (2000) "Psychological characteristics of children who speak of a previous life: a further field study in Sri Lanka." *Transcultural Psychiatry 37*, 525–544.

Inglehart, R., Basanez, M., Diez-Medrano, J., Halman, L., and Luijkx, R. (2004) *Human Beliefs and Values: A Cross-Cultural Sourcebook Based on the 1999–2002 Values Survey*. Mexico: Siglo XXI Editores.

Inglehart, R., Basanez, M., and Morendo, A. (1998) *Human Values and Beliefs: A Cross-Cultural Sourcebook*. Ann Arbor, MI: University of Michigan Press.

Karasu, T.B. (1986) "The specificity versus non-specificity dilemma: toward therapeutic indentifying change agents." *American Journal of Psychiatry 143*, 687–695.

Karasu, T.B. (1999) "Spiritual psychotherapy." *American Journal of Psychotherapy 53*, 2, 143–162.

Keil, H.J. and Tucker, J.B. (2000) "An unusual birthmark case thought to be linked to a person who had previously died." *Psychological Reports 87*, 1067–1074.

Keil, H.J. and Tucker, J.B. (2005) "Children who claim to remember previous lives: cases with written records made before the previous personality was identified." *Journal of Scientific Exploration 19*, 1, 91–101.

Kelly, E.F., Kelly, E.W., Crabtree, A., Gauld, A., Grosso, M., and Greyson, B. (2007) *Irreducible Mind: Toward a Psychology for the 21st Century.* Lanham, MD: Rowman & Littlefield.

Kuhn, T. (1962) *The Structure of Scientific Revolutions.* Chicago: University of Chicago Press.

Lee, R.V. (2000) "Doctoring to the music of time." *Annals of Internal Medicine 132*, 1, 11–17.

Masten, A.S. and Coatsworth, J.D. (1998) "The development of competence in favorable and unfavorable environments: lessons from research on successful children." *American Psychology 53*, 2, 205–220.

Mills, A., Haraldsson, E., and Keil, H.H.J. (1994) "Replication studies of cases suggestive of reincarnation by three independent investigators." *Journal of the American Society for Psychical Research 88*, 3, 207–219.

Moreira-Almeida, A. and Koenig, H.G. (2007) "Book review of *Irreducible Mind.*" *Journal of Mental and Nervous Disease. 196*, 4, 345–346.

Morse, M.L. and Neppe, V. (1991) "Near-death experiences." *Lancet 6*, 337, 8745, 858.

Newberg, A., Pourdehnad, M., Alavi, A., and d'Aquili, E.G. (2003) "Cerebral blood flow during meditative prayer: preliminary findings and methodological issues." *Perceptual and Motor Skills 97*, 2, 625–630.

Parnia, S. (2007) "Do reports of consciousness during cardiac arrest hold the key to discovering the nature of consciousness?" *Medical Hypotheses 69*, 933–937.

Pasricha, S.K., Keil, J., Tucker, J.B., and Stevenson, I. (2005) "Some bodily malformations attributed to previous lives." *Journal of Scientific Exploration 19*, 3, 359–383.

Penfield, W. (1978) *The Mystery of Mind—A Critical Study of Consciousness and the Human Brain.* Princeton, NJ: Princeton University Press.

Peres, J.F.P., Mercante, J.P., and Nasello, A.G. (2005) "Psychological dynamics affecting traumatic memories: implications in psychotherapy." *Psychology and Psychotherapy: Theory, Research and Practice 78*, 4, 431–447.

Peres, J.F.P., Moreira-Almeida, A., Nasello, A.G., and Koenig, H.G. (2007a) "Spirituality and resilience in trauma victims." *Journal of Religion and Health 46*, 343–350.

Peres, J.F.P., Newberg, A.B., Mercante, J.P., Simão, M., and Albuquerque, V.E. (2007b) "Cerebral blood flow changes during retrieval of traumatic memories before and after psychotherapy: a SPECT study." *Psychological Medicine 37*, 10, 1481–1491.

Peres, J.F.P., Simão, M., Nasello, A.G. (2007c) "Spirituality, religiousness and psychotherapy." *Revista de Psiquiatria Clinica 34*, 1, 136–145.

Prochaska, J.O., DiClemente, C.C., and Norcross, J.C. (1992) "In search of how people change: applications to addictive behaviors." *American Psychology 47*, 9, 1102–1114.

Ramachandran, V.S. and Gregory, R.L. (1991) "Perceptual filling in of artificially induced scotomas in human vision." *Nature 350*, 699–702.

Rivas, T. (2003) "Three cases of the reincarnation type in the Netherlands." *Journal of Scientific Exploration 17*, 3, 527–532.

Sayed, M.A. (2003) "Psychotherapy of Arab patients in the West: uniqueness, empathy, and 'otherness.'" *American Journal of Psychotherapy 57*, 4, 445–459.

Severino, P.R. (1994) *Life's Triumph: Research on Messages Received by Chico Xavier.* São Paulo: Editora FE.

Shafranske, E.P. (1996) *Religion and the Clinical Practice of Psychology.* Washington, DC: American Psychological Association.

Shaw, A., Joseph, S., and Linley, P.A. (2005) "Religion, spirituality, and posttraumatic growth: a systematic review." *Mental Health, Religion and Culture 8*, 1, 1–11.

Stevenson, I. (1974a) *Twenty Cases Suggestive of Reincarnation*, 2nd rev. edn. Charlottesville, VA: University Press of Virginia. (1st edn published 1966.)

Stevenson, I. (1974b) *Xenoglossy: A Review and Report of a Case.* Charlottesville, VA: University Press of Virginia.

Stevenson, I. (1975) *Cases of the Reincarnation Type, Vol. 1: Ten Cases in India.* Charlottesville, VA: University Press of Virginia.

Stevenson, I. (1977a) *Cases of the Reincarnation Type, Vol. 2: Ten Cases in Sri Lanka.* Charlottesville, VA: University Press of Virginia.

Stevenson, I. (1977b) "The Southeast Asian interpretation of gender dysphoria: an illustrative case report." *Journal of Nervous and Mental Disease 165*, 201–208.

Stevenson, I. (1977c) "Research into the evidence of man's survival after death: a historical and critical survey with a summary of recent developments." *Journal of Nervous and Mental Disease 165*, 152–170.

Stevenson, I. (1980) *Cases of the Reincarnation Type, Vol. 3: Twelve Cases in Lebanon and Turkey.* Charlottesville, VA: University Press of Virginia.

Stevenson, I. (1983a) *Cases of the Reincarnation Type, Vol. 4: Twelve Cases in Thailand and Burma.* Charlottesville, VA: University Press of Virginia.

Stevenson, I. (1983b) "American children who claim to remember previous lives." *Journal of Nervous and Mental Disease 171*, 742–748.

Stevenson, I. (1984) *Unlearned Language: New Studies in Xenoglossy.* Charlottesville, VA: University Press of Virginia.

Stevenson, I. (1986) "Characteristics of cases of the reincarnation type among the Igbo of Nigeria." *Journal of Asian and African Studies 21*, 204–216.

Stevenson, I. (1987) *Children Who Remember Previous Lives: A Question of Reincarnation.* Charlottesville, VA: University Press of Virginia.

Stevenson, I. (1993) "Birthmarks and birth defects corresponding to wounds on deceased persons." *Journal of Scientific Exploration 7*, 403–410.

Stevenson, I. (1997a) *Reincarnation and Biology: A Contribution to the Etiology of Birthmarks and Birth Defects.* Santa Barbara, CA: Praeger Scientific Publishers.

Stevenson, I. (1997b) *Where Reincarnation and Biology Intersect.* Santa Barbara, CA: Praeger Scientific Publishers.

Stevenson, I. (2000a) "The phenomenon of claimed memories of previous lives: possible interpretations and evidence." *Medical Hypotheses 54*, 4, 652–659.

Stevenson, I. (2000b) "Unusual play in young children who claim to remember previous lives." *Journal of Scientific Exploration 14*, 557–570.

Stevenson, I. (2003) *European Cases of the Reincarnation Type.* Jefferson, NC: McFarland.

Stevenson, I. and Greyson, B. (1979) "Near-death experiences: relevance to the question of survival after death." *Journal of the American Medical Association 20*, 242, 265–267.

Stevenson, I. and Samararatne, G. (1988) "Three new cases of the reincarnation type in Sri Lanka with written records made before verification." *Journal of Nervous and Mental Disease 176*, 12, 741.

Thompson, R.E. (2003) "The legacy of Ladan and Laleh." *Physician Executive 29*, 5, 52–54.

Tucker, J.B. (2005) *Life before Life: A Scientific Investigation of Children's Memories of Previous Lives.* New York: St. Martin's Press.

van Lommel, P., van Wees, R., Meyers, V., and Elfferich, I. (2001) "Near-death experience in survivors of cardiac arrest: a prospective study in the Netherlands." *Lancet 358*, 9298, 2039–2045.

Varma, V.K. (1988) "Culture, personality and psychotherapy." *International Journal of Social Psychiatry 34*, 2, 142–149.

Wallis, C. (1996) "The most intimate bond." *Time*, March 25, 60–64.

Wambach, H. (1978) *Reliving Past Lives—The Evidence Under Hypnosis.* New York: Bantam.

World Values Survey (www.worldvaluessurvey.org)

Yarrow, K., Haggard, P., and Heal, R. (2001) "Illusory perceptions of space and time preserve cross-saccadic perceptual continuity." *Nature 414*, 302–305.

Chapter 9: The Group Field

Benson, H. (1996) *Timeless Healing: The Power and Biology of Belief.* New York: Simon and Schuster.

Bragdon, E. (2006) *I Do Not Heal, God Is the One Who Heals.* Woodstock, VT: Spiritual Alliances.

Hochstätter, Z. and Coté, S. (2005) *Think About It.* Think About It Productions. Available at www.healingbioenergy.com/flashtest.htm, accessed March 21, 2011.

Zeig, S. (2008) *Soul Masters: Dr. Guo and Dr. Sha.* Ontario: 926363 Ontario Limited.

Chapter 10: Spiritual Counseling and Fellowship in Spiritist Centers

Azevedo, J.L. (1997) *Spirit and Matter: New Horizons for Medicine.* Las Vegas, NV: New Falcon Publications.

Bragdon, E. (2008) *Spiritism: Bridging Spirituality and Health.* Woodstock, VT: Old Dog Documentaries and Spiritual Alliances.

Franco, D. (1974) *Obsession.* Salvador, Brazil: Livraria Espirita Alvorada Editora.

Kardec, A. (1986) *The Mediums' Book.* Rio de Janeiro: FEB. (Original work published 1861.)

Kardec, A. (1996) *The Spirits' Book,* 2nd edn. Rio de Janeiro: FEB. (Original work published 1860.)

Kardec, A. (2004) *The Gospel According to Spiritism.* São Paulo: ISC. (Original work published 1866.)

Payas, M. and Romaquera, O. (eds) (2003) *The Gospel at Home.* Philadelphia: AKES.

Spiegel, D., Bloom, J., Kraemer, H., and Gottheil, E. (1989) "Effect of psychosocial treatment on survival of patients with metastatic breast cancer." *Lancet 2,* 888–891.

Spira, J.L. and Reed, G.M. (2002) *Group Psychotherapy for Women with Breast Cancer.* Washington, DC: American Psychological Association.

Xavier, C. and Vieira, W. (1981) *Leis de Amor.* São Paulo: FEESP.

Chapter 11: Jung, Spirits, and Madness

Boyers, R. and Orrill, R. (eds) (1971) *R.D. Laing and Anti-Psychiatry.* New York: Harper and Row.

Broch, H.B. (2001) "The villagers' reactions towards craziness: an Indonesian example." *Transcultural Psychiatry 35,* 3, 275–305.

Csordas, T. and Lewton, E. (1998) "Practice, performance and experience in ritual healing." *Transcultural Psychiatry 35,* 4, 435–512.

Ellenberger, H. (1970) *The Discovery of the Unconscious.* London: Penguin Books.

Guarnaccia, P.J., Parra, P., Deschamps, A., Milstein, G., and Argiles, N. (1992) "Si dios quiere: Hispanic families' experiences of caring for a seriously mentally ill family member." *Culture, Medicine, and Psychiatry 16,* 2, 187–215.

Hillman, J. (1977) "Some early background to Jung's ideas: notes on C.G. Jung's medium by Stephanie Zumstien-Preiswork." *Spring 18,* 136.

Hollan, D. (2000) "Culture and dissociation in Toraja." *Transcultural Psychiatry 37,* 4, 545–559.

Homans, P. (1979) *Jung in Context: Modernity and the Making of a Psychology.* Chicago: University of Chicago Press.

Jung, C.G. (1960a) *The Collected Works, Vol. 3: The Psychogenesis of Mental Disease.* New York: Bollingen Foundation.

Jung, C.G. (1960b) *The Collected Works, Vol. 8: The Structure and Dynamics of the Psyche.* New York: Bollingen Foundation.

Jung, C.G. (1965) *Memories, Dreams, Reflections.* London: Random House.

Kardec, A. (1986) *The Spirits' Book,* trans. Anna Blackwell. Rio de Janeiro: FEB. (Original work published 1860.)

Koss, J.D. (1976) "Religion and science divinely related: a case history of spiritism in Puerto Rico." *Caribbean Studies 16,* 22–43.

Koss, J.D. (1980) "The therapist–spiritist training project in Puerto Rico: an experiment to relate the traditional healing system to the public health system." *Social Science and Medicine 14,* B, 255–266.

Koss, J.D. (1986) "Symbolic transformations in traditional healing rituals: perspectives from analytical psychology." *Journal of Analytical Psychology 32,* 341–355.

Koss-Chioino, J. (1992) *Women as Healers, Women as Patients: Mental Health Care and Traditional Healing in Puerto Rico.* Boulder, CO: Westview Press.

Lévy-Bruhl, L. (1926) *How Natives Think.* London: Allen & Unwin. (Original work published 1912.)

Nietzsche, F. (1961) *Thus Spoke Zarathustra,* trans. R.J. Hollingdale. Harmondsworth: Penguin Books.

Rogler, L.H. and Hollingshead, A.B. (1965) *Trapped: Families and Schizophrenia.* New York: John Wiley and Sons.

Samuels, A. (1985) *Jung and the Post-Jungians.* London: Routledge and Kegan Paul.

Chapter 12: The Practice of Integrating Spirituality into Psychotherapy

Capra, F. (1984) *The Turning Point: Science, Society, and the Rising Culture.* New York: Bantam.

Capra, F. (2010) *The Tao of Physics.* Boston: Shambhala.

Freud, S. (1972) *Obras completas.* Rio de Janeiro: Imago.

Goswami, A. (2005) *A física da alma.* São Paulo: Aleph.

Grof, S. (2007) *Quando o impossível acontece.* São Paulo: Heresis.

Grof, S. and Grof, C. (1994) *A tempestuosa busca do ser.* São Paulo: Cultrix.

Grof, S. and Grof, C. (1995) *Emergência espiritual.* São Paulo: Cultrix.

Guitton, J., Bogdanov, G., and Bogdanov, I. (1992) *Deus e a ciência.* Rio de Janeiro: Nova Fronteira.

Kardec, A. (1968) *Obras básicas.* São Paulo: Edicel.

Koenig, H. (2005) *Espiritualidade no cuidado com o paciente.* São Paulo: Fé Editora.

Lacan, J. (1988) *O seminário, livro 3, As psicoses.* Rio de Janeiro: Jorge Zahar Editor.

Lazlo, E. (2008) *A ciência e o campo akáshico.* São Paulo: Cultrix.

Moreno, J.L. (1946) *Psychodrama,* vol. 1. New York: Beacon House.

Moutinho, M. and Melo, K.R. (2010) *Lapso de tempo.* Blumenau: Odorizzi.

Nicolescu, B. (1999) *O manifesto da transdisciplinaridade.* São Paulo: Trion.

Wallace, A. (2009) *Dimensões escondidas.* São Paulo: Peirópolis.

Wilber, K. (ed.) (1991) *O paradigma holográfico e outros paradoxos—uma investigação nas fronteiras da ciência.* São Paulo: Cultrix.

Woolger, R. (2007) *As várias vidas da alma.* São Paulo: Cultrix.

Chapter 13: When Medical Doctors Are Mediums

Bergson, H. (1984) *Correspondências, obras e outros escritos.* São Paulo: Abril Cultural.

Jung, C.G. (1991) *Tipos psicológicos.* Rio de Janeiro: Editora Vozes.

Kardec, A. (1998) *O Livro dos médiuns,* 63rd edn. Rio de Janeiro: FEB. (Original work published 1861.)

von Franz, M.L. and Hillman, J.A. (1990) *Tipologia de Jung.* São Paulo: Editora Cultrix.

Chapter 14: A Science of Understanding the Mind

Feynman, R.P. (1965) *The Character of Physical Law.* Cambridge: MIT Press.

James, W. (1912) "Radical Empiricism." In *The Will to Believe and Other Essays in Popular Philosophy.* New York: Henry Holt and Co.

James, W. (1950) *The Principles of Psychology.* New York: Dover Publications.

Treisman, A. (2009) Comments made at a Mind and Life Institute meeting with HH the Dalai Lama at the Dalai Lama's residence in Dharamsala, India, April. Conference co-organized by Alan Wallace and David Meyer.

Chapter 15: Spirit Attachment and Health

Allen, S. (2007) *Spirit Release: A Practical Handbook.* Alresford, Hampshire: O-Books.

Baldwin, W.J. (1992) *Spirit Releasement Therapy—A Technique Manual.* Falls Church, VA: Human Potential Foundation Press.

Barlow, D., Abel, G., and Blanchard, E. (1977) "Gender identity change in a transsexual: an exorcism." *Archives of Sexual Behavior 6,* 387–395.

Fiore, E. (1987) *The Unquiet Dead.* New York: Ballantine Books.

Fiore, E. (2011) "The treatment of gender dysphoria: sex change or spirit change?" Available at www.spiritrelease.com/cases/Fiore_gender.htm, accessed on 7 June 2011.

Ireland-Frey, L. (1999) *Freeing the Captives.* Newburyport, MA: Hampton Roads.

Kardec, A. (2003) *The Spirits' Book.* São Paulo: Allan Kardec Editoria. (Original work published 1860.)

Lawton, I. (2008) *The Big Book of the Soul.* Southend-on-Sea: Rational Spirituality Press.

Matthews, C. (2005) *The Psychic Protection Handbook.* London: Piatkus.

Modi, S. (1997) *Remarkable Healings.* Newburyport, MA: Hampton Roads.

Page, K. (1999) *The Heart of Soul Healing.* Cleveland, GA: Clear Light Arts.

Petrak, J. (1996) *Angels, Guides and Other Spirits.* Lenoir City, TN: Curry-Peterson.

Sagan, S. (1997) *Entity Possession.* Rochester, VT: Destiny Books.

Stevenson, I. (1984) *Unlearned Language: New Studies in Xenoglossy.* Charlottesville, VT: University Press of Virginia.

Sylvia, C., with Novak, W. (1997) *A Change of Heart.* London: Little, Brown.

Van Dusen, W. (1972) *The Natural Depth in Man.* New York: Harper and Row.

Wickland, C.A. (1974) *Thirty Years Among the Dead.* Hollywood, CA: Newcastle Publishing.

Chapter 17: Current Research on Survival of Consciousness and Mediumship

Almeder, R. (1992) *Death and Personal Survival: The Evidence for Life after Death.* Boston: Rowman & Littlefield.

Beischel, J. (2007) "Contemporary methods used in laboratory-based mediumship research." *Journal of Parapsychology 71*, 37–68.

Beischel, J. and Rock, A.J. (2009) "Addressing the survival vs psi debate through process-focused mediumship research." *Journal of Parapsychology 73*, 71–90.

Braude, S.E. (2003) *Immortal Remains: The Evidence for Life after Death.* Lanham, MD: Rowman & Littlefield.

Cook, E.W. (1987) "The survival question: impasse or crux?" *Journal of the American Society for Psychical Research 81*, 2, 125–139.

Dodds, E.R. (1934) "Why I do not believe in survival." *Proceedings of the Society for Psychical Research 42*, 147–178.

Ducasse, C.J. (1969) "Paranormal phenomena, science and life after death." *Parapsychological Monographs no. 8.* New York: Parapsychology Foundation.

Eisenbeiss, W. and Hassler, D. (2006) "An assessment of ostensible communications with a deceased grandmaster as evidence for survival." *Journal of the Society for Psychical Research 70*, 2, 65–97.

Fontana, D. (2005) *Is There an Afterlife? A Comprehensive Overview of the Evidence.* Oakland, CA: O Books.

Gauld, A. (1961) "The 'super-ESP' hypothesis." *Proceedings of the Society for Psychical Research 53*, 226–246.

Gauld, A. (1982) *Mediumship and Survival: A Century of Investigations.* London: Heinemann.

Griffin, D.R. (1997) *Parapsychology, Philosophy and Spirituality.* Albany, NY: State University of New York Press.

Grosso, M. (1999) "Survival research: evidence, problems and paradigms." *Human Nature Magazine*, August, 11–25.

Hodgson, R.A. (1898) "A further record of observations of certain phenomena of trance." *Proceedings of the Society for Psychical Research 13*, 284–582.

James, W. (1956) *Will to Believe.* New York: Dover Publications. (Original work published 1896.)

James, W. (2009) *The Varieties of Religious Experience: A Study in Human Nature.* Des Moines, IA: Library of America. (Original work published in 1902.)

Kelly, E.F., Kelly, E.W., Crabtree, A., Gauld, A., Grosso, M., and Greyson, B. (2006) *Irreducible Mind: Toward a Psychology for the 21st Century.* Lanham, MD: Rowman and Littlefield.

Kelly, E.W. (2010) "Some directions for mediumship research." *Journal of Scientific Exploration 24*, 2, 247–282.

Lodge, O. (1935) "Foreword." In N. Walker, *Through a Stranger's Hands.* London: Hutchinson.

Myers, F.W.H. (1903) *Human Personality and Its Survival of Bodily Death.* London: Longmans Green.

Neppe, V.M. (2007) "A detailed analysis of an important chess game: revisiting Maroczy versus Korchnoi." *Journal of the Society for Psychical Research 71*, 3, 129–147.

O'Keeffe, C. and Wiseman, R. (2005) "Testing alleged mediumship: methods and results." *British Journal of Psychology 96*, 165–179.

Playfair, G.L. and Keen, M. (2004) "A possibly unique case of psychic detection." *Journal of the Society for Psychical Research 68*, 1, 1–17.

Rock, A.J., Beischel, J., and Cott, C.C. (2009) "Psi vs. survival: a qualitative investigation of medium's phenomenology comparing psychic readings and ostensible communication with the deceased." *Transpersonal Psychology Review 13*, 2, 76–89.

Roy, A.E. and Robertson, T.J. (2001) "A double-blind procedure for assessing the relevance of a medium's statements to a recipient." *Journal of the Society for Psychical Research 65*, 161–174.

Roy, A.E. and Robertson, T.J. (2004) "Results of the application of the Robertson–Roy protocol to a series of experiments with mediums and participants." *Journal of the Society for Psychical Research 68*, 18–34.

Schiebeler, W. (1988) *Der Tod, die Brücke zu neuem Leben. Die Silberschnur.* Melsbach, Germany: Neuwied.

Schwartz, G. and Russek, L. (2001) "Evidence of anomalous information retrieval between two mediums: telepathy, network memory resonance, and continuance of consciousness." *Journal of the Society for Psychical Research 65*, 257–275.

Schwartz, G., Russek, L., and Barentsen, C. (2002) "Accuracy and replicability of anomalous information retrieval: replication and extension." *Journal of the Society for Psychical Research 66*, 144–156.

Schwartz, G., Russek, L., Nelson, L.A., and Barentsen, C. (2001) "Accuracy and replicability of anomalous after-death communication across highly skilled mediums." *Journal of the Society for Psychical Research 65*, 1–25.

Schwartz, G., Russek, L.G., Watson, D., Campbell, L., *et al.* (1999) "Potential medium to departed to medium communication of pictorial information: exploratory evidence consistent with psi and survival of consciousness." *Noetic Journal 2*, 283–294.

Chapter 18: The Power of "Magnetized" Water

Ball, P. (2008) "Water as an active constituent in cell biology." *Chemical Reviews 2008 108*, 1, 74–108.

Batmanghelidj, F. (1995) *Your Body's Many Cries for Water.* Falls Church, VA: Global Health Solutions.

Bell, I., Lewis, D.A., and Brooks, A.J. (2003) "Ultramolecular doses of homeopathic medications under blinded controlled conditions." *Journal of Alternative and Complementary Medicine 9*, 25–37.

Chai, B., Yoo, H., and Pollack, G.H. (2009) "Effect of radiant energy on near-surface water." *Journal of Physical Chemistry B 113*, 13953–13958.

Davenas, E., Beauvais, F., Amara, J., Oberbaum, B., *et al.* (1988) "Human basophil degranulation triggered by very dilute antiserum against IgE." *Nature 333*, 816–818.

Del Giudice, E. and Preparata, G. (1998) "A New QED Picture of Water: Understanding a Few Fascinating Phenomena." In E. Sassoroli, Y. Srivastava, J. Swain, and A. Widom (eds) *Macroscopic Quantum Coherence.* Hackensack, NY: World Scientific Publishing Co.

Emoto, M. (2004) "Healing with water." *Journal of Alternative and Complementary Medicine 10*, 1, 19–21.

Endler, P.C. and Schulte, J. (1994) *Ultra High Dilution: Physiology and Physics.* Dordrecht: Kluwer Academic Publishers.

Huang, K.C., Yang, C.C., and Hsu, S.P. (2006) "Electrolyzed-reduced water reduced hemodialysis-induced erythrocyte impairment in end-stage renal disease patients." *Kidney International 70*, 391–398.

Kim, M.-J., Kyung, H.J., and Uhm, Y.K. (2007) "Preservative effect of electrolyzed reduced water on pancreatic beta-cell mass in diabetic db/db mice." *Biological & Pharmaceutical Bulletin 30*, 2, 234–236.

Korotkov, K.G. (2002) *Human Energy Field: Study with GDV Bioelectrography.* Fair Lawn, NJ: Backbone Publishing Co.

Montagnier, L. (2010) "DNA, waves, and water." Presentation at Water Conference, Mt Snow, VT, October 22, 2010.

Piccardi, G. (1962) *The Chemical Basis of Medical Climatology.* Springfield, IL: Thomas Press.

Popp, F.A., Warnke, U., Koenig, H.L., and Peschka, W. (1989) *Electromagnetic Bio-Information.* Baltimore, MD: Urban and Schwartzenberg.

Preparata, G. (1995) *QED Coherence in Matter.* Singapore: World Scientific Publishing.

Roy, R., Tiller, W.A., Bell, I., and Hoover, M.R. (2005) "The structure of liquid water; novel insights from materials research; potential relevance to homeopathy." *Material Research Innovations 9*, 4, 577–708.

Rubik, B. (1997) "The unifying concept of information in acupuncture and other energy medicine modalities." Proceedings of the 1996 Medical Acupuncture Research Foundation Symposium on the Physiology of Acupuncture. *Journal of Alternative and Complementary Medicine 3*, Suppl. 1, S-67–S-76.

Rubik, B. (2007) Unpublished data from the Institute for Frontier Science, Emeryville, California.

Rubik, B. (2010) "Studies and observations on frequency-treated water, electrolyzed water, and human blood." Presentation at Water Conference, Mt Snow, VT, October 24, 2010.

Rubik, B., Brooks, A., and Schwartz, G. (2006) "In vitro effect of reiki treatment on bacterial cultures: role of experimental context and practitioner wellbeing." *Journal of Alternative and Complementary Medicine 12*, 1, 7–13.

Savieto, R.M. and da Silva, M.J. (2004) "Efeitos do toque terapêutico na cicatrização de lesões da pele de cobaias [Therapeutic touch for the healing of skin injuries in guinea pigs]." *Revista Brasileira de Enfermagem 57*, 3, 340–343.

Schiff, M. (1995) *The Memory of Water: Homeopathy and the Battle of Ideas in the New Science.* London: Thorsons/HarperCollins.

Shirahata, S., Kabayama, S., and Nakano, M. (1997) "Electrolyzed-reduced water scavenges active oxygen species and protects DNA from oxidative damage." *Biochemical and Biophysical Research Communications 234*, 269–274.

Smith, C.W. (1994a) "Electromagnetic and Magnetic Vector Potential Bio-Information and Water." In P.C. Endler and J. Schulte (eds) *Ultra High Dilution: Physiology and Physics.* Dordrecht: Kluwer Academic.

Smith, C.W. (1994b) "Coherence in living biological systems." *Neural Network World 3*, 379–388.

Smith, C.W. (2004) "Quanta and coherence effects in water and living systems." *Journal of Alternative and Complementary Medicine 10*, 1, 69–78.

Szent-Gyorgyi, A. (1979) In W. Drost-Hansen and J.S. Clegg (eds) *Cell-Associated Water.* New York: Academic Press.

Tiller, W. (1997) *Science and Human Transformation.* Walnut Creek, CA: Pavior Press.

Tiller, W. (2001) *Conscious Acts of Creation.* Walnut Creek, CA: Pavior Press.

Ye, J., Li, Y., and Hanasaki, T. (2008) "Inhibitory effect of electrolyzed reduced water on tumor angiogenesis." *Biological & Pharmaceutical Bulletin 31*, 1, 19–26.

Zheng, J.M. and Pollack, G.H. (2006) "Solute Exclusion and Potential Distribution Near Hydrophilic Surfaces." In G.H. Pollack, I.L. Cameron, and D.N. Wheatley (eds) *Water and the Cell.* Dordrecht: Springer.

Chapter 19: The Positive Potential of Dissociative States of Consciousness

American Psychiatric Association (1994) *Diagnostic and Statistical Manual of Mental Disorders, Fourth Edition.* Washington, DC: American Psychological Press.

Atwater, F.H. (2001) *Captain of My Ship, Master of My Soul.* Charlottesville, VA: Hampton Roads Publishing.

Beahrs, J. (1982) *Unity and Multiplicity.* New York: Brunner/Mazel.

Beauregard, M. and O'Leary, D. (2007) *The Spiritual Brain.* New York: Harper Collins.

Binet, A. (1890) *On Double Consciousness.* Chicago: Open Court.

Braude, S. (1995) *The First Person Plural: Multiple Personality and the Philosophy of Mind.* Lanham, MD: Rowman and Littlefield.

Braude, S. (2002) "The creativity of dissociation." *Journal of Trauma and Dissociation 3*, 5–26.

Buchanan, L. (2003) *The Seventh Sense: Secrets of Remote Viewing.* New York: Paraview Pocket Books.

Cline, J.D. (1997) *Silencing the Voices: One Woman's Triumph over Multiple Personality Disorder.* New York: Berkeley Books.

Crabtree, A. (1985) *Multiple Man: Explorations in Possession and Multiple Personality.* London: Holt Rinehart and Winston.

Crabtree, A. (1993) *From Mesmer to Freud: Magnetic Sleep and the Roots of Psychological Healing.* New Haven, CT: Yale University Press.

Crabtree, A. (2006) "Automatism and Secondary Centers of Consciousness." In E.F. Kelly, E.W. Kelly, A. Crabtree, A. Gauld, M. Grosso, and B. Greyson (eds) *Irreducible Mind: Toward a Psychology for the 21st Century.* Lanham, MD: Rowman and Littlefield.

Dunne, B. and Jahne, R. (1982) *Margins of Reality.* Princeton, NJ: Princeton University Press.

Evan, H. (1989) *Alternate States of Consciousness.* Wellingborough, England: Aquarium Press.

Gabbard, G.O. and Twemlow, S.W. (1985) *With the Eyes of the Mind: Empirical Analysis of the Out of Body State.* New York: Praeger.

Gauld, A. (2006) "Memory." In E.F. Kelly, E.W. Kelly, A. Crabtree, A. Gauld, M. Grosso, and B. Greyson (eds) *Irreducible Mind: Toward a Psychology for the 21st Century.* Lanham, MD: Rowman and Littlefield.

Gazzaniga, M.S. (1989) "The organization of the human brain." *Science 245*, 492, 947–952.

Gazzaniga, M.S. (2008) *Human: The Science of What Makes Us Unique.* New York: HarperCollins.

GoForth, A. (2011) "The disparity of a standard of care for spirit mediumship as a permissible behavioral health care profession." *Paranthropology,* January.

GoForth, A. and Gray, T. (2009) *The Risen: Dialogues of Love, Grief and Survival Beyond Death. 21st Century Reports from the Afterlife Through Contemplative, Intuitive, and Physical Mediumship.* New York: Tempestina Teapot Books.

Greyson, B. (2006) "Near Death Experiences." In E.F. Kelly, E.W. Kelly, A. Crabtree, A. Gauld, M. Grosso, and B. Greyson (eds) *Irreducible Mind: Toward a Psychology for the 21st Century.* Lanham, MD: Rowman and Littlefield.

Hilgard, E. (1977) *Divided Consciousness: Multiple Controls in Human Thought and Action.* New York: John Wiley and Sons.

Holmes, E.A., James, E.L., Kilford, E.J., and Deeprose, C. (2010) "Key steps in developing a cognitive vaccine against traumatic flashbacks: visuo-spatial tetris versus verbal pub quiz." *PLoS ONE 5,* 11, e13706 DOI.

Janet, P. (1901) *The Mental State of Hystericals: A Study of Mental Stigmas and Mental Accidents.* New York: G.P. Putnam.

Journal of Conscientiology: International Institute of Conscientiology and Projectiology. Foz do Iguacu PR Brazil (www.iipc.org).

Krippner, S. and Powers, S.M. (1997) *Broken Images, Broken Selves: Dissociative Narratives in Clinical Practice.* Washington, DC: Brunner/Mazel.

Morse, M.L. (1994a) *Transformed by the Light.* New York: Harper Collins.

Morse, M.L. (1994b) "Near death experiences and death related visions in children: implications for clinicians." *Current Problems in Pediatrics 24,* 55–83.

Morse, M.L. (2002) *Where God Lives: Paranormal Science and How Our Brains Are Connected to the Universe.* New York: HarperCollins.

Morse, M.L., Castillo, P., and Venecia, D. (1986) "Children's near death experiences." *American Journal of Diseases of Children 140,* 110–114.

Mosher, C., Beischel, J., and Boccuzzi, M. (2010) "The potential therapeutic benefit of mediumship readings in the treatment of grief." Poster at Science of Consciousness, University of Arizona, Tucson, Arizona. Available at www.consciousness.arizona.edu/documents/AbstractBook2010_v12full.pdf, accessed on April 23, 2011.

Myers, F.W.H. (1885) "Automatic writing, or the rationale of planchette." *Contemporary Review 47,* 233–249.

Peres, J. (2009) Lecture at Second British Spiritist Medical Conference, London, England, November 8.

Shapiro, F. (2001) *Eye Movement Desensitization and Reprocessing: Basic Principles, Protocols and Procedures,* 2nd edn. New York: Guilford Press.

Sperry, R.W. (1974) "Lateral Specialization in the Surgically Separated Hemispheres." In F.O. Schmitt and F.G. Worden (eds) *The Neurosciences: The Third Study Program.* Cambridge, MA: MIT Press.

Sperry, R.W. (1993) "The impact and promise of the cognitive revolution." *American Psychologist 48,* 878–885.

Spiritist Medical Association of the USA (2010) "What is Spiritism?" Available at www.sma-us.org, accessed on November 15, 2010.

Spitzer, C., Barnow, S., Freyberger, H.J., and Grabe, H.J. (2006) "Recent developments in the theory of dissociation." *World Psychiatry 5,* 2, 82–86.

Stapp, H. (2007) *Mindful Universe: Quantum Mechanics and the Participating Observer.* New York: Springer.

Targ, R. and Puthoff, H. (1974) "Information transmission under conditions of sensory shielding." *Nature 251,* 602–607.

van Lommel, P. (2010) *Consciousness Beyond Life: The Science of the Near Death Experience.* New York: HarperCollins.

van Lommel, P., van Rees, R., Myers, V., and Elferich, I. (2001) "Near death experiences in survivors of cardiac arrest: a prospective study." *Lancet 358*, 9298, 2039–2045.

Whinnery, J.E. (1989) "Methods for describing and quantifying +Gz induced loss of consciousness." *Aviation, Space and Environmental Medicine 60*, 589–593.

Whinnery, J.E. and Whinnery, A.M. (1990) "Acceleration induced loss of consciousness." *Archives of Neurology 47*, 764–776.

Chapter 20: Compassionate Intention as a Therapeutic Intervention by Partners of Cancer Patients

Achterberg, J., Cooke, K., Richards, T., Standish, L.J., Kozak, L., and Lake, J. (2005) "Evidence for correlations between distant intentionality and brain function in recipients: a functional magnetic resonance imaging analysis." *Journal of Alternative and Complementary Medicine 11*, 6, 965–971.

Astin, J.A., Harkness, E., and Ernst, E. (2000) "The efficacy of 'distant healing': a systematic review of randomized trials." *Annals of Internal Medicine 132*, 903–910.

Barnes, P., Powell-Griner, E., McFann, K., Nahin, R., *et al.* (2004) "Advance Data Report #343." *Complementary and Alternative Medicine Use Among Adults: United States.* May 27.

Benson, H., Dusek, J.A., Sherwood, J.B., Lam, P., *et al.* (2006) "Study of the therapeutic effects of intercessory prayer (STEP) in cardiac bypass patients: a multicenter randomized trial of uncertainty and certainty of receiving intercessory prayer." *American Heart Journal 151*, 4, 934–942.

Blair, R.C. and Karniski, W. (1993) "An alternative method for significance testing of waveform difference potentials." *Psychophysiology 30*, 518–524.

Brady, M., Peterman, A.H., Fitchett, G., Mo, M., and Cella, D.A. (1999) "A case for including spirituality in quality of life measurement in oncology." *Psycho-Oncology 8*, 417–428.

Braud, W. (2000) "Wellness implications of retroactive intentional influence: exploring an outrageous hypothesis." *Alternative Therapies in Health and Medicine 6*, 37–48.

Cella, D.F., Tulsky, D.S., Gray, G., Sarafian, B., *et al.* (1993) "The Functional Assessment of Cancer Therapy (FACT) scale: development and validation of the general measure." *Journal of Clinical Oncology 11*, 570–579.

Chodron, P. (1996) *Awakening Loving-Kindness.* Boston, MA: Shambhala.

Davis, A. (ed.) (1997) *Meditation from the Heart of Judaism.* Woodstock: Jewish Lights.

Duane, T.D. and Behrendt, T. (1965) "Extrasensory electroencephalographic induction between identical twins." *Science 150*, 367.

Grinberg-Zylberbaum, J., Delaflor, M., Attie, L., and Goswami, A. (1994) "The Einstein–Podolsky–Rosen paradox in the brain: the transferred potential." *Physics Essays 7*, 422–427.

Hudson, W.W. (1997) *The WALMYR Assessment Scales Scoring Manual.* Tallahassee, FL: WALMYR Publishing.

Kiecolt-Glaser, J.K., McGuire, L., Robles, T.F., and Glaser, R. (2002) "Psychoneuroimmunology and psychosomatic medicine: back to the future." *Psychosomatic Medicine 64*, 15–28.

Krieger, D. (1993) *Accepting Your Power to Heal.* Rochester: Bear and Co.

Krucoff, M.W., Crater, S.W., Gallup, D., Blankenship, J.C., *et al.* (2005) "Music, imagery, touch, and prayer as adjuncts to interventional cardiac care: the Monitoring and Actualization of Noetic Trainings (MANTRA) II randomized study." *Lancet 366*, 9481, 211–217.

Krucoff, M.W., Crater, S.W., Green, C.L., Maas, A.C., *et al.* (2001) "Integrative noetic therapies as adjuncts to percutaneous intervention during unstable coronary syndromes: Monitoring and Actualization of Noetic Training (MANTRA) feasibility pilot." *American Heart Journal 142*, 5, 760–769.

Leibovici, L. (2001) "Effects of remote, retroactive intercessory prayer on outcomes in patients with bloodstream infection: randomized controlled trial." *British Medical Journal 323*, 1450–1451.

Lerner, M. (1995) *Jewish Renewal: A Path to Healing and Transformation.* San Francisco: Perennial.

Lin, J.C. (ed.) (2005) *Advances in Electromagnetic Fields in Living Systems, Volume 4.* New York: Springer Science and Business Media.

May, E.C., Paulinyi, T., and Vassy, Z. (2005) "Anomalous anticipatory skin conductance response to acoustic stimuli: experimental results and speculation about a mechanism." *Journal of Alternative and Complementary Medicine 11*, 4, 587–588.

McCraty, R., Atkinson, M., and Bradley, R.T. (2004a) "Electrophysiological evidence of intuition: Part 1. The surprising role of the heart." *Journal of Alternative and Complementary Medicine 10*, 133–143.

McCraty, R., Atkinson, M., and Bradley, R.T. (2004b) "Electrophysiological evidence of intuition: Part 2. A system-wide process." *Journal of Alternative and Complementary Medicine 10*, 325–336.

McNair, D.M., Lorr, M., and Droppleman, I.F. (1971) *Profile of Mood States.* San Diego: Education and Industrial Testing Service.

Radin, D.I. (1997) "Unconscious perception of future emotions: an experiment in presentiment." *Journal of Scientific Exploration 11*, 2, 163–180.

Radin, D.I. (2004a) "Event related EEG correlations between isolated human subjects." *Journal of Alternative and Complementary Medicine 10*, 315–324.

Radin, D.I. (2004b) "Electrodermal presentiments of future emotions." *Journal of Scientific Exploration 18*, 253–274.

Radin, D.I. (2006) *Entangled Minds.* New York: Simon and Schuster.

Radin, D.I. and Schlitz, M.J. (2005) "Gut feelings, intuition, and emotions: an exploratory study." *Journal of Alternative and Complementary Medicine 11*, 1, 85–91.

Radin, D.I., Machado, F., and Zangari, W. (2000) "Effects of distant healing intention through time and space: two exploratory studies." *Subtle Energies and Energy Medicine 11*, 207–240.

Richards, T.L., Kozak, L., Johnson, L.C., and Standish, L.J. (2005) "Replicable functional magnetic resonance imaging evidence of correlated brain signals between physically and sensory isolated subjects." *Journal of Alternative and Complementary Medicine 11*, 6, 955–963.

Rinpoche, S. (1994) *The Tibetan Book of Living and Dying.* San Francisco: HarperSanFrancisco.

Rosenthal, R. (1994) "Parametric Measures of Effect Size." In H. Cooper and L.V. Hedges (eds) *The Handbook of Research Synthesis.* New York: Russell Sage Foundation.

Schlitz, M. and Braud, W.G. (1997) "Distant intentionality and healing: assessing the evidence." *Alternative Therapies in Health and Medicine 3*, 6, 62–73.

Schlitz, M., Radin, D.I., Malle, B.F., Schmidt, S., Utts, J., and Yount, J.L. (2003) "Distant healing intention: definitions and evolving guidelines for laboratory studies." *Alternative Therapies in Health and Medicine 9*, A31–A43.

Schlitz, M., Wiseman, R., Watt, C., and Radin, D.I. (2006) "Of two minds: skeptic-proponent collaboration within parapsychology." *British Journal of Psychology 97*, 313–322.

Schmidt, S., Schneider, R., Utts, J., and Walach, H. (2004) "Distant intentionality and the feeling of being stared at: two meta-analyses." *British Journal of Psychology 95*, 235–247.

Schwartz, S.A. (2007) *Opening to the Infinite.* Nemoseen Media: www.nemoseen.com.

Sloan, R.P. and Ramakrishnan, R. (2005) "The MANTRA II study." *Lancet 366*, 1769–1770.

Spottiswoode, S.J.P. and May, E.C. (2003) "Skin conductance prestimulus response: analyses, artifacts and a pilot study." *Journal of Scientific Exploration 17*, 4, 617–641.

Standish, L.J., Kozak, L., Johnson, L.C., and Richards, T.J. (2004) "Electroencephalographic evidence of correlated event-related signals between the brains of spatially and sensory isolated human subjects." *Journal of Alternative and Complementary Medicine 10*, 2, 307–314.

Wackermann, J., Seiter, C., Keibel, H., and Walach, H. (2003) "Correlations between brain electrical activities of two spatially separated human subjects." *Neuroscience Letters 336*, 60–64.

Walach, H. (2005) "Generalized entanglement: a new theoretical model for understanding the effects of complementary and alternative medicine." *Journal of Alternative and Complementary Medicine 11*, 3, 549–559.

Wallis, C. (1996) "Faith and healing." *Time Magazine*, June 24, 58–64.

Webster, K., Odom, L., Peterman, A., Lent, L., and Cella, D. (1999) "The functional assessment of chronic illness therapy (FACIT) measurement system: validation of version 4 of the core questionnaire." *Quality of Life Research 8*, 7, 604.

Wiseman, R. and Schlitz, M. (1997) "Experimenter effects and the remote detection of staring." *Journal of Parapsychology 61*, 197–207.

Chapter 21: The Pineal Gland and Its Influence on Body–Mind–Soul Integration

Brainard, G.C. (1978) "Pineal research: the decade of transformation." *Journal of Neural Transmission Suppl. 13*, 3–10.

Brendel, H., Niehaus, M., and Lerchl, A. (2000) "Direct suppressive effects of weak magnetic fields (50 Hz and 16 2/3 Hz) on melatonin synthesis in the pineal gland of Djungarian hamsters (Phodopus sungorus)." *Journal of Pineal Research 29*, 4, 228–233.

Bruis, E., Crasson, M., and Legros, J.J. (2000) "Mélatonine: Physiologie de la secretion." *Revue Medical de Liege 55*, 8, 785–792.

Commentz, J.C., Stegner, H., Winkler, P., Helmke, K., *et al.* (1986) "Pineal calcification does not affect melatonin production." *Journal of Neural Transmission 21*, 418.

Demaine, C. and Semm, P. (1985) "The avian pineal gland as an independent magnetic sensor." *Neuroscience Letters 20, 62*, 1, 119–122.

Douglas, C.R. (2000) *Tratado de Fisiologia Aplicada à Ciência da Saúde*, 4th edn. São Paulo: Ed. Robe.

Gerber, R. (2001) *Vibrational Medicine*, 3rd edn. Rochester, VT: Bear and Co.

Gould, J.L. (1984) "Magnetic fields sensitivity in animals." *Annual Review of Physiology 46*, 585–598.

Hacker, G.W., Pawlak, E., Pauser, G., Tichy, G., *et al.* (2005) "Biomedical evidence of influence of geopathic zones on the human body: scientifically traceable effects and ways of harmonization." *Forsch Komplementärmed Klass Naturheilkd 12*, 6, 315–327.

Harvalik, Z.V. (1978) "Anatomical localization of human detection of weak electromagnetic radiation: experiments with dowsers." *Physiological Chemistry and Physics 10*, 6525–6534.

Janjoppi, L., Silva de Lacerda, A.F., Scorza, F.A., Amado, D., *et al.* (2006) "Influence of pinealectomy on the amygdala kindling development in rats." *Neuroscience Letters 392*, 1–2, 150–153.

Jansen, R., Metzdorf, R., van der Roest, M., Fusani, L., ter Maat, A., and Gahr, M. (2005) "Melatonin affects the temporal organization of the song of zebra finch." *FASEB Journal 19*, 7, 848–850.

Jockers, R. and Petit, L. (1998) "Structure et fonction des récepteurs de la mélatonine." *Comptes Rendus des Séances de la Sociétè de Biologie et de Ses Filiales 192*, 4, 659–667.

Kanta, S., Dhall, U., Misha, D.S., and Dhall, A. (1996) "Age-related incidence of normal pineal calcification: evaluation by computed tomography." *Journal of the Anatomical Society of India 45*, 2, 93–96.

Karasek, M., Woldanska-Okonska, M., Czernicki, J., Zylinska, K., and Swietoslawski, J. (1998) "Chronic exposure to 2.9 mT, 40 Hz magnetic field reduces melatonin concentrations in humans." *Journal of Pineal Research 25*, 4, 240–244.

Mazzucchelli, C., Pannacci, M., Nonno, R., Lucini, V., *et al.* (1996) "The melatonin receptor in the human brain." *Molecular Brain Research 39*, 117–126.

Rosen, L.A., Barber, I., and Lyle, D.B. (1998) "A 0.5 G, 60 Hz magnetic field suppresses melatonin production in pinealocytes." *Bioelectromagnetics 19*, 2, 123–127.

Schmid, G., Uberbacher, R., Samaras, T., Tschabitscher, M., and Mazal, P.R. (2007) "The dielectric properties of human pineal gland tissue and RF absortion due to wireless communication devices in the frequency range 400–1850 MHz." *Physics in Medicine and Biology 52*, 17, 5457–5468.

Semm, P., Schneider, T., and Vollrath, L. (1980) "Effects of earth-strength magnetic fields on electrical activity of pineal cells." *Nature 288*, 607–608.

Sengupta, A. and Kumar Maitra, S. (2006) "The pineal gland, but not melatonin, is associated with the termination of seasonal testicular activity in an annual reproductive cycle in rose-ringed parakeet Psittacula krameri." *Chronobiology International 23*, 5, 915–933.

Tunç, A.T., Aslan, H., Turgut, M., Ekici, F., Odaci, E., and Kaplan, S. (2007) "Inhibitory effect of pinealectomy on the development of cerebellar granule cells in the chick: a stereological study." *Brain Research 1138*, 214–220.

Tunç, A.T., Turgut, M., Aslan, H., Sahin, B., Yurtseven, M.E., and Kaplan, S. (2006) "Neonatal pinealectomy induces Purkinje cell loss in the cerebellum of the chick: a stereological study." *Brain Research 1067*, 1, 95–102.

Turgut, M., Turkkani-Tunc, A., Aslan, H., Yazici, A.C., and Kaplan, S. (2007) "Effect of pinealectomy on the morphology of the chick cervical spinal cord: a stereological and histopathological study." *Brain Research 1129*, 1, 166–173.

Walcott, C., Gould, J.L., and Lednor, A.J. (1988) "Homing of magnetized and demagnetized pigeons." *Journal of Experimental Biology 134*, 27–41.

Xavier, F. (2009) *Missionários da Luz/Missionaries of Light*. Brasilia: IEC. (Original work published 1945.)

Zimmerman, R.A. and Bilaniuk, L.T. (1982) "Age-related incidence of pineal calcification detected by Computed Tomography." *Radiology 142*, 659–662.

Editor's Note for Part IV

Moore, D.W. (2005) "Three in four Americans believe in paranormal." Available at www.gallup.com/poll/16915/Thee-Four-Americans-Believe-Paranormal.aspx, accessed on April 4, 2011.

Newport, F. (2010) "Near-record high see religion losing influence in America." Available at www.gallup.com/poll/145409/Near-Record-High-Religion-Losing-Influence-America.aspx, accessed on March 25, 2011.

Robinson, B.A. (2007a) "Comparing U.S. religious beliefs with those in other mainly Christian countries." Available at www.religioustolerance.org/rel_comp.htm, accessed on March 25, 2011.

Robinson, B.A. (2007b) "Religious beliefs of Americans: about ghosts, Satan, Heaven, Hell, etc." Available at www.religioustolerance.org/chr_poll3.htm, accessed on April 4, 2011.

Chapter 22: What Spiritist Centers Offer Outside Brazil

Fenwick, P. (2008) *The Art of Dying*. New York: Continuum.

Xavier, C. (2007) *Two Thousand Years Ago*. Philadelphia: AKES.

Chapter 23: Contributions of Brazilian Spiritist Treatments to the Global Improvement of Mental Health Care

Almeida, A.M. de, Almeida, T.M. de, and Gollner, A.M. (2000) "Cirgurgia espiritual: uma investigacao [Spiritual surgery: an investigation]." *Journal of the Medical Research Association of Brazil 46*, 194–200.

Bragdon, E. (2002) *Spiritual Alliances: Discovering the Roots of Health at the Casa de Dom Inácio*. Woodstock, VT: Lightening Up Press.

Mary, F. (1999) *Padre Pio: The Wonder Worker*. Fort Collins, CO: Ignatius Press.

Pellegrino-Estrich, R. (1997) *The Miracle Man*. Australia: Triad Books.

Savaris, A.A. (1997) *Curas Paranormais Realizadas por João Teixeira de Farias [Paranormal Cures Performed by João Teixeira de Farias]*. Curitiba, Brazil: Curitiba Press.

Chapter 24: Training Mediums Who Treat Psychiatric Patients

Kardec, A. (1986) *The Mediums' Book*. Rio de Janeiro: FEB. (Original work published 1861.)

Kardec, A. (1987) *The Gospel According to Spiritism*. London: Headquarters Publishing Co. (Original work published 1864.)

Kardec, A. (1996) *The Spirits' Book*, 2nd edn. Rio de Janeiro: FEB. (Original work published 1860.)

Schubert, S.C. (2008) *Obsessão/Desobsessão [Obsession/Disobsession]*. Rio de Janeiro: FEB.

Xavier, F. (2008) *The Messengers*. Brasilia: FEB.

Chapter 25: Teaching Health Professionals How to Support Personal Transformation in Patients

Franco, D. (1995) *O Ser Consciente*. Salvador: LEAL.

Jung, C.G. (1982) *Aion—Estudo Sobre o Simbolismo do Si-mesmo.* Petropolis: Editora Vozes.

Jung, C.G. (1994) "A dinâmica do inconsciente." *Obras Completas*, vol. VIII. Petropolis: Editora Vozes.

Kardec, A. (1985) *The Spirits' Book*, 2nd edn. Rio de Janeiro: FEB.

Moore, T. (2010) *Writing in the Sand: Jesus, Spirituality, and the Soul of the Gospels.* Carlsbad, CA: Hay House.

Moreira-Almeida, A. (2010) "The growing impact of publications in spirituality and health and the role of Revista de Psiquiatria Clínica." *Revista de Psiquiatria Clínica [Journal of Clinical Psychiatry]* 37, 2, 41–42.

Saad, M. and de Medeiros, R. (2008) "Espiritualidade e saúde." *Einstein: Educação Continuada em Saúde 6*, 135–136.

World Health Organization (2003) *Bulletin of the World Health Organization 81*, 6. Geneva, Switzerland: WHO.

Xavier, F. (1991) *Nos Domínios da Mediunidade.* Rio de Janeiro: FEB.

Xavier, F. and Vieira, W. (1999) *Mechanisms of Mediumship.* Rio de Janeiro: FEB.

Editor's Note for Chapter 26

Lake, J. and Spiegel, D. (eds) (2007) *Complementary and Alternative Treatments in Mental Health Care.* Washington, DC: American Psychiatric Publishing, Inc.

Chapter 26: Researching the Invisible

Achterberg, J., Cooke, K., Richards, T., Standish, L.J., Kozak, L., and Lake, J. (2005) "Evidence for correlations between distant intentionality and brain function in recipients: a functional magnetic resonance imaging analysis." *Journal of Alternative and Complementary Medicine 11*, 965–971.

Beischel, J. (2007–2008) "Contemporary methods used in laboratory-based mediumship research." *Journal of Parapsychology 71*, 37–68.

Beischel, J. and Rock, A.J. (2009) "Addressing the survival vs. psi debate through process-focused mediumship research." *Journal of Parapsychology 73*, 71–90.

Beischel, J. and Schwartz, G.E. (2007) "Anomalous information reception by research mediums demonstrated using a novel triple-blind protocol." *Explore: The Journal of Science and Healing 3*, 1, 23–27.

Benor, D.J. (1992) "Intuitive diagnosis." *Subtle Energies 3*, 2, 41–64.

Benor, D.J. (n.d.) "Intuitive assessments: an overview." Available at www.wholistichealingresearch.com/intuitiveassessmentsoverview.html, accessed on 16 June 2011.

Benor, D.J. (n.d.) "Spiritual healing and psychotherapy." Available at www.wholistichealingresearch.com/spiritualhealingandpsychotherapy.html, accessed on 16 June 2011.

Braud, W. (2000) "Wellness implications of retroactive intentional influence: exploring an outrageous hypothesis." *Alternative Therapies in Health and Medicine 6*, 1, 37–48.

Braud, W. (2002) "Psi Favorable Conditions." In V.W. Rammohan (ed.) *New Frontiers of Human Science.* Jefferson, NC: McFarland.

Braud, W. (2003) *Distant Mental Influence: Its Contributions to Science, Healing, and Human Interactions.* Charlottesville, VA: Hampton Roads Publishing.

Braud, W. (2008) "Patanjali Yoga and Siddhis: Their Relevance to Parapsychological Theory and Research." In K.R. Rao, A.C. Paranjpe, and A.K. Dalal (eds) *Handbook of Indian Psychology.* New Delhi, India: Cambridge University Press (India)/Foundation Books.

Braud, W. (2009) "Dragons, spheres, and flashlights: appropriate research approaches for studying workplace spirituality." *Journal of Management, Spirituality & Religion 6*, 1, 59–75.

Braud, W. and Anderson, R. (1998) *Transpersonal Research Methods for the Social Sciences: Honoring Human Experience.* Thousand Oaks, CA: Sage.

Braud, W. and Associates (2007) "Extending positive psychology's 'broaden-and-build' theory to a spiritual context." Paper presented at the 115th Annual Convention of the American Psychological Association, San Francisco, CA, August.

Braud, W., Shafer, D., McNeill, K., and Guerra, V. (1995) "Attention focusing facilitated through remote mental interaction." *Journal of the American Society for Psychical Research 89*, 2, 103–115.

Dean, D., Mihalasky, J., Ostrander, S., and Schroeder, L. (1974) *Executive ESP*. Englewood Cliffs, NJ: Prentice-Hall.

Dossey, L. (2008) "Healing research: what we know and don't know." *Explore: The Journal of Science and Healing 4*, 6, 341–352.

Fontana, D. (2005) *Is There an Afterlife? A Comprehensive Overview of the Evidence*. Oakland, CA: O Books.

Gauld, A. (1984) *Mediumship and Survival: A Century of Investigations*. Chicago: Academy Chicago Publishers.

Grad, B. (1965) "Some biological effects of the 'laying on of hands': A review of experiments with animals and plants." *Journal of the American Society for Psychical Research 59*, 95–127.

Krippner, S. and Achterberg, J. (2000) "Anomalous Healing Experiences." In E. Cardena, S.J. Lynn, and S. Krippner (eds) *Varieties of Anomalous Experience: Examining the Scientific Evidence*. Washington, DC: American Psychological Association.

Mills, A. and Lynn, S.J. (2000) "Past-Life Experiences." In E. Cardena, S.J. Lynn, and S. Krippner (eds) *Varieties of Anomalous Experience: Examining the Scientific Evidence*. Washington, DC: American Psychological Association.

Murphy, M. and White, R.A. (1995) *In the Zone: Transcendent Experiences in Sports*. New York: Penguin/Arkana.

Palmer, G. and Braud, W. (2002) "Exceptional human experiences, disclosure, and a more inclusive view of physical, psychological, and spiritual well-being." *Journal of Transpersonal Psychology 34*, 29–61.

Palmer, G. and Braud, W. (2010) "Psychical experiences and their life and work impacts for members of a professional academic transpersonal community." Unpublished manuscript.

Radin, D. (1997) *The Conscious Universe*. San Francisco, CA: HarperSanFrancisco.

Radin, D. (2006) *Entangled Minds*. New York: Paraview/Simon & Schuster.

Schouten, S.A. (1994) "An overview of quantitatively evaluated studies with mediums and psychics." *Journal of the American Society for Psychical Research 88*, 221–254.

White, R.A. (1992) "Review of approaches to the study of spontaneous psi experiences." *Journal of Scientific Exploration 6*, 2, 93–126.

White, R.A. (1997) "Dissociation, Narrative, and Exceptional Human Experience." In S. Krippner and S. Powers (eds) *Broken Images, Broken Selves: Dissociative Narratives in Clinical Practice*. Washington, DC: Brunner-Mazel.

Subject Index

Note: page numbers in *italics* indicate figures and tables

abortion 180
affect bridge 182
agoraphobia 185–6
alcohol abuse 177–8
alkaline water, drinking 202–4, *203*
André Luiz Hospital *see* Hospital Éspírita André Luiz
animism 273
animistic obsession 50–1
anxiety *see* panic attacks
apparitions 42–3
attention
    goals of training 162
    refining 160–1
aura *see* magnetism anatomy of human
autism, Spiritist therapy for 17
automatic writing 194, 217
    developing 274–5

blindness 182–3
body scan 170
Bragdon, Emma
    exploring a resource in Brazil 12–13
    I Do Not Heal, God is the One Who Heals 14
    reflections on value of Spiritist therapies 263–4
    Resources for Extraordinary Healing: Schizophrenia, Bipolar and Other Serious Mental Illnesses 66, 72
    Spiritism: Bridging Spirituality and Health 14
    Spiritual Alliances: Discovering the Roots of Health at the Casa de Dom Inacio 14, 259–60
brain
    functional dysregulation of 2
    "god spot"/"spiritual brain" 214–16
    left vs. right 214

brain sand 238
    melatonin, mediumship and 238–9
    prevalence 240
Brazilian Spiritist Federation (FEB) 116, 119
Britain *see* United Kingdom

cancer 114, 223–8
    see also case studies; distant healing intention; Krippner, Stanley
Caritas, Prayer of 68–9
Casa de Dom Inácio de Loyola (House of St. Ignatius of Loyola) 66, 69, 113–15, 121, 257–60
    see also John of God
Casa do Padre Pio 261–2
Casas Éspiritas *see* Spiritist Houses/Spiritist Centers
case studies 141–2, 146–7, 215, 237, 276
    Alice 182–3
    Barbara/Miria 185–6
    Carol 177–8
    case worker in USA 62–5
    Christine 177
    Ernesto 78–80
    Gerry 59–62
    Gillian 180–1
    Helen 186–8
    Janet 186
    Joan and Ted 179–80
    Louise 62–5
    M.A. 111
    Marcel 56–7
        from mental illness to mediumship 57–9
    Marie 80–1
    Pat 183–4
    Peter 181–2
    P.L. 111
    Rosemary and Tessa 178–9
    Sally 181
    Tony 64–5
    see also Hospital Éspírita André Luiz; psychotherapy
Catholic Church 24

chakras 244
channeling 84, 274–6
    see also automatic writing; mediumship; *specific topics*
Chinese medicine 5
collective unconscious 126
consciousness
    Jung's views on 126
        compared with Spiritists' views 130–2
    paradigms of 142–4
    see also research
controlled remote viewing (CRV)/controlled out-of-body perceptions 217
corrente *see* Current rooms
cultural psychiatry
    historical perspectives and lessons for 136–7
    Jung and 136–8
Current rooms 113, 121, 259

Damo, Bartolo 57
Damo, Vania 58
dark-field microscopy *202*, 202–4, *203*
de Queiroz, Luiz Augusto 260–2
death-related sensory experiences (DRSEs) 250
    see also near-death experiences
Deep Memory Process 143
delusions, content of 42
"demons," souls of 186
depression, case studies of 177, 180, 181, 183–4
Descartes, René 238
diagnosis 264
diathesis-stress model 38
Dirac Sea 243
direct knowing
    research on 286–8
    see also medical intuition; super-psi/super-ESP hypothesis
direct mental influence 288
discarnates 289, 291

disobsession 43, 124–5, 276
　books on 271, 298
　dynamics of 53
　see also spirit release
dissociation 126, 220
　case report 215
　current view of 212, 214
　as normal state of
　　consciousness 214–15
　spectrum of 213
dissociative experiences 132–3
　non-local perceptions and
　　215–16
　used to transform and heal the
　　mind 216–17
dissociative identity disorder
　(DID) 168, 218, 220
distant healing intention (DHI)
　221–2, 235
　study on cancer patients and
　　their partners 222–35
Domancic, Zdenko 114
Down syndrome, Spiritist
　therapy for 17
dreams, soul 188
dualism, interactionist 38, 39

ego 176
Eisenbeiss, W. 194–200
empathy 18
empiricism, William James'
　radical 159–60
entanglement 289
epileptic disorders, Spiritist
　therapy for 17
ethics
　Spiritism and a new ground
　　for 33–4
　see also morality
Euripides Barsanulfo Hospital
　56–7
exceptional human experiences
　(EHEs) 292
　benefits 293
　psychiatric and psychological
　　relevance 293–4
　risks 292
exorcism see spirit release
experiential regression therapy
　de Peres (TRVP) 218
extrasensory perception (ESP)
　see super-psi/super-ESP
　hypothesis

eye movement desensitization
　and reprocessing (EMDR)
　215, 217–18

fascination and obsession 40
Foundation for Energy Therapies
　69n5
Fox, Kate 22, 24
Fox, Maggie 22, 24
Frederic, Dr. (Frederic von Stein)
　260, 263
Frei Luiz Shrine 260–1

Galileo Galilei 156
"god spot" (brain) 214–16
Gospel According to Spiritism, The
　(Kardec) 23, 91, 123–4
group field 113–15

Hahnemann, Christian Friedrich
　Samuel 98
hallucination 42–3, 135
healing analog studies 288
health, Spiritist vision of 47–8
HeartMath, Institute of 16
homeopathy 24, 209–10
Hospital Éspírita André Luiz
　(HEAL)
　available patient care 74
　case studies 78–81
　history 73–4
　Spiritual Assistance
　　Department (DAE) 74–6
　spiritual guidance sessions
　　76–7
Hospital of Porto Alegre (HEPA)
　continuing education for
　　professionals 86–7
　current profile 82–4
　history 82
　organizational structure 84
　program for training and
　　supervising mediums
　　85–6
　results of therapies 86
　Spiritual Assistance Programs
　　(DAE) 84–5
hospitalization, spiritual help
　during 88
hospitals, Spiritist psychiatric
　international role of 27–8
　see also specific topics
House of Padre Pio see Casa do
　Padre Pio

House of St. Ignatius of Loyola
　see Casa de Dom Inácio de
　Loyola
humors 39

I Do Not Heal, God is the One Who
　Heals (film) 14
Ignatius of Loyola 117
　see also Casa de Dom Inácio de
　Loyola
imagination 42
individuation 131
informational body see subtle
　body
integration of spirituality and
　psychiatry
　organizations supporting
　　300–1
　see also psychotherapy
integrative model of health care
　6–7, 14–15
　an accessible path for growth
　　and well-being and an
　　13–14
　books on 298
　emerging paradigm 5–6
　see also psychotherapy
intelligent principle 243–4
intentional influence see direct
　mental influence
introspection 160, 162–3
intuition 150–3
　see also medical intuition
ionized water, drinking 202–4,
　203

James, William 26, 156
　radical empiricism 159–60
Jesus 43, 55–6
João de Deus see John of God
João Evangelista Hospital (HOJE)
　88–90
　day hospital 92
　expanding knowledge and
　　understanding 93–4
　intake 90–1
　Programe de Integração Saúde
　　Mental e Espiritualidade
　　(PRISME) 90, 92
　research 95
　treatment modalities 91–2
　treatment results 94–5
　volunteers 92–3

John of God (João de Deus) 14,
    60, 61, 66, 257–9, 263
    see also Casa de Dom Inácio de
        Loyola
Jung, Carl Gustav 126–8, 136–8
    cultural psychiatry and 136–8
    notions of the unconscious
        126
        early influences on 128–30
        on psychogenesis and
            psychosis 133–4
        and Spiritists' views on
            consciousness 130–2

karma 147, 279
    see also past lives; reincarnation
Korchnoi, Viktor 194, 195, 198,
    200
Krippner, Stanley
    journey 257–62
    reflections 263

laying-on of hands 85–6, 102,
    268–70
    healing effects 16
    magnetism and 86, 97, 100,
        101, 124, 275–6
life after death *see* past lives;
    reincarnation; survival
    hypothesis/survivalism
lightbody infusion/light
    infusion 261, 262
live blood analysis *202*, 202–4,
    203
Luiz, André 87, 99–102, 271,
    278–80
    observations about pineal
        gland 244–6

magnetic action 100–1
    manners of 100
magnetic passes *see* laying-on of
    hands
magnetism 97–8
    anatomy of human 98–100
    see also water
Maróczy, Géza 194–8
materialism 157, 159
medical intuition 69n2, 264,
    286–7
    see also mediumship
medium and healer, working as
    a 268–9

mediums 31
    education and training 85–6,
        252–3
    examples of concrete results
        275–6
    physicians as 152–3
    as psychotherapists 219
    treating psychiatric patients
        challenges 269
        discipline 269–70
        healing at a distance 270–3
        role of group leader 274
        self-care 273–4
    as a valuable resource 190
mediumship 31, 119, 149–50
    and being an intuitive
        physician 152–3
    chess game with deceased
        grandmaster 194–200
    defined 49–50
    intuition and 150–3
    mental disorder and 52, 57–9
    in psychotherapy 218
        examples of 218–19
    repressed 52
    research on
        challenges in current 191–2
        importance of current
            190–1
        laboratory 193
    see also Spiritist Houses/
        Spiritist Centers
mediumship abilities and
    dysfunction 49–50
memory of water 209–10
mental disorders
    etiology 38–9
    treatment 43–4
    see also specific topics
mental health
    religious and spiritual beliefs
        and 3
    spiritual practices and 4
    see also integrative model of
        health care
mental illness
    causes of 14–16, *66*, 66–7
    differing views of 5
    paths to emerging from *66*,
        66–8
    potential outcomes of severe
        66, 66–7
    Spiritist perspective on cure
        for 14–16

mental perception 158
    refining 158–9
mental retardation, Spiritist
    therapy for 17
Mesmer, Franz Anton 97–8
mind-body dualism 38, 39
mind-body relationship 107–8
mindfulness 162
mirror scan 170
"monster soul" 219
morality 278–80
    mind and 280–1
    see also ethics
multiple personality disorder
    see dissociative identity
        disorder
Myers-Briggs Type Indicator
    (MBTI) *see* psychological
        types

near-death experiences (NDEs)
    48, 146, 212, 215
    see also death-related sensory
        experiences
neurotheology 286
non-local interconnectedness
    289
non-local perceptions 216
    see also distant healing
        intention
Nostradamus 238

obsession(s) 40–1, 67
    books on 271, 298
    defined 40
    forms of 50–2
    levels of severity of 40
    treatment 43
    see also disobsession
Occam's razor 158, 164n2, 200
orthomolecular psychiatry 61,
    69n3
Ouija boards 167

panic attacks 185
    Spiritist therapy for 17,
        185–6
Paracelsus 97
paranoid psychosis 147
    see also psychosis;
        schizophrenia
passé *see* laying-on of hands

past life memories, children's 105–6, 110
  positive and false-positive cases 106–7
  see also reincarnation
past lives 41–2, 147, 290
  delusions and 42
  schizophrenia and 59
  spirit release from 185–6
  see also case studies; reincarnation
perceptual changes
  in the realm of vision 42–3
  see also mental perception
perispirit 15
  defined 15, 69n4
personality and reincarnation 107–8
pharmacologic treatment 10–11
  appropriate and reasonable uses 2
  limitations 2–3, 10–11
  as sole treatment 11
phobias 181–2, 185–6
pineal gland 237–8
  and the intelligent principle 243–4
  maturation, aging, and 241
  melatonin, brain sand, mediumship, and 238–9
  observations of André Luiz 244–6
  soul, chakras, and 244
  spirit, cosmos, and 242–3
  time, the fourth dimension, and 242
Pio of Pietrelcina (Padre Pio) 260–2
Pocket Ranch 66
poltergeist 51
possession-trance 132
  see also spirit possession
post-traumatic stress disorder (PTSD) 109–10, 220
  treatment 215, 217, 218
prayer 4, 101–3, 124, 221
Prayer of Caritas 68–9
Programe de Integração Saúde Mental e Espiritualidade (PRISME) 90, 92
psi 287
  see also super-psi/super-ESP hypothesis
"Psi Man," supported through group activity 281–3

psychic reservoir hypothesis 191–2
psychic surgery 16, 257–9
  see also John of God
psychodrama 176
psychokinesis 288
psychological types 151
psychosis
  as challenge to psychiatry 146–7
  due to obsession vs. organic origin 41, 42
  Puerto Rican Spiritists and 134–5
  see also schizophrenia
psychotherapist mediums 219
  see also mediums
psychotherapy 175–6
  case studies
    connecting with soul 177–8
    "demons" have souls too 186
    healing for two souls 182–3
    release of earthbound spirit 183–4
    a reunion of souls 179–80
    a soul dream 178
    a soul remembers 181–2
    soul retrieval 181
    a soul that never got born 180–1
    soul to soul 178–9
    soul trauma 186–8
    soul wisdom 176–7
    spirit release from a past life 185–6
    suicide and spirit attachment 184–5
    treasuring the soul 177–8
    see also case studies
  integrating spirituality into 140–2, 148
  paradigms of consciousness and 142–4
  psychosis and 146–7
  therapeutic techniques and 144–5
  and unusual capacities of the mind 145–6
  see also integration of spirituality and psychiatry; integrative model of health care

reincarnation and 109–12
  see also spirit release; Spiritist therapy
Puerto Rican Spiritists and madness 134–5

quantum entanglement 234

R agents (mental radiations) 51, 53
rational emotive therapy (RET) 26–7
Rational Spirituality 174
reincarnation 104–5, 111–12, 147
  clinical cases 110–11
  psychotherapy and 109–12
  research on 105–6
  and the riddle of personality 107–8
  see also case studies; past lives
relaxation 18
religion
  in Brazil 24
  mental health and 3
  ways of experiencing 128–9
remote communication 169
remote viewing 217, 287
repetition compulsion 147
repressed mediumship 52
research 95, 173
  current consciousness 48–9
  on direct knowing 286–8
  on direct mental influence 288–9
  need for additional support and 294
  need for expanded approaches to 291–2
  on reincarnation 105–6
  on survival hypothesis 191–3
research institutes 301
Resources for Extraordinary Healing: Schizophrenia, Bipolar and Other Serious Mental Illnesses (Bragdon) 66, 72
Revue Spirite—Journal d'Études Psychologiques 37–8
right brain 214
Rollans, Robert 194

sarcoid 182–3
Sauer, Maria Lucia 261

schizophrenia 135–7
  causes 59, 62, 127, 135
  Jung on 126–7, 133–5, 137,
    138
  treatment 17, 56–9, 136,
    138, 171, 298
  see also psychosis
science
  significant points in the
    history of 156–8
  spirituality and 31–3, 162–4
self, sense of 283
self-discovery 282–3
Sergio Felipe de Oliveira 238–9
sexual abuse and past lives 147
sexuality 245
shared obsession 51
Smith, Jeff 215
Society for Psychical Research
  (SPR) 189–90
soul connection 177–9
Soul Masters: Dr. Guo and Dr. Sha
  (film) 114
soul medicine 18
soul retrieval 27, 181
soul-centered therapy see
  psychotherapy
soul(s) 15–16, 175, 176
  case of a soul that never got
    born 180–1
  see also psychotherapy, case
    studies
"special energy system" 244
spirit 175, 286
spirit attachment
  assessing the different
    approaches to 172
  and the cycle of rebirth 166–7
  diagnosis 168
  effects 168
  identifying and typing the
    attached spirit 169
  need for research on 173
  phenomenology 167
  protection from 172–3
  suicide and 184–5
  treatment 170–1
    effects of 171–2
  uncovering techniques 170
  vulnerability to 167
  see also spirit possession; spirit
    release
spirit possession 40–1, 52
  see also case studies, Gerry;
    spirit attachment

spirit release 165
  assessing different approaches
    to 172
  dangers 172
  "demons" and 186
  of earthbound spirit 183–4
  future of 174
  historical perspective on
    165–6
  from a past life 185–6
  see also disobsession; spirit
    attachment
Spiritism 255–6
  history and development
    22–5, 30–1
  international impact 247–8
  knowledge of, in international
    community 26–7
  original texts on 23, 298–9
  as prophylaxis 44–5
  as unique integrative model of
    care 6–7
  see also specific topics
Spiritism: Bridging Spirituality and
  Health (film) 14
Spiritist healing
  is done without charge 24
  see also specific topics
Spiritist Houses/Spiritist Centers
  12–13, 116, 123–5,
    264–6
  Current rooms 113, 121, 259
  discipline at 119–20
  fellowship 117–19
  guidance offered 253–4
  orientation 123
  personal transformation
    ("reforma intima") 117
  shadow and negative
    influences in 119
  spiritual counseling 121–2
  spiritual healing techniques
    120–1
  study at 24–5, 116–17
  studying the meaning of life
    254–5
  see also Casa de Dom Inácio de
    Loyola
Spiritist hypothesis 30
Spiritist Medical Association
  (AME) 26
Spiritist philosophy 24
Spiritist principles and practices,
  parapsychological and
  related parallels to 286

past life considerations 290
research on direct knowing
  286–8
research on direct mental
  influence 288–9
spirituality considerations 286
subtle, spiritual realm 291
survival evidence 290–1
work with mediums 289–90
Spiritist Psychiatric Hospital of
  Porto Alegre see Hospital of
  Porto Alegre
Spiritist Review—Journal of
  Psychological Studies 37–8
Spiritist therapy 55
  results of 17
  see also psychotherapy; specific
    topics
Spiritist treatment 53
  effects of 53–4
  see also specific topics
Spiritist-medical paradigm 48–9
Spiritists, types of 25
spirits
  as components of natural
    world 31–3
  of the deceased see discarnates
  see also specific topics
Spiritual Alliances: Discovering the
  Roots of Health at the Casa de
  Dom Inacio (Bragdon) 14
Spiritual Assistance Programs
  (DAE) 74–6, 84–5
Spiritual Care Registry (SCR/
  RAE) 94
spiritual development 131–2
spiritual emergency 55–6, 59
spiritual reality 45, 281–2
spiritual transformation
  a call for 34–5
  three elements of inner 283
  three operational levels for
    284
SpiritualAlliances.com 69n5
Spiritualism and Spiritualists
  23, 129
spirituality 286
  defined 286
Spirituality and Mental Health
  Integration Program see
  Programe de Integração
  Saúde Mental e
  Espiritualidade
Stein, Frederic von ("Dr.
  Frederic") 260, 263

Steiner, Rudolf 56
Stevenson, Ian 290
subjugation 40
subtle body 15, 16, 264
    see also perispirit
suicide 172
    reasons to refrain from 45
    spirit attachment and 184–5
"super-normal" processes 191–2
super-psi/super-ESP hypothesis
    191–2, 196, 198–9
survival hypothesis/survivalism
    (life after death) 194, 198,
    199
    research on
        current challenges in 191–2
        laboratory 193

Teixera de Farias, João *see* John
    of God
telekinesis *see* psychokinesis
telepathic obsession 51
telepathy *see* super-psi/super-ESP
    hypothesis
temperament 39
traditional Chinese medicine
    (TCM) 5
transformation *see* spiritual
    transformation
trauma
    soul 186–8
    see also post-traumatic stress
        disorder

unconscious 126
United Kingdom (UK)
    Spiritism in 249–52
utilitarianism 34

vampirism 51
van Helmont, Jan Baptist 97
vision, types of perceptual
        changes in the realm of
        42–3
visions 42
    true 42–3
volunteerism 93, 265

water 201, 211
    healer interactions with
        210–11
    health, biological terrain,
        and energized drinking
        201–4

imbued with frequencies
    205–7
"magnetized" 86, 124, 201,
    210, 211
memory of 209–10
a new science of 208–9
with sentience 207–8
studies on 201–7
will 103
Windbridge Institute for Applied
    Research in Human
    Potential 193

Xavier, Chico 254–6

Author Index

Abel, G. 171
Achterberg, J. 4, 222, 288, 289
Allen, S. 166
Almeder, R. 199
Almeida, A.A.S. 37
Almeida, A.M. 37, 52
American Psychiatric Association 212
Anderson, J. 4
Anderson, L. 4
Anderson, R. 292
Andrade, H.G. 51, 106, 107
André, J. 204
Aspect, A. 49
Astin, J.A. 4, 222
Athappilly, G.K. 106
Atkinson, M. 235
Atwater, F.H. 217
Aubrée, M. 29, 30
Azari, N.P. 109
Azevedo, J.L. 72, 125

Bagiella, E. 4
Baldwin, W. 166
Ball, P. 208
Barber, I. 239
Barentsen, C. 193
Barlow, D. 171
Barnes, P. 221
Basanez, M. 109
Batmanghelidj, F. 202
Beahrs, J. 214
Beauregard, M. 108, 109, 215
Behrendt, T. 222
Beischel, J. 191–3, 219, 290
Bell, I. 205, 210
Benor, D.J. 288
Benson, H. 18, 47, 114, 222
Benveniste, J. 210
Berger, W. 11
Bergner, R.M. 104, 110
Bergson, H. 152
Binet, A. 214
Birks, J. 11
Blair, R.C. 227
Blanchard, E. 171
Blau, S. 26–7
Boccuzzi, M. 219

Bogdanov, G. 143
Bogdanov, I. 143
Bohart, A.C. 110
Bradley, R.T. 235
Brady, M. 228
Bragdon, E. 14, 59, 72, 122, 260
Brainard, G.C. 237
Braud, W.G. 4, 222, 233, 286–8, 292
Braude, S.E. 190, 199, 214, 216
Breggin, P. 18
Brendel, H. 239
Broch, H.B. 137
Brooks, A. 207
Brooks, A.J. 205
Bruis, E. 239
Brune, M. 109
Buchanan, L. 217
Bucklin, M.A. 29
Burgess, P. 110
Bushwick, B. 3, 4

Cadoret, R.J. 107
Capra, F. 47, 142
Cardeña, E. 52
Castillo, P. 215
CEI (Conselho Espírita Internacional—International Spiritist Council) 30
Cella, D.F. 228
Chai, B. 210
Chibeni, S.S. 32
Chodron, P. 223
Church, D. 12, 16, 18
Cline, J.D. 219
Coatsworth, J.D. 110
Commentz, J.C. 239
Connor, K.M. 109–10
Cook, E.W. 192
Coté, S. 114
Cott, C.C. 192
Crabtree, A. 214
Crasson, M. 239
Crawford, C.C. 4
Creamer, M. 110
Csordas, T. 137

da Silva, M.J. 210
D'Aquili, E.G. 4
Data Folha 109
Davenas, E. 210
Davidson, J.R. 109–10
Davis, A. 223
de Medeiros, R. 277
Dean, D. 287
Del Giudice, E. 208, 209
Demaine, C. 242
DiClemente, C.C. 110
Dixon, L.B. 11
Dodds, E. 190
Dossey, L. 26, 28, 289
Douglas, C.R. 242
Droppleman, I.F. 228
Duane, T.D. 222
Ducasse, C.J. 200
Dunne, B. 220

Eisenbeiss, W. 194–200
Ellenberger, H. 37, 127, 129, 136
Elliott, G. 3
Ellis, A. 26–7
Emoto, M. 201
Endler, P.C. 209
Ernst, E. 4, 222
Evan, H. 212

Felsenthal, G. 4
Fenwick, P. 48, 250
Fernandes, W.L.N. 33
Fernyhough, C. 38
Ferreira, I. 17, 53–4
Feynman, R. 163
Fiore, E. 166, 171
Flynn, C.P. 48
Fontana, D. 190, 290
Fountoulakis, K.N. 11
Fournier, J.C. 11
Fowler, P. 107
Franco, D.P. 37, 39, 41–4, 125, 283
Freud, S. 146, 148

Gabbard, G.O. 220
Gauld, A. 29, 190, 192, 199, 216, 290
Gazzaniga, M.S. 214
Gerber, R. 241
GoForth, A. 219
Goswami, A. 47, 142
Gould, J.L. 239, 242
Grad, B. 288
Gregory, R.L. 110
Grey, M. 48
Greyson, B. 48, 106, 216
Griffin, D.R. 199
Grinberg-Zylberbaum, J. 222
Grof, C. 144
Grof, S. 144
Grosso, M. 199
Guarnaccia, P.J. 134–5
Guitton, J. 143

Hacker, G.W. 244
Haggard, P. 110
Hahnemann, S. 98
Hamburg, D. 3
Hanasaki, T. 204
Haraldsson, E. 42, 105–7, 109, 110
Harkness, E. 4, 222
Harner, M. 27
Harvalik, Z.V. 239
Harvey, R.J. 11
Hassler, D. 194, 196–200
Heal, R. 110
Hebert, R.S. 3
Hervé, I. 17
Hess, D. 37
Hilgard, E, 214
Hillman, J. 127
Hillman, J.A. 151
Hochstätter, Z. 114
Hodgson, R. 190
Hollan, D. 126, 137, 139
Hollingshead, A.B. 134
Holmes, E.A. 217
Homans, P. 128, 129
Hsu, S.P. 204
Huang, K.C. 204
Hudson, W.W. 228
Hufford, D.J. 29
Hyman, S. 11

Igreja, V. 52
Ingerman, S. 27
Inglehart, R. 109

Institute of HeartMath 16
Ireland-Frey, L. 167

Jahne, R. 220
James, W. 26, 159–61, 189, 190
Janet, P. 37, 212
Janjoppi, L. 241
Jansen, R. 240
Jockers, R. 240
Jonas, W.B. 4
Jones, S.R. 38
Joseph, S. 112
Jung, C.G. 126–34, 138, 151–2, 279–81

Kabayama, S. 204
Karasek, M. 239
Karasu, T.B. 104, 110
Kardec, A. 15–16, 23–5, 29–45, 49, 50, 57, 91, 100, 101, 119, 123, 136, 140, 145, 150, 165, 255, 258, 272, 273, 278, 282
Karniski, W. 227
Katzman, M.A. 11
Keen, M. 193
Keil, H.J. 105–7
Kelly, E.F. 108, 200, 216
Kendler, K. 11
Kiecolt-Glaser, J.K. 221
Kim, M.-J. 204
King, D. 3, 4
King, M.B. 3
Kirsch, I. 11
Koenig, H.G. 3, 26–8, 45, 47, 104
Korotkov, K.G. 205
Koss-Chioino, J. 131, 135, 137, 139
Krelly, E.W. 192
Krieger, D. 223
Krippner, S. 22, 212, 289
Krucoff, M.W. 222
Kübler-Ross, Elisabeth 48
Kuhn, T. 104, 106
Kumar Maitra, S. 240
Kyung, H.J. 204

Lacan, J. 146
Lacasse, J. 11
Lake, J. 285
Lam, R.W. 11
Laplantine, F. 29, 30
Larson, D.B. 45, 47

Larson, S.S. 45
Lawton, I. 174
Lazlo, E. 143
Lednor, A.J. 242
Lee, L.C. 109–10
Lee, R.V. 110
Legros, J.J. 239
Leibovici, L. 233
Lerchl, A. 239
Lerner, M. 223
Levin, J. 3
Lévy-Bruhl, L. 127
Lewis, D.A. 205
Lewton, E. 137
Li, Y. 204
Lin, J.C. 233
Linley, P.A. 112
Lodge, O. 190
Lorr, M. 228
Lotufo Neto, F. 30, 37
Lyle, D.B. 239
Lynn, S.J. 290

Machado, F. 233
MacLean, C.D. 3
Mary, F. 261
Masten, A.S. 110
Matthews, C. 173
May, E.C. 235
Mazzucchelli, C. 240
McCraty, R. 235
McCullough, M.E. 47
McFarlane, A.C. 110
McNair, D.M. 228
Melo, K.R. 143
Mercante, J.P. 110
Michaelus 97, 98
Miller, W. 47
Mills, A. 107, 290
Mitchell, L. 3
Modi, S. 166, 171
Montagnier, L. 210
Moody, R. 48
Moore, D. 248
Moore, T. 96, 278
Moreira, A. 17
Moreira-Almeida, A. 17, 30, 32, 37, 39, 104, 277
Morendo, A. 109
Moreno, J.L. 145
Morse, M.L. 26, 48, 106, 214–16
Mosher, C. 219
Moutinho, M. 143

Murphy, M. 287
Myers, F.W.H. 29, 190, 214

Nakano, M. 204
Nasello, A.G. 110
Neeleman, J. 3
Neihaus, M. 239
Neppe, V. 106
Neppe, V.M. 195–6, 198–200
Neto, L.F. 52
Newberg, A. 109
Newberg, A.B. 4
Newport, F. 248
Nicolescu, B. 147
Nobre, M. 50–3
Norcross, J.C. 110
Novak, W. 167

O'Keeffe, C. 193
O'Leary, D. 215
Olive, K. 4

Page, K. 166
Paquette, V. 109
Parnia, S. 48, 108
Parron, D. 3
Pasricha, S.K. 105–7
Paulinyi, T. 235
Payas, M. 123
Penfield, W. 108
Peres, J.F.P. 109–10, 112, 218
Periyannanpillai, V. 107
Perry, P. 26
Petit, L. 240
Petrak, J. 168
Piccardi, G. 209
Playfair, G.L. 193
Pollack, G.H. 208, 210
Popp, F.A. 207
Powell, T. 4
Powers, S.M. 212
Preparata, G. 208, 209
Prochaska, J.O. 110
Puchalski, C. 26, 47
Puthoff, H. 220

Radin, D.I. 222, 233–5, 287–9
Ramachandran, V.S. 110
Ramakrishnan, R. 221, 234
Reed, G.M. 117–18
Richards, T.L. 222
Ring, K. 48
Rinpoche, S. 223
Rivas, T. 106

Robertson, T.J. 193
Robinson, B.A. 247
Robinson, J.M. 56
Rock, A.J. 191, 192, 290
Rogler, L.H. 134
Romans, S. 3
Romaquera, O. 123
Romer, A. 47
Rosen, L.A. 239
Rosenthal, R. 222, 223
Roy, A.E. 193
Roy, R. 209
Rubik, B. 204, 206–7
Russek, L. 193

Saad, M. 277
Sabom, M. 48
Sagan, S. 166, 167
Sageman, S. 3
Samano, E.S. 4
Samararatne, G. 110
Sampaio, J.R. 30
Samuels, A. 128
Sathya Sai Baba 27
Savaris, A.A. 260
Savieto, R.M. 210
Sayed, M.A. 109, 110
Schiebeler, W. 199
Schiff, M. 209
Schlitz, M. 4, 221–2, 234
Schmid, G. 239
Schmidt, S. 222
Schneider, T. 239
Schouten, S.A. 290
Schubert, S.C. 271
Schulte, J. 209
Schwartz, G. 193, 207
Schwartz, G.E. 290
Schwartz, S.A. 233
Semm, P. 239, 242
Sengupta, A. 240
Severino, P.R. 106
Shafranske, E.P. 112
Shapiro, F. 217
Shaw, A. 112
Shealy, N. 12, 16, 18
Shirahata, , S. 204
Shoenfelt, J.L. 11
Sloan, R.P. 4, 221, 234
Smith, C.W. 208, 209
Sogyal Rinpoche see Rinpoche, S.
Sperry, R.W. 214
Spiegel, D. 117, 118, 285
Spira, J.L. 117–18

Spiritist Medical Association
    (Associacao Medico-
    Espirita) 26, 27
Spiritist Medical Association of
    the USA 220
Spitzer, C. 212
Spottiswoode, S.J.P. 235
Sri Sathya Sai Institute of Higher
    Medical Sciences 27
Standish, L.J. 4, 222
Stapp, H. 216
Stark, M. 47
Stevenson, I. 42, 105–7, 110,
    170
Stoll, S.J. 30
Sullivan, W.P. 3
Swyers, J.P. 47
Sylvia, C. 167
Szent-Gyorgyi, A. 208

Tajima, K. 11
Tandon, A. 10
Targ, R. 220
Thase, M.E. 11
Thompson, R.E. 108
Tiller, W. 210
Treisman, A. 157, 158
Tucker, J.B. 42, 105–7
Tunç, A.T. 241
Turgut, M. 241
Twemlow, S.W. 220

Uhm, Y.K. 204
US Department of Health and
    Human Services 10

Van Dusen, W. 168
van Lommel, P. 48, 215, 216
Varma, V.K. 104, 109
Vassy, Z. 235
Venecia, D. 215
Venkataramaiah, V. 52
Vieira, W. 48, 49, 123–4, 279
Villoldo, A. 22
Vollrath, L. 239
von Franz, M.L. 151

Wackermann, J. 222
Walach, H. 222
Walcott, C. 242
Wallace, A. 27, 142, 144
Wallis, C. 108, 221
Wambach, H. 106
Webster, K. 228

Weisberg, B. 22
Weston, C.G. 11
Whinnery, J. 215
Whitaker, R. 10–11, 15
White, R.A. 287, 291, 292
Wickland, C. 166
Wilber, K. 143
Wiseman, R. 193, 234
Woolger, R. 143
World Health Organization
    (WHO) 277

Xavier, F.C. 48–52, 99–103,
    123–4, 241, 244–6, 254,
    255, 271, 278–80

Yang, C.C. 204
Yankelovich Partners Inc. 4
Yarrow, K. 110
Ye, J. 204
Yoo, H. 210

Zangari, W. 233
Zeig, S. 114
Zheng, J.M. 208